SURGERY
ON CALL

□ □ □ □ □
□ □ □ □ □

Second Edition

Associate Editors

Douglas L. Fraker, MD
Associate Professor of Surgery
Head, Division of Surgical Oncology
University of Pennsylvania
Philadelphia, Pennsylvania

Eric A. Wiebke, MD
Assistant Professor, Department of Surgery
Indiana University
Indianapolis, Indiana

Consulting Editors

Marianne Billeter, PharmD
Assistant Professor of Clinical Pharmacy
College of Pharmacy
Xavier University of Louisiana
New Orleans, Louisiana

Alan Schuricht, MD
Assistant Professor, Department of Surgery
Jefferson Medical College
Thomas Jefferson University
Philadelphia, Pennsylvania

John Kairys, MD
Assistant Professor, Department of Surgery
Jefferson Medical College
Thomas Jefferson University
Philadelphia, Pennsylvania

SURGERY ON CALL

□　□　□　□　□
□　□　□　□　□

Second Edition

Edited by

Leonard G. Gomella, MD
The Bernard W. Goodwin Jr. Associate Professor
Department of Urology
Jefferson Medical College
Thomas Jefferson University
Philadelphia, Pennsylvania

Alan T. Lefor, MD
Associate Professor of Surgery and Oncology
Department of Surgery and the University of Maryland
  Cancer Center
University of Maryland School of Medicine
Baltimore, Maryland

APPLETON & LANGE
Stamford, Connecticut

0-8385-8746-1

96 97 98 99 / 10 9 8 7 6 5 4 3 2 1

Prentice Hall International (UK) Limited, *London*
Prentice Hall of Australia Pty. Limited, *Sydney*
Prentice Hall Canada, Inc., *Toronto*
Prentice Hall Hispanoamericana, S.A., *Mexico*
Prentice Hall of India Private Limited, *New Delhi*
Prentice Hall of Japan, Inc., *Tokyo*
Simon & Schuster Asia Pte. Ltd., *Singapore*
Editora Prentice Hall do Brasil Ltda., *Rio de Janeiro*
Prentice Hall, *Englewood Cliffs, New Jersey*

ISBN: 0-8385-8746-1
ISSN: 1044-4033

Acquisitions Editor: Shelley Reinhardt
Production Service: Spectrum Publisher Services
Cover Designer: Mary Skudlarek

PRINTED IN THE UNITED STATES OF AMERICA

To our families, who understand the demands of medicine and the extra demands that writing about medicine brings

Contents

Contributors

Tiffany Bee, MD
Resident in General Surgery
University of Maryland Medical Center
Baltimore, Maryland

Marianne Billeter, PharmD
Assistant Professor of Clinical Pharmacy
College of Pharmacy
Xavier University of Louisiana
New Orleans, Louisiana

Robert B. Cameron, MD
Chief, General Thoracic Surgery
Department of Surgery
University of California, San Francisco
and UCSF/Mount Zion Cancer Center, San Francisco

Steven Canfield
Class of 1996
Jefferson Medical College
Philadelphia, Pennsylvania

Murray Cohen, MD
Associate Director, Division of Trauma, Department of Surgery
Jefferson Medical College
Thomas Jefferson University
Philadelphia, Pennsylvania

Douglas L. Fraker, MD
Associate Professor of Surgery
Head, Division of Surgical Oncology
University of Pennsylvania
Philadelphia, Pennsylvania

Kelly Fritz, MD
Senior Resident in General Surgery
University of Maryland Medical Center
Baltimore, Maryland

Leonard G. Gomella, MD
The Bernard W. Goodwin Jr. Associate Professor
Department of Urology
Jefferson Medical College
Thomas Jefferson University Medical Center
Philadelphia, Pennsylvania

Steven Haist, MD
Associate Professor, Department of Medicine
University of Kentucky College of Medicine
Lexington, Kentucky

Ira R. Horowitz, MD
Associate Professor, Department of Obstetrics and Gynecology
Emory College of Medicine
Atlanta, Georgia

Alan T. Lefor, MD
Associate Professor of Surgery and Oncology
Department of Surgery and the University of Maryland
Cancer Center
University of Maryland School of Medicine
Baltimore, Maryland

Tracy Magnuson, MD
Chief Resident in General Surgery
University of Maryland Medical Center
Baltimore, Maryland

John A. Morris, MD
Director, Division of Trauma, Section of Surgical Sciences
Vanderbilt University Medical Center
Nashville, Tennessee

Nicholas A. Pavona, MD
Assistant Professor, Department of Surgery
Benjamin Franklin University Medical Center
Sewell, New Jersey

Gail H. Rosen, PharmD
Director, Nutrition Support Services, Department of Pharmacy
Clinical Instructor, Department of Medicine
Clinical Assistant Professor, School of Pharmacy
University of Maryland Medical Center
Baltimore, Maryland

Robin Smith, MD
U.S.Q.A. Managed Care Fellow
Jefferson Medical College
Thomas Jefferson University Medical Center
Philadelphia, Pennsylvania

Eric Strauch, MD
Fellow in Pediatric Surgery
Johns Hopkins Hospital and University of Maryland
Medical Center
Baltimore, Maryland

Stephen R. Strup, MD
Fellow, Surgery Branch
National Cancer Institute
National Institutes of Health
Bethesda, Maryland

Walter M. Sartor, MD
Senior Resident in General Surgery
University of Maryland Medical Center
Baltimore, Maryland

Kurt Wehberg, MD
Resident in General Surgery
University of Maryland Medical Center
Baltimore, Maryland

Eric A. Wiebke, MD
Assistant Professor, Department of Surgery
Indiana University College of Medicine
Indianapolis, Indiana

Preface

We are grateful to be able to bring to you the second edition of *Surgery On Call*. The first edition of *Surgery on Call* was the initial book in the "On Call" series developed by Appleton & Lange. The series is based on Dr. Tricia Gomella's concept that first appeared in 1988 in her book *Neonatology: Basic Management, On-call Problems, Diseases, and Drugs*. The idea is a simple one: house officers are not usually presented with a diagnosis when on-call, but with a specific complaint or problem that requires action and ultimately leads to a diagnosis. Most medical books approach diseases from the diagnosis and disease perspective. Medical education requires a careful synthesis of the practicality of dealing with patient issues on a day-to-day basis with the essentials of medicine. We hope that this manual will provide the house officer and student with the tools to provide the patient with well thought out initial care. This initial care should be followed by a more detailed study of the patient's problem available in standard text books of surgery.

All sections of the book have been updated from the original edition to reflect the ever-changing practice of medicine. In general, the problems reflect that of the adult population, with consideration to pediatric surgical issues supplied where appropriate. Contributions of house staff are invaluable in identifying the issues addressed while on call on a given surgical service. We take great pride in the fact that this book is designed to reflect generally accepted practices from medical centers around the country.

We would like to acknowledge our contributors for their efforts, Appleton & Lange for their encouragement and patience, and Nancy Desimone for her outstanding administrative assistance. Please contact us with any suggestions you may have so that the book will be able to provide our readership with the essential skills needed to make the all important on-call experience one of efficient patient care and a sound educational opportunity.

Leonard G. Gomella, MD
Alan T. Lefor, MD

Philadelphia and Baltimore
December 1995

I. On-Call Problems

1. ABDOMINAL DISTENTION

I. Problem. A 42-year-old female patient is complaining of abdominal bloating.

II. Immediate Questions

A. Was the patient recently operated upon? Immediate postoperative abdominal distention is common and may be related to ileus or gastric distention. Retroperitoneal surgery may also cause an ileus.

B. Is a nasogastric tube in place? Nasogastric tubes can relieve gastric distention, but will be of little use in draining colonic gas. Verify the tube is functioning (see Problem 55, page 185).

C. What medication is the patient taking? Certain medications such as narcotics (eg, codeine, morphine) and anticholinergics (eg, atropine, belladonna) will slow intestinal motility. Diuretic (eg, furosemide) induced hypokalemia may also cause decreased motility.

D. What previous operations has the patient had? The cause of the distention may be obstruction from adhesions or tumor.

E. What are the vital signs? Abdominal distention may restrict pulmonary function and cause tachypnea. Fever may suggest an infectious process such as peritonitis or pneumonia, which may cause a reflex ileus.

F. When was the most recent bowel movement or flatus? Bowel movements and the passage of flatus are useful indicators of bowel activity. Their absence suggests ileus, which can be mechanical (obstruction) or functional (adynamic ileus) in origin.

G. Has the patient been vomiting? Vomiting is often a sign of obstruction. The characteristics of the material may aid in diagnosing the site of obstruction. In gastric outlet obstruction, there is little, if any, bile in the vomitus, whereas distal small bowel obstruction tends to be bilious.

III. Differential Diagnosis

A. Gastrointestinal Tract Obstruction

1. Stomach. Gastric outlet obstruction by tumor, or ulcer or gastric atony secondary to surgery can lead to gastric dilatation and a sensation of bloating.

2. **Small intestine.** Adhesions after previous surgery and other mechanical causes such as intraluminal obstruction (foreign body, gallstone, etc) or extraluminal obstruction from tumors commonly cause small bowel obstruction. Internal hernias, or strangulated/incarcerated external hernias can also cause small bowel obstruction.

3. **Large intestine.** Causes include tumors, volvulus and fecal impaction (particularly in elderly, bedridden patients).

4. **Nongastrointestinal tract.** Rarely, gynecologic tumors, retroperitoneal sarcomas, lymphomas or genitourinary tumors (as well as others) may cause obstruction.

B. **Intestinal Ischemia.** Usually diagnosed by acidosis, elevated WBC, and "pain out of proportion to physical findings."

C. **Paralytic Ileus (adynamic ileus).** This can be secondary to intra-abdominal infection (peritonitis), or inflammatory processes (pancreatitis, cholecystitis). This is frequently seen in the postoperative period after abdominal or retroperitoneal surgery, after blunt abdominal trauma and can also be caused by medications (see page 1). "Reflex" ileus is often associated with pneumonia or urinary tract infection (pyelonephritis).

D. **Intussusception.** Occurs most often at the ileocecal valve and can be a result of tumors as the lead point, which leads to obstruction.

E. **Organomegaly.** Massive hepatomegaly and splenomegaly may be confused with distention.

F. **Intra-abdominal Mass.** A variety of lesions, such as cysts (mesenteric, ovarian, renal), tumors, aneurysms, or even an unrecognized pregnancy can lead to complaints of distention.

G. **Bladder Distention.** Bladder outlet obstruction, most often because of prostatic enlargement or neurogenic bladder (spinal cord injury, diabetic) may cause massive bladder distention.

H. **Abdominal Wall or Groin Hernia.** These may cause an obstructed loop of bowel that may also be strangulated and thus ischemic.

I. **Hirschsprung's Disease.** Also known as aganglionic megacolon, is usually diagnosed early in life and causes intermittent constipation with bloating and vomiting.

J. **Ascites.** Usually a chronic condition related to liver diseases (alcoholic cirrhosis) or carcinoma (malignant ascites). Inquire about any history of alcohol abuse.

K. **Ogilvie's Syndrome.** Pseudoobstruction of the colon in the absence of an obstructing lesion, usually seen in bedridden patients with severe extra-abdominal diseases such as respiratory or renal insufficiency or vertebral fractures.

IV. Database

A. Physical Exam Key Points

1. **Vital signs.** Fever suggests an inflammatory process, and tachypnea may represent respiratory compromise.
2. **Heart.** Atrial fibrillation, which can lead to intestinal embolization and ischemia.
3. **Lungs.** Auscultation may reveal evidence of pneumonia.
4. **Abdomen.** Perform auscultation, percussion, inspection, and palpation. Direct special attention to the left upper quadrant for evidence of gastric distention such as tympany, evaluate for the presence of bowel sounds (usually absent with peritonitis, increased and high pitched with small bowel obstruction). Note any old surgical scars and palpate for any tenderness to suggest peritoneal irritation (generalized with peritonitis, or localized with other causes of an acute abdomen such as cholecystitis (see Problem 2, page 5). Abdominal wall herniation may be present. Costovertebral angle tenderness suggests an inflammatory process involving the diaphragm, liver, spleen, or kidney. A fluid wave is seen in ascites.
5. **Rectal exam.** Digital exam may reveal fecal impaction, or rectal tenderness. Determine the presence of occult blood on a fecal sample.
6. **Inguinal.** Check for hernias in groin and femoral areas.
7. **Skin.** Changes consistent with alcohol abuse, such as spider angiomata; palmar erythema may go along with ascites.
8. **Peripheral vascular.** Sign of embolization that may have accompanying abdominal emboli leading to intestinal ischemia (ie, absent pulses in the lower extremities).
9. **Pelvic exam**. Adnexal masses or tenderness may suggest ovarian tumors as a cause of ascites or pelvic inflammatory disease.

B. Laboratory Data

1. **Hemogram.** Left shift and leukocytosis may suggest an infectious process.
2. **Serum electrolytes.** Severe hypokalemia may cause an ileus.
3. **Liver function tests.** These can evaluate for liver disease and include bilirubin, alkaline phosphatase, ALT, AST.
4. **Urinalysis.** White cells and positive leukocyte esterase suggest a urinary tract infection.
5. **Serum amylase.** Typically elevated with pancreatitis, it may also be elevated with a perforated viscus, intestinal obstruction or mesenteric ischemia.
6. **Arterial blood gas.** Acidosis may help diagnose ischemic intestine.

C. Radiologic and Other Studies

1. **Abdominal x-rays.** Supine and upright abdominal x-rays are ordered in patients with abdominal distention. (***Note:*** An up-

right chest x-ray should also always be included in the evaluation; see below). A "ground glass" appearance is seen with ascites, air fluid levels on the upright film are seen with ileus and a large gastric bubble may suggest postoperative gastric atony or gastric outlet obstruction. If the cecum is markedly dilated (>10–12 cm across), cecal perforation may result and emergent intervention is needed.

2. **Chest x-ray.** An upright chest x-ray is often the best film to detect free air under the diaphragm. Free air may be normal in the immediate postoperative period after a laparotomy, otherwise this suggests a perforation. Pneumonia may also be diagnosed. Pleural effusion directs attention to a sub-diaphragmatic inflammatory process.

3. **Barium studies.** These should **not** be obtained if obstruction is suspected, without very careful consideration. In the case of an intussusception, however, a barium enema may be curative as well (in infants only). These studies are particularly hazardous in the presence of a perforation, because extravasated barium is a terrible complication ("barium peritonitis"). Water soluble contrast media (meglumine diatrizoate [Gastrografin]) are a good alternative if there is any chance of perforation.

4. **Ultrasound and CT scan.** This can help establish the diagnosis especially if a tumor, ascites, or organomegaly is suspected. Cholelithiasis with resulting cholecystitis may be detected on ultrasound.

V. Plan. Relieve the distention first and then identify and treat the underlying cause. Excessive distention of the cecum can lead to perforation. Gastric distention can lead to vomiting with pulmonary aspiration, dehydration, electrolyte abnormalities or forceful emesis, which may cause esophageal rupture. Thus, distention can lead to serious consequences.

A. Initial Management. In most cases, keeping the patient NPO with adequate intravenous hydration is acceptable initial therapy while the workup is in progress (see Section IV, page 337).

B. Nasogastric Intubation. When gastrointestinal obstruction is the cause or severe vomiting is present, a functioning nasogastric tube is essential. In the absence of gastric distention, a nasogastric tube may be less useful at relieving distention, but should be used empirically (see Section III, page 311).

C. Fluid Balance. Carefully monitor fluid intake and output, especially if a nasogastric tube is in place.

D. Specific Treatment Plans. The underlying cause must be clearly identified and appropriately treated. Common treatment plans include:

1. Correct any electrolyte abnormalities, especially hypokalemia. Use IV potassium chloride (see page 152).
2. Review medications and dosing intervals for any agents that may slow intestinal motility, and adjust accordingly.
3. Fecal impaction should be cleared with gentle digital extraction.
4. Ascites is usually managed medically (sodium restriction, spironolactone) with paracentesis used therapeutically if respiratory compromise is present.
5. Postoperative ileus usually clears spontaneously, unless complications such as infection intervene.
6. Operative intervention in many cases of abdominal distention including bowel ischemia, obstructing hernia, perforation or mechanical obstruction. Sometimes, there is no other choice since a specific lesion cannot be diagnosed preoperatively.

2. ABDOMINAL PAIN

I. **Problem.** Seven days after a 40% burn, the patient, a 60-year-old man, complains of pain in the right upper quadrant.

II. Immediate Questions

A. **What are the vital signs?** Fever indicates an inflammatory process. Hypotension and tachycardia may indicate shock owing to sepsis or hemorrhage. Fever may be absent in the elderly or in those patients receiving immunosuppressive or antipyretic medications.

B. **Where is the pain located?** This is only a general guide to the diagnosis of abdominal pain, since early in the course of the illness, pain may be "shifted" away from the actual site of pathology, and late in the course pain may become generalized. The classic example is appendicitis, where discomfort is initially periumbilical or epigastric and later localized in the right lower quadrant. If the process goes unchecked, generalized abdominal pain (peritonitis) may result. Referred pain to the groin can be seen with ureteral colic, and referred back pain with pancreatitis or a ruptured abdominal aneurysm (Figures I–1 and I–2).

C. **When did it start?** Acute, explosive pain is typical of a perforated viscus, ruptured aneurysm or abscess or ectopic pregnancy. Pain intensifying over 1–2 hours is typical of acute cholecystitis, acute pancreatitis, strangulated bowel, mesenteric thrombosis, proximal small bowel obstruction or renal or ureteral colic. Vague pain that increases over several hours is most often seen with acute ap-

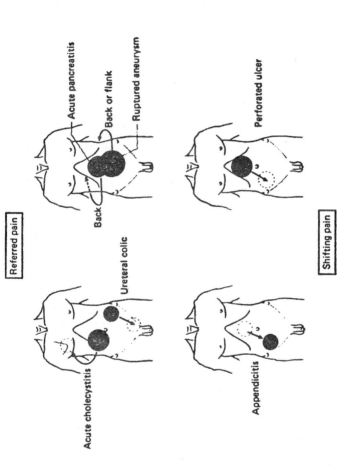

Figure I–1. Referred and shifting pain in the acute abdomen. Solid circles indicate the site of maximum pain, and dashed circles show the sites of lesser pain. *(Reproduced, with permission, from Boey JH: Acute Abdomen. In: Current Surgical Diagnosis & Treatment, 10/e. Way LW (editor). Appleton & Lange, 1994.)*

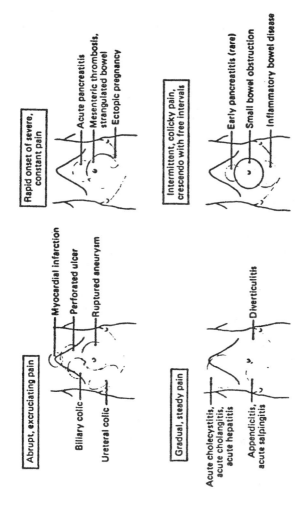

Figure I–2. The location and character of the pain are useful in the differential diagnosis of the acute abdomen. (*Reproduced, with permission, from Boey JH: Acute Abdomen. In: Current Surgical Diagnosis & Treatment, 10/e. Way LW (editor). Appleton & Lange, 1994.*)

pendicitis, distal small bowel and large bowel obstructions, uncomplicated peptic ulcer disease, and various gynecologic and
genitourinary conditions (Figure I–2).

D. What is the quality of the pain (dull, sharp, intermittent, constant, worst in life, burning)? Classically described patterns include "burning" (eg, peptic ulcer disease), "searing" (eg, ruptured aortic aneurysm), "intermittent" (eg, renal or ureteral colic) (Figure I–2). Have the person scale the severity of the pain from 1 (least painful) to 10 (most painful). This gives a guide to follow the course more objectively.

E. What makes the pain better or worse? Pain that increases with deep inspiration is associated with diaphragmatic irritation (eg, pleurisy or inflammatory lesions of upper abdomen). Food often relieves the pain of peptic ulcer disease. Narcotics relieve colic, but are of little relief in pain because of strangulated bowel or mesenteric thrombosis. Bending forward often relieves the pain of pancreatitis.

F. What are the associated symptoms, if any? Vomiting with the onset of pain is seen in peritoneal irritation or perforation of a hollow viscus and is a prominent feature of upper abdominal diseases such as Boerhaave's syndrome, acute gastritis or pancreatitis. In distal small bowel or large bowel obstruction, nausea is usually present long before vomiting begins. Hematemesis suggests upper GI bleeding (ulcer disease, Mallory-Weiss syndrome). Diarrhea, if severe and associated with abdominal pain, suggests infectious gastroenteritis, and if bloody, may represent ischemic colitis, ulcerative colitis, Crohn's disease or amebic dysentery. Constipation alternating with diarrhea may be seen with diverticular disease. Although constipation is often nonspecific, obstipation (absence of passage of both stool and flatus) is strongly suggestive of mechanical bowel obstruction. Hematuria suggests a genitourinary cause.

G. What are the characteristics of the vomitus? (see Problem 53, page 179.)

H. When did the patient eat last? Allows an assessment of the time course of the illness and particularly important if anesthesia is planned.

I. What is a female patient's menstrual history? Missed or late period may suggest an ectopic pregnancy. Mittelschmerz is pain due to a ruptured ovarian follicle.

J. What is the patient's medical and surgical history? Knowledge of a history of ulcers, gallstones, alcohol abuse, or previous operations along with a list of current medications aids in establishing the cause. A history of blunt abdominal trauma 1–3 days before the onset of the pain may signify subcapsular hemorrhage of the liver, spleen, or kidney.

III. Differential Diagnosis. Abdominal pain has both intra-abdominal and extra-abdominal sources and can be associated with both medical and surgical diseases. The list is too long to reproduce in its entirety here, but listed are some of the more frequently encountered causes.

A. Intra-abdominal

1. **Hollow viscera.** Hollow viscera can perforate in the face of obstruction and perforation represents an acute surgical emergency.

   a. **Upper abdominal:** esophagitis, gastritis, peptic ulcer disease, cholecystitis.

   b. **Mid gut:** small bowel obstruction or infarction. Obstruction may be a result of adhesions (benign and malignant), hernias (internal and external), or volvulus.

   c. **Lower abdominal:** inflammatory bowel disease, appendicitis, mesenteric lymphadenitis, obstruction.

   d. **Gastroenteritis, colitis.**

2. **Solid organs.**

   a. **Liver:** Hepatitis.

   b. **Pancreas:** Pancreatitis.

   c. **Spleen:** Splenic infarction.

   d. **Kidney:** Stones, pyelonephritis, abscess.

3. **Pelvic.**

   a. Pelvic inflammatory disease.

   b. Ectopic pregnancy (rupture is a surgical emergency).

   c. **Other:** Fibroid torsion, cysts, endometriosis.

4. **Vascular.** Vascular catastrophes are surgical emergencies.

   a. Ruptured aneurysm.

   b. Dissecting aneurysm.

   c. Mesenteric thrombosis or embolism.

   d. Splenic or hepatic rupture. Usually posttraumatic.

B. Extra-abdominal. Pathology in extra-abdominal diseases may rarely present as referred abdominal pain. The most important to remember are sickle cell crisis, pneumonia (especially lower lobe), myocardial infarction, and rarely, diabetic ketoacidosis.

C. Other

1. **Trauma patient.** Blunt trauma may cause injuries to solid viscera (spleen, liver, kidney, pancreas) or to fixed structures such as the duodenum. Penetrating trauma may injure any intra-abdominal structure.

2. **Postoperative.** Postoperative abdominal pain usually improves significantly in uncomplicated cases during the first 2–3 postoperative days. Persistent pain may indicate a problem, such as obstruction or abscess formation. Uncomplicated postoperative pain is derived from both visceral fibers, because of surgical injury to peritoneal linings and to somatic fibers innervating the abdominal wall.

3. **Critically ill patient.** Patients suffering severe stress from such serious insults as multiple trauma or burns, often complicated by sepsis, may suffer from potentially life-threatening intra-abdominal events.
   a. Acute stress gastritis (usually manifested as massive upper GI bleeding).
   b. Curling's ulcer with or without perforation (after burn).
   c. Acalculous cholecystitis and cholestasis from chronic use of total parenteral nutrition.

IV. Database
A. Physical Exam Key Points
1. **Overall appearance.** Writhing in agony is typical of colic, whereas a motionless patient is suggestive of peritoneal irritation.
2. **Lungs.** Listen for basilar rales or rhonchi indicating possible pneumonia. Dullness to percussion may represent pleural effusion or consolidation.
3. **Heart.** Look for evidence of cardiac decompensation (distended neck veins, S3 gallop, peripheral edema), especially in the patient with preexisting coronary disease, which may direct attention towards a myocardial infarction or atrial fibrillation to suggest emboli.
4. **Abdomen.**
   a. **Inspection:** Note presence of distention (obstruction, ileus, ascites), scaphoid (perforated ulcer) flank ecchymoses (hemorrhagic pancreatitis), caput medusae (portal hypertension), surgical scars (adhesions, tumor).
   b. **Auscultation:** Listen for bowel sounds (absent or occasional tinkle with obstruction or ileus; hyperperistaltic with gastroenteritis; rushes with small bowel obstruction).
   c. **Percussion:** Tympany is associated with distended loops of bowel; dullness and a fluid wave with ascites; loss of liver dullness is associated with free air.
   d. **Palpation:** Guarding, rigidity, and rebound tenderness are hallmarks of peritonitis. Localized tenderness is often seen with cholecystitis, appendicitis, salpingitis, and diverticulitis. Costovertebral angle tenderness is common with pyelonephritis. Murphy's sign is inspiratory arrest while palpating the gallbladder in acute cholecystitis. Pain with active hip flexion (psoas sign) can represent a retrocecal appendix or psoas abscess. The obturator sign (pain on internal and external rotation of the flexed thigh) can be found with a retrocecal appendix or obturator herniation. Masses may also be detected.

5. **Rectal exam.** A mass suggests a rectal carcinoma, a fissure indicates Crohn's disease, unilateral tenderness suggests appendicitis (usually retrocecal) or an abscess. If stool is present, evaluate for occult blood (see page 285).
6. **Pelvic exam.** Examine for cervical motion tenderness and purulent cervical discharge that suggests pelvic inflammatory disease (salpingitis, tuboovarian abscess). Other masses may be felt (ectopic pregnancy, ovarian cyst, or neoplasm).
7. **Extremities.** Evaluate for asymmetric pedal pulses, pain, pallor, and paresthesia for evidence of ischemia that may be associated with embolic phenomenon.
8. **Skin.** Look for jaundice and spider angiomata seen with liver disease. Cool and clammy skin from peripheral vasoconstriction is an ominous sign of severe hypotension.

B. **Laboratory Data**
   1. **Hemogram.** Anemia may indicate hemorrhage from an ulcer, colon cancer, or leaking aneurysm. Leukocytosis indicates presence of inflammation. A low white count is more typical of viral infections such as gastroenteritis or mesenteric adenitis.
   2. **Serum electrolytes, BUN, creatinine.** Bowel obstruction with vomiting can cause hypokalemia, dehydration, or both (BUN/creatinine ratio > 20:1).
   3. **Bilirubin, AST, ALT, alkaline phosphatase.** Hepatitis, cholecystitis and other liver diseases may be diagnosed through these tests.
   4. **Amylase.** Markedly elevated levels are associated with pancreatitis. Amylase can also be elevated with perforated ulcer and small bowel obstruction; occasionally, a pseudocyst or hemorrhagic pancreatitis may result in a normal amylase level.
   5. **Arterial blood gases.** Hypoxia is often an early sign of sepsis. Acidosis may be present in ischemic bowel.
   6. **Pregnancy test.** Premenopausal women should be tested to rule out ectopic pregnancy, whether they use birth control or not.
   7. **Urinalysis.** Hematuria may indicate urolithiasis; pyuria and hematuria can be present in urinary tract infections or rarely in appendicitis.
   8. **Cervical culture.** Send specimen specifically for gonorrhea (anaerobic) if pelvic inflammatory disease is suspected.

C. **Radiologic and Other Studies**
   1. **Flat and upright abdominal films.** If the patient is debilitated, a left lateral decubitus film may be substituted for the upright. Observe for the following key elements: gas pattern, bowel dilatation, air-fluid levels, presence of air in rectum, pancreatic calcifications, loss of psoas margin, displacement of hollow viscera, gall and renal stones, portal vein air, or aortic calcifications.

2. **Chest film.** May reveal pneumonia, widened mediastinum (dissecting aneurysm), pleural effusion, or elevation of a hemidiaphragm (subdiaphragmatic inflammatory process). Free air under diaphragm suggests a perforation and is most often seen on the upright chest film.
3. **Ultrasound.** May reveal gallstones, ectopic pregnancy, other pathology.
4. **Electrocardiogram.** Rule out myocardial infarction as cause of upper abdominal distress and nausea.
5. **Other studies as clinically indicated:**
   a. IVP (excretory urogram is helpful in the workup of urolithiasis).
   b. Abdominal CT scan.
   c. Biliary scintigraphy.
   d. **Contrast bowel studies:** Upper GI swallow and enemas (barium, dilute barium, Gastrografin).
   e. **Endoscopic studies:** Esophagogastroduodenoscopy (EGD), colonoscopy, endoscopic retrogradcholangiopancreatography (ERCP).
   f. Arteriography.
   g. Peritoneal lavage (page 323) or paracentesis (page 319).

V. **Plan.** Abdominal pain in any patient can present a diagnostic dilemma, but even more so in patients at the extremes of age or in those unable to communicate. The surgeon's goal is to determine if abdominal pain requires surgical treatment in order to prevent further morbidity. In rough terms, pain that is present 6 or more hours and does not improve is likely to have a cause requiring surgical intervention. Many cases of abdominal pain have no definite diagnosis before laparotomy. A brief period of observation may ultimately point to the cause, but operation is safer in most cases. The use of analgesics remains controversial, but most clinicians now believe moderate doses of pain medicine will not mask symptoms and will make the patient much more comfortable. Specific types of therapy and operations for each possible diagnosis cannot be described here but can be found in surgical and medical textbooks. It is essential to recognize that certain conditions are life threatening and usually require urgent operation (Table I–1).

A. **Observation.** With the exception of catastrophes that require urgent surgical exploration (Table I-1), most cases of abdominal pain require close observation, medical management, and occasionally analgesics. In the case of postoperative abdominal pain, analgesics are used most frequently.
   1. Keep patient NPO and consider nasogastric suction, especially if vomiting is present.
   2. Intravenous hydration (see Section IV, page 337), with careful attention to intake and output.

TABLE I–1. INDICATIONS FOR URGENT OPERATION IN PATIENTS WITH ACUTE ABDOMEN.

Physical findings

Involuntary guarding or rigidity, especially if spreading
Increasing or severe localized tenderness
Tense or progressive distention
Tender abdominal or rectal mass with high fever or hypotension
Rectal bleeding with shock or acidosis
Equivocal abdominal findings along with—
    Septicemia (high fever, marked or rising leukocytosis, mental changes, or increasing
        glucose intolerance in a diabetic patient)
    Bleeding (unexplained shock or acidosis, falling hematocrit)
    Suspected ischemia (acidosis, fever, tachycardia)
    Deterioration on conservative treatment

Radiologic findings

Pneumoperitoneum
Gross or progressive bowel distention
Free extravasation of contrast material
Space-occupying lesion on scan, with fever
Mesenteric occlusion on angiography

Endoscopic findings

Perforated or uncontrollably bleeding lesion

Paracentesis findings

Blood, bile, pus, bowel contents, or urine

(Reproduced, with permission, from Boey JH: Acute Abdomen. In: Current Surgical Diagnosis and Treatment, 10/e. LW Way (editor). Appleton & Lange, 1994.)

   3. Parenteral analgesics are used carefully to avoid masking pathologic processes.
   4. Serial physical exams by the same examiner will be very useful in determining progression of symptoms and aid in securing the diagnosis.
 B. Surgery. Vascular catastrophes, perforated viscus, most causes of bowel obstruction, many splenic and hepatic injuries, ruptured ectopic pregnancies, and appendicitis require emergency surgery. Indications for urgent operation without a precise preoperative diagnosis are outlined in Table I–1.

3. ACIDOSIS

(See also Section II, page 245)

 I. Problem. A patient with fulminant acute pancreatitis and accompanying ARDS requires intubation and mechanical ventilation. The initial arterial blood gas following intubation reveals a pH of 7.14.

II. Immediate Questions

A. Is the acidosis respiratory, metabolic, or a combination of both? Often the report of the blood gas will give the calculated base excess/deficit at the end of the report (eg, Po_2/Pco_2/pH/bicarbonate/base excess). If the base excess is negative (or a positive deficit), the acidosis is at least partially metabolic. If the base excess is not reported with the results of the ABG, the differentiation between metabolic and respiratory can still be quickly made. If the $Pco_2 < 40$, then the acidosis is metabolic, possibly with respiratory compensation. If the $Pco_2 > 40$, the acidosis is at least partially respiratory. Every 10 torr that the Pco_2 is greater than 40, the pH will be lowered by 0.08 in normal circumstances. For example, if the Pco_2 is 60, one would expect an acidosis of 7.24, any additional acidosis can be attributed to metabolic causes.

B. What is the volume status of the patient? A common cause of metabolic acidosis in the acute setting is lactic acidosis due to poor perfusion of the tissues. Examine the patient, look at the recent urine output, and the cardiac filling pressures (if available) to gauge the intravascular volume of the patient. Volume contraction, usually diuretic induced, is often associated with alkalosis.

C. Is there any problem with the ventilator circuitry? In a nonintubated patient with a respiratory acidosis, there is usually apparent difficulty with breathing. In a patient on a ventilator a respiratory acidosis may not be clinically apparent in a sedated or obtunded patient. Check the ventilator circuitry, the exhaled volume, and check the settings on the ventilator to make certain there is no technical explanation for the acidosis. Verify the position of the endotracheal tube on chest x-ray because it can slip distally into the right mainstem bronchus.

D. Are there any arrhythmias or ectopy? With a profound acidosis of any cause there may be disturbances of the cardiac rhythm or ventricular ectopy. Obtain an ECG and monitor the patient style.

III. Differential Diagnosis. As previously mentioned, the most important initial distinction in diagnosing the cause of acidosis is between respiratory and metabolic causes. In the acutely ill surgical patient both causes may be present as in the patient example above.

A. Respiratory Acidosis. By definition, this is alveolar hypoventilation.

1. Pulmonary conditions

a. Asthma: If an asthmatic has progressed to a respiratory acidosis, they have very severe disease and usually require prompt intubation.

        b. Mechanical upper airway obstruction: A foreign body or laryngospasm may be the cause.

        c. Space-occupying lesions: Pneumothorax, pleural effusion, or hemothorax may result in respiratory compromise.

        d. Severe pulmonary edema: As in congestive heart failure.

        e. Pneumonia: Usually with baseline respiratory compromise such as COPD.

  2. Drugs/toxins

        a. Alcohol ingestion.

        b. Narcotics/sedative overdose.

        c. Neuromuscular blocking agents (eg, curare).

  3. Neuromuscular conditions

        a. Myasthenia gravis

        b. Pickwickian syndrome

        c. Cerebrovascular accident

        d. Guillain-Barré syndrome

B. Metabolic Acidosis. This can be subdivided into conditions with a normal anion gap and those with an increased anion gap implying an elevated unmeasured anion. The anion gap is calculated by $[Na] - ([Cl] + [HCO_3])$. The normal range is 8–12 mEq/L.

  1. Normal anion gap

        a. Loss of bicarbonate: Usually from the GI tract as diarrhea, small bowel fistula, pancreatic-cutaneous fistula, or a large amount of external biliary drainage.

        b. Renal tubular acidosis

  2. Elevated anion gap

        a. Lactic acidosis: Poor perfusion with interference with the normal oxidative metabolism.

        b. Diabetic ketoacidosis

        c. Alcoholic ketoacidosis

        d. Chronic renal insufficiency: Elevated unmeasured anions include sulfates and phosphates.

        e. Drugs and poisoning: Overdosage of aspirin or ingestion of methyl alcohol, ethylene glycol, or paraldehyde.

IV. Database

A. Physical Exam Key Points

  1. Vital signs. Look for evidence of hypoventilation, hypotension, tachycardia, or fever. Sepsis can cause shock—a common cause of acidosis.

  2. Skin. Cool, clammy, and mottled skin on extremities as in shock with clamped down peripheral perfusion.

  3. HEENT. Ketosis or fruity odor on breath suggests diabetic ketoacidosis. Look for tracheal shift from a space occupying lesion or venous distention (eg, CHF or tension pneumothorax).

4. **Pulmonary.** Evaluate for absent or decreased breath sounds, stridor in upper airway obstruction, wheezes, or rales.
5. **Abdomen.** Peritoneal signs indicate an acute abdomen, and marked distention may inhibit respiration.
6. **Neuromuscular.** Generalized weakness or focal neurologic signs, depressed level of consciousness, obtundation, or coma should be noted.

B. **Laboratory Data**
1. **Hemogram.** Leukocytosis is seen with sepsis and anemia is common with chronic renal insufficiency.
2. **Electrolytes, BUN and creatinine.** An elevated serum chloride in nonanion gap metabolic acidosis. Calculate the anion gap from the electrolytes (see page 15). Renal insufficiency may be present.
3. **Blood glucose, ketone levels.** Elevations are associated with diabetic ketoacidosis.
4. **Lactate levels.** Levels are elevated with sepsis and poor perfusion.
5. **Arterial blood gas.** Repeat the ABG to follow therapeutic interventions.

C. **Other Studies**
1. **Chest x-ray.** To evaluate for infiltrates, pulmonary edema, effusions, and endotracheal tube position (ideal position is approximately 2 cm above the carina).
2. **ECG with rhythm strip.** To evaluate for arrhythmias.
3. **EMG.** This and other specialized neurology tests may be needed to diagnose primary neurologic conditions.

V. **Plan.** In general for both respiratory and metabolic acidosis, treatment of the underlying cause of the acidosis is the primary goal. In emergent situations, the two methods to reverse the acidosis are to administer sodium bicarbonate intravenously and to hyperventilate the patient. Be sure to check serial pH values to monitor the progress of therapy.

A. **Metabolic Acidosis**
1. **Bicarbonate therapy.** In general, administer IV bicarbonate if the pH < 7.20.
   a. Calculate the total body bicarbonate need:

   Patient's weight (in kg) $\times$ 0.40 $\times$ (24 − [HCO_3]) = total number of mEq of HCO_3 needed.

   b. Give 50% of this amount over the first 12 hours as a mixture of bicarbonate with D5W.
   c. Complications of bicarbonate therapy include:
      i. Hypernatremia
      ii. Volume overload
      iii. **Hypokalemia:** Caused by intracellular shifts of potassium as the pH increases.

    2. Treat underlying causes
      a. Volume resuscitate in sepsis, hemorrhagic shock and other causes of lactic acidosis.
      b. Insulin and saline for diabetic ketoacidosis (see page 453).
      c. Dialysis as needed for renal failure.

B. Respiratory Acidosis. The main goal is to treat the underlying cause.

    1. If necessary, intubate the patient and treat with mechanical ventilation. If a patient is already intubated and has a significant respiratory acidosis, then increase alveolar ventilation by either increasing tidal volume (up to 10–15 ml/kg) while following peak inspiratory pressures or increasing the respiratory rate.

    2. In an emergent situation disconnect the patient from the ventilator and hyperventilate by hand using the bag device. The importance of good pulmonary toilet, ie, suctioning of secretions, cannot be overemphasized. Sedation is often a necessary adjunct to mechanical ventilation (see page 225).

4. ALKALOSIS

(See also Section II, page 245)

I. Problem. A 47-year-old female is on a ventilator in the ICU and has a pH of 7.56 one day after thoracotomy for a Belsey anti-reflux procedure.

II. Immediate Questions

A. Is the patient on a ventilator and if so, what is the respiratory rate and tidal volume? Alkalosis may be a result of over ventilation. The minute ventilation is what is important. Thus, rate (IMV or Assist Control) as well as volume for each delivered breath (tidal volume) are important. The tidal volume should be set at 10–15 mL/kg. Minute ventilation = rate × tidal volume, so a change in either parameter will affect the minute ventilation.

B. What medication is the patient taking? Thiazide diuretics can result in a "contraction" alkalosis and excess bicarbonate and bicarbonate precursors (such as acetate in hyperalimentation solutions) can cause a metabolic alkalosis.

C. What is the composition of IV fluids? Be sure there is no added bicarbonate (avoid Ringer's lactate) and make sure the patient is receiving sufficient chloride (80–100 mEq/d as NaCl, plus losses).

D. Is there a nasogastric tube in place, or is there vomiting? The nasogastric tube drainage of HCl from the GI tract is a common cause of hypochloremic alkalosis in surgical patients.

III. Differential Diagnosis. The key differential point here is similar to acidosis—is the origin of the disturbance metabolic or respiratory?

    A. Metabolic Alkalosis. This is seen usually as an elevated serum bicarbonate. The compensation is usually by hypoventilation and increased renal excretion of bicarbonate. It is diagnosed by an increased pH, with a normal or increased arterial Pco_2.

        1. Loss of HCl (chloride responsive)
            a. Nasogastric suction, vomiting
            b. Villous adenoma (potassium wasting)
            c. Diuretics (especially thiazides)
            d. Posthypercapnia
        2. Chloride resistant
            a. Bicarbonate administration (oral and parenteral)
            b. Chronic hypokalemia
            c. Primary hyperaldosteronism
            d. Cushing's syndrome, exogenous steroids

    B. Respiratory Alkalosis. Hyperventilation results in a decreased Pco_2 and the compensatory mechanism is through increased renal bicarbonate excretion.

        1. Anxiety.
        2. Hypermetabolic states (eg, fever, early sepsis).
        3. Iatrogenic. Ventilator rate set for too many breaths, or tidal volume is too high.
        4. Pregnancy.
        5. Cirrhosis.
        6. Cardiac disease (refer to Problem 12, page 47).
        7. Pulmonary disease (refer to Problem 26, page 97).
        8. Brain stem lesion (refer to Problem 14, page 60).
        9. Salicylate intoxication (alkalosis early, with metabolic acidosis later).

IV. Database

    A. Physical Exam Key Points

        1. Vital signs. Pay particular attention to the respiratory rate. Tachypnea may signify a respiratory cause.
        2. Lungs. Check for signs of pulmonary edema (rales).
        3. Skin. Look for changes associated with alcohol abuse such as palmar erythema, spider angiomata, etc. Signs of sepsis or decreased perfusion may be present.

    B. Laboratory Data. Obtain simultaneous arterial blood gases and electrolytes.

        1. Arterial blood gases. As noted above.
        2. Serum electrolytes. Pay particular attention to hypokalemia, which may accompany alkalosis. (Low serum H^+ balanced by exchange of K^+).

3. **Serum salicylate levels.** If aspirin intoxication is suspected.
4. **Spot urine electrolytes for chloride.** This is most helpful in the diagnosis and treatment of metabolic alkalosis. If the urine chloride is < 10 mEq/L, this represents a "chloride responsive" alkalosis (caused by diuretics or GI tract losses) that can often be corrected by administration of chloride-containing IV fluids. If the urine chloride is > 10 mEq/L, this represents a "chloride resistant" alkalosis (caused by adrenal diseases, exogenous steroid use) and usually cannot be corrected by chloride infusion.

V. Plan. It is essential to identify the cause of alkalosis and treat it.

A. **Discontinue Exogenous Bicarbonate.** Bicarbonate precursors such as the acetate salts (amino acids) found in hyperalimentation solutions should also be evaluated. If hyperalimentation is essential, attempt to increase the chloride salts in the solution, and the amino acid content may need to be reduced.

B. **IV Replacement.** For alkalosis resulting from the loss of HCl, give NaCl as normal saline IV. For alkalosis that is chloride resistant, give KCl IV.

C. **Sedation.** Sedate for anxiety on ventilated patients that may be causing respiratory alkalosis with agents such as diazepam, lorazepam, or midazolam.

D. **Increase $Fico_2$.** Use a rebreathing mask in the nonintubated patient for respiratory alkalosis, or decrease the minute ventilation by decreasing the rate or the tidal volume. Be sure that the tidal volume is set for 10–15 mL/kg.

E. **Treat Hypokalemia.** Use KCl supplementation.

F. **Replace Volume Losses.** Replace fluid volume lost through the nasogastric tube or vomiting, usually using D5 ½ NS with 20 mEq KCl/L.

5. ANAPHYLAXIC REACTION (DRUG REACTIONS)

Immediate Actions

1. Stop administration of allergen
2. Assess airway, intubate if necessary
3. Check breathing, administer o_2
4. Assure adequate IV access (14 or 16 gauge IV) and begin fluids (LR 500 ml bolus)
5. Treat with epinephrine, Benadryl, steroids, aminophylline (see following section, "Plan").

I. Problem. A postoperative patient has developed severe dyspnea and a generalized rash after receiving intravenous penicillin.

II. Immediate Questions. The respiratory distress and hypotension can be life-threatening and the patient should be seen immediately.

   A. What are the patient's vital signs? Tachycardia is a common finding and could represent the response to hypoxia, fear, hypotension or arrhythmia. Hypotension requires immediate treatment in this setting.

   B. Can the patient communicate appropriately? Appropriate answers to simple questions indicate cerebral oxygenation is adequate. Inability to speak suggests severe respiratory deterioration or to upper airway obstruction from laryngospasm or laryngeal edema.

   C. What medication is the patient taking? Many medications can cause anaphylaxis, but the most common in this setting are penicillin, other β-lactamase antibiotics (cephalosporins), and intravenous contrast materials. Aspirin and other nonsteroidal anti-inflammatory drugs (NSAIDs) may cause reactions in sensitive patients. Transfusion reactions are discussed in Problem 68, page 217. Insect stings are another cause and essentially managed the same way.

III. Differential Diagnosis. Anaphylaxis technically refers to the signs and symptoms caused by an antigen mediated release of IgE induced mediators. It can be localized (as in allergic rhinitis) or systemic and life-threatening.

   A. Acute Allergic Reaction (Anaphylaxis). In the hospital setting, most often caused by medications noted in Section II-C above. Less frequently, anaphylaxis may be caused by food, environmental agents (dust, pollen) or insects.

   B. Upper Airway Obstruction. May be caused by a foreign body or laryngeal edema and classically presents as stridor.

   C. Acute Asthmatic Attack. Wheezing with a history of asthma is usually present.

   D. Pulmonary Embolus. Especially in the postoperative setting, this must be considered in the acutely short of breath patient.

   E. Others. Other causes for this constellation of symptoms are discussed in other sections: Dyspnea (Problem 26, page 97) Hypotension (Problem 47, page 159), Pruritus (Problem 60, page 197) and Wheezing (Problem 75, page 236).

IV. Database. Knowledge of patient allergies and current medications is essential. Relationship of medication administration to onset of symptoms is also important, because anaphylaxis usually occurs several minutes after administration of the medication.

A. Physical Exam Key Points
   1. **Vital signs.** Hypotension must be recognized early.
   2. **Lungs.** Listen for wheezing (suggests bronchospasm), stridor (suggests laryngospasm), and adequacy of air movement.
   3. **Skin.** Generalized rash, urticaria, and pruritus often accompany an acute anaphylactic reaction.
   4. **Extremities.** Look for evidence of cyanosis.
   5. **Mental status.** Somnolence in this setting demands immediate respiratory support and is frequently indicative of severe hypercapnia.

B. Laboratory Data
   1. **Arterial blood gas.** Determine level of hypoxia or hypercapnia, but usually the problem must be treated before results are available.

C. Radiologic and Other Studies
   1. **Chest x-ray.** When time permits, a chest x-ray will rule out other causes of respiratory distress (CHF, pneumonia, etc).
   2. **Electrocardiogram.** Acute myocardial infarction can present as pulmonary edema with severe dyspnea. Right ventricular strain can be seen in pulmonary embolus. Myocardial infarction may result from severe hypotension in anaphylaxis.

V. Plan. Treatment should be initiated quickly based on clinical findings and before performing other studies and lab exams. Be prepared to initiate cardiopulmonary resuscitation.

A. Oxygen. Oxygen by face mask should be instituted for moderate to severe dyspnea. Intubation may be required if the patient is severely somnolent, unable to manage their own secretions, or if arterial blood gases reveal elevated Pco_2 or a low Po_2.

B. Epinephrine. Epinephrine 1:1000 solution 0.3–0.5 mL subcutaneously should be given immediately for laryngospasm, with dramatic improvement often seen. Repeat the dose in 5–10 minutes as needed. The epinephrine used for CPR is a 1:10,000 solution given IV and should **not** be used in this situation. Use epinephrine with caution in patients over 40 years of age.

C. Diphenhydramine (Benadryl). Benadryl 25–50 mg IM should follow epinephrine to reduce effects of histamine release, although its usefulness is primarily for lesser degrees of anaphylactic reaction, such as mild urticaria. This may be given intravenously in patients with a moderate reaction or in the elderly where epinephrine should be used with caution, if at all.

D. **High Dose Glucocorticoids.** Hydrocortisone 100 mg IV may be needed if the patient fails to respond to epinephrine and diphenhydramine.

E. **Blood Pressure.** Normally responds to correction with epinephrine and Benadryl, however, normal saline with volume repletion and occasionally pressors (dopamine) are needed to support pressure.

F. **Monitoring.** Resolution of the respiratory distress associated with anaphylaxis is usually so dramatic that ICU monitoring after the episode is often unnecessary. However, clinical judgment is needed, and exceptions include the elderly or severely ill patients, patients who experience arrhythmias or appear near to respiratory arrest before treatment.

6. ANEMIA

I. **Problem.** A patient admitted for a varicose vein stripping has a hematocrit of 19% on preoperative laboratory evaluation.

II. **Immediate Questions**

A. **Is the patient hemodynamically stable?** A patient with a chronic anemia is usually somewhat compensated for volume loss. The evaluation and treatment of those patients can proceed in an orderly fashion. Patients with a low hematocrit secondary to an acute bleed may need urgent volume resuscitation. However, those patients almost always present with clinically apparent bleeding as opposed to being diagnosed on a routine lab. Tachycardia and determination of postural hypotension are sensitive signs of hypovolemia.

B. **Is the patient's stool positive for occult blood?** On a surgical service, a patient with a new decreased hematocrit should be assumed to have GI bleeding until proven otherwise. Check the indices (MCV, MCH, MCHC) on the CBC, and if they show a microcytic, hypochromic anemia (see Section II, page 245), chances are even greater that the cause is GI blood loss. Ask about melena (tarry stools) or change in bowel habits. Even if the stool is negative on first check, obtain 2–3 more specimens at different times for a more thorough evaluation.

C. **Does the patient have a history of anemia?** Review the chart or clinic records to find the most recent hematocrit. Ask if the patient has knowledge of an anemia or if there is a family history of anemia.

D. Is the low hematocrit result correct? If the lab result is unexpected or if it does not correlate with the clinical appearance of the patient, question the validity of the test. Sources of lab error regarding a low hematocrit include (1) the sample is from a different patient; (2) a technical problem with the machine; and (3) blood drawn proximal to an open IV line. Incorrect laboratory results are unusual, but it is worth repeating the test before embarking on an extensive workup. This is true regarding any lab result that does not correlate with the clinical situation.

E. Is there blood available in the blood bank? If emergency transfusion is considered, call the blood bank to determine whether blood is already set-up for the patient. If not, obtain the specimens needed to type and cross-match blood. Do not transfuse the patient unless clinically indicated (hemodynamically unstable, etc) or before completing the initial evaluation, confirming the validity of the result, and drawing blood specimens for the laboratory tests discussed below.

III. Differential Diagnosis. Anemia is present in many disease states. It can be categorized as inadequate red blood cell production or excessive red blood cell loss or destruction.

A. Inadequate Red Blood Cell Production
  1. Deficient hemoglobin production
   a. Iron deficiency: Usually a result of chronic blood loss or inadequate intake.
   b. Folate deficiency: A megaloblastic anemia, common with poor diet (alcoholics, etc).
   c. Vitamin B_{12}: A megaloblastic anemia can be associated with ileal resection or sprue.
   d. Thalassemias: These are inherited deficits in hemoglobin synthesis.
  2. Inadequate red blood cell production
   a. Marrow aplasia: Caused by drug or chemical exposure.
   b. Marrow replacement: Because of neoplasia or fibrosis.
   c. Chronic disease: Systemic illnesses can lead to a normochromic, normocytic anemia. Chronic renal failure represents a separate category for this type of anemia owing to the absence of erythropoietin production by the kidneys.

B. Destruction of Red Blood Cells
  1. Intracorpuscular defects
   a. Hereditary spherocytosis
   b. Enzyme deficiencies
   c. Sickle cell disease

  2. Extracorpuscular defects
   a. Hemolytic anemias: May be caused by autoimmune reactions that are often drug-induced and may be part of a systemic autoimmune disease.
   b. Hemolysis due to prosthetic heart valves.
 C. Acute Blood Loss. Caused by bleeding either from GI tract, GU tract (including menstrual and dysfunctional uterine bleeding in women), retroperitoneal, external bleeding, or postoperative.

IV. Database
A. Physical Exam Key Points
  1. Vital signs. Orthostatic hypotension and tachycardia indicate hemodynamically significant anemia.
  2. Skin. Pallor, pale conjunctiva and nail beds correlate with the degree of anemia reported by the lab.
  3. Abdomen. Splenomegaly is present in hemolytic anemias, in disorders with intracorpuscular defects leading to RBC destruction, and myeloid metaplasia. A mass may be present with malignancy.
  4. Rectal exam. Pay close attention to any mass or the presence of occult blood.
  5. Dressings, drains, and surgical sites should be inspected.
B. Laboratory Data (see Section II, page 245 for more details)
  1. Hemogram. Aside from the hematocrit, look at the white blood count and platelet count for evidence of general bone marrow depression or leukemia.
  2. Red blood cell indices. MCV and MCHC allow a classification of anemia according to RBC size (microcytic, normocytic, or macrocytic) and hemoglobin content (hypochromic or normochromic). Iron deficiency anemia is microcytic and hypochromic, whereas megaloblastic anemia is typically macrocytic.
  3. Peripheral blood smear. This can also be used to look at the actual size of red cells where the indices may be misleading. For example, if a microcytic and a macrocytic process were occurring together, the MCV may be normal owing to a mixed population of red cells. Examining the shape of the cells (spherocytosis, elliptocytosis, RBC fragments) is sometimes helpful.
  4. Reticulocyte count. This gives a measure of the production of red cells at the level of the marrow. A low reticulocyte count suggests inadequate production of red cells whereas an increased count is associated with increased destruction of red cells.
  5. Serum chemistries, BUN, and creatinine. This may show evidence of renal failure, or elevated indirect bilirubin in hemolytic anemias.

    6. Iron, total iron binding capacity (TIBC). In iron deficiency, serum iron is decreased and TIBC is increased. In anemia of chronic disease, serum iron is decreased or normal and TIBC is decreased.

    7. Haptoglobin. Often decreased in hemolytic anemia.

    8. Folate, Vitamin B$_{12}$ levels. These levels measure deficiencies of specific metabolites.

    9. Coombs' test. This measures IgM and IgG antibodies in hemolytic anemias.

  C. Radiologic and Other Studies

    1. Bone marrow biopsy. If reticulocyte count is low, this assesses erythrocyte precursors, iron stores, and bone marrow replacement by infiltrative disease processes.

    2. GI workup. May include UGI series, barium enema, upper endoscopy, colonoscopy, angiography, or tagged red blood cell nuclear scans if workup indicates GI source of anemia.

    3. Ultrasound and CT scans. May be adjunctive in the evaluation for a tumor.

V. Plan. Notify senior staff as elective operations will often be postponed when an anemia is identified.

  A. Acute Management. If hemodynamically significant anemia is present, start a large bore IV (18 gauge or larger and draw necessary blood samples for the lab and blood bank at the same time) and begin fluid resuscitation if hypovolemia is evident. Check stools for occult blood and if heme-positive, consider passing a nasogastric tube as an initial diagnostic maneuver to check for an upper GI source of bleeding.

  B. Evaluation. Continue with GI workup as described above. If anemia is due to causes other than acute blood loss, gather laboratory data as discussed above, along with a hematology consultation.

  C. Specific Treatments

    1. Iron deficiency. Ferrous sulfate or gluconate 325 mg three times a day given with a stool softener (eg, Colace) because iron pills cause constipation. Inform patient that the stools will be darkened by the iron.

    2. Folate deficiency. 1 mg PO or mixed with IV every day.

    3. Vitamin B$_{12}$ deficiency. 1000 μg IM daily for 14 days, then 1000 μg IM monthly.

    4. Hemolytic anemia. Often treated with glucocorticoids such as prednisone 60–100 mg/d and may require splenectomy.

    5. Intracorpuscular red blood cell defect. Often splenectomy will be helpful.

    6. Transfusions as needed.

    7. Operation may be needed depending on GI tract evaluation.

    8. H$_2$-receptor blockers (eg, Tagamet or Zantac) and antacids for ulcer disease.

7. ARTERIAL LINE PROBLEMS

(The technique for arterial line placement is discussed in Section III, page 295).

I. Problem. The arterial line is not functioning in a 65-year-old patient on the first postoperative day after pulmonary lobectomy.

II. Immediate Questions

A. What is the appearance of the tracing? An absent tracing may indicate clotting of the catheter. A normal tracing at least says that there is adequate arterial flow in the catheter. A dampened tracing may indicate either air in the system or a clot.

B. Is the extremity distal to the line compromised? Be sure that the extremity is not ischemic. If there is any question, the line should be removed.

C. Can blood be drawn back through the catheter? Even if the catheter cannot be used to draw blood, it can often function as a blood pressure monitor.

D. Does the arterial pressure measured correlate with a cuff pressure? Find out how well arterial pressure was measured when the catheter did work. In general, cuff measurements should be within 10–15 mm Hg of the arterial line reading.

III. Differential Diagnosis

A. Mechanical

1. **Kinked catheter.** Can be diagnosed by a lack of a tracing on the monitor as well as inability to draw blood.
2. **Clotted catheter.** Often caused by insufficient heparin in the flush solution.
3. **Faulty monitor or transducer.** The ICU staff will be helpful in this problem. It may represent a connector, electrical, or transducer malfunction or air in the system.
4. **Cracked catheter.** Bleeding, air on drawing back through the line, or lack of a tracing may be present. Replacing the line over a guidewire is often successful.
5. **Positional catheter.** This is often a problem with the way the catheter was sutured in place or the positioning of the extremity on the armboard.

B. Vascular

1. **Thrombosed vessel.** Check the pulse proximally, using a Doppler probe if necessary. Risk factors include (1) hypoten-

sion, (2) mechanical pressure to control bleeding at the site, (3) use of a catheter too large for the vessel, and (4) the longer time interval a catheter is left in place.

  2. Torn artery around the catheter causing bleeding. Most common after a problematic cut-down. Application of pressure, as in any bleeding, should control the problem. Failure to prevent a large periarterial hematoma may result in a pseudoaneurysm later.

IV. Database

A. Physical Exam Key Points

1. Examine the insertion site for signs of infection or bleeding. Check the suture securing the catheter.
2. The distal extremity (hand or foot) should be examined for evidence of ischemia.
3. The entire tubing, transducer, and monitor system should be checked for problems including kinking, disconnections, air in the system, and insufficient pressure in the pressure infusion bag.

B. Laboratory Data.
The only useful laboratory data is in the setting of bleeding from the site. PT/PTT, platelets, and fibrin split products are helpful if diffuse bleeding is present. Hematocrit is essential if bleeding was excessive.

V. Plan.
Check the pressure tracing against a standard blood pressure cuff measurement. Verify the acceptable withdrawal of arterial blood. Occasionally, a catheter may be used to withdraw arterial blood but not provide reliable pressure monitoring and vice-versa. A highly subjective decision will often need to be made depending on physician preference and patient condition whether to remove or change the site.

A. Bleeding

1. Apply direct pressure or a pressure dressing if bleeding from the site is a problem. Bleeding from other sites may signify disseminated intravascular coagulation.
2. After a catheter is removed, pressure should be applied to the site for at least 10 minutes to prevent bleeding with resultant hematoma and later pseudoaneurysm formation.

B. Mechanical Problems

1. The use of an armboard along with the arterial line will help prevent many mechanical problems. Positional catheter problems may be solved with an armboard or resuturing the catheter.
2. Kinked or clotted catheters usually must be replaced.
   a. If a catheter clots, verify that there is sufficient heparin in the flush bag (usually 2–4 U heparin/mL).

   b. Continuous flushing systems are preferred over intermittent
   flush systems.
   c. If the vessel appears undamaged, consider changing the
   catheter over a guidewire using sterile technique. Be sure to
   carefully suture it in place to avoid kinking the catheter.
   3. A dampened wave form usually indicates air in the transducer
   system or a clot in the catheter. Air bubbles can usually be
   flushed clear.
   4. Line leaks or connection problems can usually be solved by the
   ICU nursing staff.
   C. Reading Errors. As previously mentioned the difference between
   the cuff and arterial line pressure should be less than 10–15 mm
   Hg. Using an appropriate sized BP cuff, keeping tubing lengths as
   short as possible and verifying there is a properly "zeroed" transducer and no air in the system should minimize the differences.
   D. Thrombosis. Usually requires removal of the catheter and observation for ischemic changes.

8. ASPIRATION

   I. Problem. An obtunded patient in the emergency room being evaluated for a head injury vomits and develops acute respiratory distress.

   II. Immediate Questions
   A. What are the vital signs? Significant respiratory distress may indicate massive aspiration of gastric contents. Fever may indicate
   underlying infectious process. Hypertension and bradycardia may
   reflect a rise in intracranial pressure.
   B. Is the airway protected? If the patient cannot protect his or her
   airway then intubation is indicated.
   C. Is the patient cyanotic? Cyanosis and tachypnea after pulmonary aspiration usually require intubation.
   D. What is the patient's neurologic status? Patients who are unconscious or obtunded are at higher risk for pulmonary aspiration.

   III. Differential Diagnosis
   A. Aspiration Pneumonitis. Risk factors include (1) altered mental
   status, (2) reflux disease, (3) nasogastric tube placement, and
   (4) tracheostomy. Emergency intubation has a high incidence of
   aspiration. Emergent intubation for pregnant patients, patients
   who recently ate, or patients with bowel obstruction requires rapid
   sequence induction with cricoid pressure to reduce aspiration risk.
   Most frequently, aspiration of acidic gastric contents causes bron-

chospasm and respiratory distress. Large food particles may cause obstruction, milder forms may result in pneumonia or lung abscess formation.

B. Asthma. Wheezing from aspiration, especially chronic aspiration, can mimic asthma.

C. Pneumonia. May precede aspiration or be caused by aspiration.

D. Pulmonary Embolus and Infarction. Acute dyspnea and respiratory failure is a common presentation of pulmonary embolus (refer to Problem 26, page 97).

E. Foreign Body Aspiration. A problem in children for the most part. Older patients with poor dentition may aspirate loose teeth.

IV. Database. History of asthma should be ruled-out. Evaluate for risk factors of pulmonary embolus (birth control pills, recent operation with prolonged bedrest, previous deep venous thrombosis).

A. Physical Exam Key Points
1. **Vital signs.** Pay close attention to respiratory rate.
2. **HEENT**. Check dentition for loose or missing teeth. If a nasogastric (NG) or feeding tube is present, check its position.
3. **Neck.** Evidence of tumor involvement of the pharynx, tracheostomy, surgery of the head and neck, and radiation to the head and neck should be sought.
4. **Lungs.** Wheezing occurs when airways are irritated by acid stomach contents. Decreased breath sounds from air trapping can occur with foreign body aspiration.
5. **Skin.** Look for cyanosis to suggest hypoxia.
6. **Extremities.** Look for evidence of deep vein thrombosis (DVT).
7. **Neurologic exam.** Careful evaluation of mental status and presence of gag reflex are important.

B. Laboratory Data
1. **Arterial blood gas.** Intubation should be performed if adequate oxygenation cannot be maintained.
2. **Hemogram.** Pay particular attention to the white count.
3. **Sputum Gram's stain and culture.** Pathogenic organisms may grow in cases of chronic aspiration or in acute aspiration pneumonia.

C. Radiologic and Other Studies
1. Chest radiograph may show:
   a. Air trapping ("hyperaeration") on side of foreign body aspiration.
   b. Infiltrate in area of superior segment of lower lobes (mid-lung fields) with aspiration in bedridden patients. These segmental bronchi take off directly posteriorly and are thus most dependent in the supine patient. Infiltrates may not be seen immediately after aspiration.

      c. Wedge-shaped infarct in some cases of pulmonary embolus.

      d. Clear fields in uncomplicated asthma.

      e. Aspiration can result in infiltrates in any portion of either lung or none at all depending on quantity and quality of the material aspirated.

      f. Lung abscess formation may have associated air-fluid levels. Usually a late finding or associated with chronic aspiration.

  2. Other Studies. Ventilation/perfusion scan if venous thrombosis or pulmonary emboli suspected.

V. Plan. Aspiration should be suspected in patients who may be unable to protect their airway, with neurologic or oncologic disease affecting swallowing and coughing and with depressed mental status, obtundation, or absent gag reflex (eg, head trauma or alcohol intoxication), and in those patients who have required intubation on a full stomach. Patients undergoing gavage feedings are also at increased risk. The goal should be to recognize the at risk population and prevent aspiration.

  A. Prevention

    1. For emergent intubation, it may be advisable to administer IV agents such as cimetidine to attempt to increase gastric pH along with rapid induction and cricoid pressure.

    2. For patients being gavage fed, gastric emptying should be confirmed and the head of the bed elevated.

    3. Unconscious patients should be placed in a lateral, slightly head down position whenever possible.

  B. Oxygenation. Supplemental oxygen is usually given by mask initially. Carefully monitor oxygenation with a transcutaneous oxygen saturation monitor, or repeat arterial blood gases.

  C. Intubation and Pulmonary Toilet. These will be needed if oxygenation is poor or in the obtunded or unconscious patient to prevent recurrence.

  D. Remove Nasogastric Tube. Remove tube if possible, because gastric contents can "wick" up the tube as well as interfere with effective coughing.

  E. Replace Metal Tracheostomy. Use a cuffed tracheostomy tube. Metal tubes are used rarely now, but may be found in patients with old tracheostomies.

  F. Medications

    1. Corticosteroids and prophylactic antibiotics are **not** generally indicated in the acute management of aspiration, but there is some debate about this. Some clinicians feel hydrocortisone 30 mg/kg/d should be given for 3 days.

    2. Start antibiotics based on culture results when there is evidence of established pneumonia. Acute aspiration pneumonia may be aerobic or mixed anaerobic-aerobic flora.

   3. Anaerobic organisms are more likely with poor dentition. If empiric antibiotic therapy is chosen for an out of the hospital aspiration, penicillin G (2–6 million units/d) is recommended; for hospitalized patients, tobramycin with ticarcillin is a reasonable initial choice, pending culture results.

G. Rigid Bronchoscopy. Performed when foreign body aspiration is suspected or in those patients who aspirated particulate gastric material that cannot be adequately suctioned.

H. Chest Tube. May be needed later for drainage of an empyema. Chronic aspiration pneumonia may be necrotizing with formation of a lung abscess or progression to empyema.

9. BRADYCARDIA

I. Problem. A postoperative hernia patient is found to have a heart rate of 42 on a routine vital signs check.

II. Immediate Questions

A. What is the patient's blood pressure, and is the patient alert and oriented? The initial questions define the severity of the problem. Because the clinical relevance of a significant bradycardia is reduced perfusion pressure, the rapid assessment of perfusion—the blood pressure and the mental status—should be ascertained.

B. What is the patient's normal resting heart rate? The range of normal heart rates is wide and a rate of 42 in a resting patient may not be abnormal in some people such as highly conditioned athletes.

C. Are there any associated symptoms of chest pain or pressure, dyspnea, diaphoresis, or nausea? A new bradydysrhythmia may be a manifestation of an acute cardiac event such as an inferior myocardial infarction. Question the patient about any concurrent symptoms.

D. Has the patient felt dizzy or lightheaded in the recent past? The clinical presentation of sinus node dysfunction is frequently episodic syncope or near-syncope.

E. What medication is the patient taking, and does the patient have a pacemaker? Certain medications, such as β-blockers (propranolol, etc), verapamil, digitalis, and others can lead to bradycardia. A patient with a pacemaker may be suffering from pacer malfunction.

F. Does the patient have a history of cardiovascular disease? This may further clarify the nature of the slow heart rate.

III. Differential Diagnosis. Disturbances in the cardiac conduction pathway leading to bradydysrhythmias are due to dysfunction at the level of the sinus node or at the level of the atrioventricular (AV) node/His Purkinje system. Within these two categories a variety of conditions exist defined by characteristic ECG patterns and associated with particular clinical conditions.

A. Sinus Node Disease
   1. Sinus bradycardia
      a. Vasovagal syncope
      b. High vagal tone: More common in conditioned athletes and in the elderly.
      c. Increased intracranial pressure: Cushing's reflex results in bradycardia.
   2. Sinus node dysfunction. Sick sinus syndrome and tachycardia-bradycardia syndrome are variants of sinus node disease characterized by intermittent sinus pauses.
      a. Ischemic cardiomyopathy
      b. Hypertensive cardiomyopathy
      c. Hypothyroidism
      d. Hypothermia
      e. Infiltrative diseases (amyloidosis, etc)

B. Atrioventricular Node Disease
   1. First-degree AV block. PR interval > 0.2 seconds.
   2. Second-degree AV block Mobitz type 1 (Wenckebach). Successive prolongation of the PR interval with eventual dropped ventricular beat.
      a. Inferior myocardial infarction
      b. Drug toxicity: Frequently implicated: digoxin, β-blockers (propranolol), calcium channel blockers (verapamil).
   3. Second-degree AV block Mobitz type II. Intermittent missed ventricular beat. Associated conditions are the same as for third-degree AV block and this condition may progress to third-degree AV block.
   4. Third-degree AV block. Also called "AV dissociation."
      a. Myocardial infarction: Most common sites are anteroseptal or inferior.
      b. Primary degenerative disease of the conducting system.
      c. Infiltrative conditions: Sarcoidosis, amyloidosis, neoplasms.
      d. Infectious diseases: Viral myocarditis, acute rheumatic fever, Lyme disease.

IV. Database. The primary focus to diagnose a bradycardia is the 12-lead ECG and rhythm strip, which should be obtained concurrently with the initial history and physical exam.

A. Physical Exam Key Points

1. **Vital signs.** Note heart rate, blood pressure, respiratory rate. Hypotension < 90 mm Hg requires emergent treatment.
2. **Lungs.** Listen for evidence of failure (rales).
3. **Cardiac.** Note any new murmurs or gallops. Note if the rhythm is regular or irregular.
4. **Skin.** Pallor, cool, moist skin as evidence of poor perfusion or increased vagal tone.
5. **Neurologic.** Look for evidence of elevated intracranial pressure (papilledema). Decreased mental status is a measure of inadequate perfusion pressure.

B. Laboratory Data

1. **Electrolytes, calcium.** Hypokalemia can potentiate digoxin toxicity and hypocalcemia can result in a prolonged QT interval and bradycardia.
2. CPK with isoenzymes to evaluate myocardial injury (see Section II, page 245).
3. Digoxin level if indicated. Toxicity is often manifested as bradycardia. Toxic levels usually > 2.5 ng/mL.
4. **Thyroid hormone levels.** Hypothyroidism can cause bradycardia.
5. Arterial blood gases if indicated by respiratory distress or dyspnea.

C. Radiologic and Other Studies

1. **ECG.** This should be analyzed systematically looking for atrial rate (lead II is good), ventricular rate, PR interval, relation of P waves to QRS complexes, and evidence of ischemia (inverted T waves, ST segment depression).
2. **Chest x-ray.** Change in cardiac silhouette and lung fields may be associated with myocardial dysfunction.
3. Specialized tests conducted by cardiologists include electrophysiologic mapping to define the precise location of blocks and complete autonomic blockade (using atropine and propranolol) to determine the intrinsic heart rate and document the contribution of vagal tone to the bradycardia.

V. Plan. The treatment plan will be dictated by the type and degree of bradycardia and any underlying clinical condition. Remember that not all bradycardia is clinically significant. Use extreme caution, especially in the elderly, when treating bradycardia. In urgent situations treat with atropine IV, apply oxygen, and obtain an ECG as soon as possible.

Critical management can be found in the advanced cardiac life support (ACLS) algorithm for bradycardia (see Figure I–8, page 48).

A. Critical Symptomatic Bradycardia. Should be used in cases of acute, clinically significant bradycardia usually associated with hypotension in the following sequence:

    1. Atropine 0.5–1.0 mg IV (0.01 mg/kg). May be repeated every 5–10 minutes to a total dose of 2 mg.

    2. Transcutaneous pacing if available.

    3. Dopamine 5–20 μg/kg/min

    4. Epinephrine 2–10 μg/min

    5. Isoproterenol (Isuprel) 1–3 μg/min IV continuous infusion (low dose).

B. Treat the Underlying Condition

    1. Myocardial ischemia. Should be treated with nitrates (such as sublingual nitroglycerin) and oxygen.

    2. Increased intracranial pressure. Maneuvers to decrease pressure include mannitol diuresis, elevate the head of the bed, intubation and mechanical hyperventilation.

C. Pacemaker Therapy. If the bradydysrhythmia does not respond to medical therapy or in certain critical situations listed below, then a temporary ventricular pacer wire should be passed to treat the bradycardia. If this option is needed, contact the cardiology consultant.

    1. Indications for temporary pacemaker

        a. Transient second-degree AV block with an inferior myocardial infarction.

        b. AV block as a result of drug toxicity.

        c. As temporizing measure before permanent pacemaker.

    2. Indications for permanent pacemaker

        a. Sinus node dysfunction: Must be documented to be symptomatic.

        b. Second or third degree AV block associated with an acute myocardial infarction.

        c. Symptomatic Mobitz type II and third degree AV block.

D. Digoxin Toxicity. Check level, hold medication, and consider digoxin antibody (Digibind) 60 mg per 1 mg digoxin, IV.

10. BRIGHT RED BLOOD PER RECTUM (HEMATOCHEZIA)

I. Problem. You are called to see a 60-year-old female patient who is passing red blood per rectum 3 days after undergoing a modified radical mastectomy.

II. Immediate Questions

    A. What are the vital signs? Look for signs of hemodynamically significant blood loss such as tachycardia, hypotension.

    B. What volume of blood has been passed and over what time period? The volume of blood may help assess the significance of the bleed, as the hematocrit may not decrease until later.

C. **What was the most recent hematocrit?** A baseline value is needed to assess the amount of bleeding.

D. **What is the nature of the stool?** Coating of the stool often indicates an anal process such as hemorrhoids, but may also suggest a lower GI tumor. Bright red blood is more likely to be from the distal left colon. Melena usually signifies bleeding proximal to the right colon. However, the color of the stool is more likely determined by the length of time the blood has been in the bowel. Occasionally, bright red rectal blood can be a result of an upper GI source and rapid transit through the bowel.

E. **What medication is the patient taking, and is there any history of alcohol abuse?** Alcoholism may suggest varices; ulcerogenic medications include aspirin and other nonsteroidal anti-inflammatory agents; overuse of warfarin (Coumadin) may cause GI tract bleeding.

F. **Has the patient had recent GI tract surgery?** It is common to have some bloody bowel movements immediately after GI tract surgery.

G. **Are there any associated symptoms?** Crampy abdominal pain or fever suggests an infectious cause, inflammatory bowel disease, or diverticulitis. A change in bowel habits or decreased caliber of stools may indicate a neoplasm, whereas polyps and angiodysplasia are usually free of other symptoms.

III. Differential Diagnosis

A. **Diverticular Disease.** A common cause (up to 70%) of massive lower gastrointestinal bleeding and usually left-sided.

B. **Angiodysplasia.** These are usually right-sided lesions and thus most often associated with melena. The natural history of bleeding from angiodysplasia usually includes rebleeding. This is usually venous or capillary bleeding as contrasted with the arterial bleeding associated with diverticula.

C. **Polyps.** Villous adenomas can also cause potassium loss.

D. **Carcinoma.** Usually large intestinal adenocarcinoma.

E. **Inflammatory Bowel Disease.** Ulcerative colitis is more frequently associated with bloody diarrhea than Crohn's disease.

F. **Hemorrhoids.** While their presence may be common, this does not preclude the presence of simultaneous tumor or angiodysplasia.

G. **Mesenteric Thrombosis.** This may lead to ischemic bowel.

H. **Meckel's Diverticulitis**

I. **Anal Fissures**

J. **Excessive Anticoagulation.** Be sure to review medications the patient is taking. Check clotting studies as needed.

K. Massive Upper GI Bleed. Results in rapid intestinal transit and resulting hematochezia (see Problem 34, page 118). Blood is an excellent cathartic. Remember that lower GI bleeding can originate anywhere in the GI tract.

IV. Database

A. Physical Exam Key Points

1. **Vital Signs.** Look for evidence of hypovolemia (tachycardia and hypotension). Fever may represent inflammatory bowel disease or an infectious gastroenteritis.
2. **Abdomen.** Palpation for masses or tenderness. Left lower quadrant mass that may be associated with diverticulitis or right lower quadrant mass often associated with Crohn's disease. Bowel sounds may be hyperactive because blood is a cathartic.
3. **Rectal.** Hemorrhoids, fissures, or masses may be detected.
4. Is bleeding present at other sites to suggest a systemic cause?
5. Check for signs of cirrhosis (palmar erythema, caput medusae) to suggest a possible upper GI source.

B. Laboratory Studies

1. **Hemogram.** Serial hematocrit checks are helpful because a massive bleed may not reflect itself in a change in hematocrit for some time. Microcytic and hypochromic indices are indicative of chronic blood loss.
2. **Clotting studies.** PT/PTT and platelet count may reveal a coagulation disorder.
3. **Blood bank.** Obtain a type and cross-match.

C. Radiologic and Other Studies

1. **Nasogastric tube.** Pass a nasogastric tube to rule out upper GI bleeding.
2. **Angiography.** Is indicated for the diagnosis of lower GI bleeding in any patient who requires more than 2 units of blood to maintain their hematocrit or becomes hypotensive. Remember that angiography is impossible with barium in the gut. To be helpful, bleeding must usually be > 0.5–1.0 mL/min. Selective embolization or vasopressin infusion may be possible to control bleeding.
3. **Radiolabeled red cell study (Usually ^{99m}Tc).** This can sometimes localize lesions in the GI tract, especially with slower rates of bleeding than needed for angiography (0.2 mL/min).
4. **Sigmoidoscopy.** This will detect a low lying source of bleeding. Colonoscopy is occasionally used and may allow fulguration bleeding sites, eg, angiodysplasia.
5. **Upper GI Endoscopy (esophagogastroduodenoscopy [EGD]).** While a nasogastric tube can usually rule out upper GI

sources of bleeding, an inconclusive workup for lower GI bleeding necessitates a definitive look at the upper GI tract.

V. Plan. Approximately 80% of patients with lower GI bleeding stop bleeding spontaneously. Acute, severe hemorrhage is potentially life-threatening and should be treated first.

   A. Acute Intervention. Large-bore IVs (16 gauge) should be placed for repletion of volume. Use crystalloid or blood if there is a low hematocrit. Attempt to keep hematocrit > 30%. A Foley catheter will allow more accurate assessment of volume status. Consider a central venous pressure (CVP) line if there is any instability and in the elderly patient.

   B. Diagnosis and Treatment. A suggested algorithm for the diagnosis and treatment of acute lower GI bleeding is outlined in Figure I–3.

   1. Treatment is directed at the cause. If a bleeding diverticulum is found, initial therapy is the intra-arterial infusion of vasopressin rather than resection.

   2. The combined approach of angiography and colonoscopy can usually localize the bleeding site. In those extreme cases where the site cannot be identified, subtotal colectomy is usually indicated.

   3. Surgery may eventually be needed to treat lesions such as carcinoma, polyps, hemorrhoids, and the lesions of inflammatory bowel disease.

   4. Local care for hemorrhoids includes sitz baths, stool softeners (DOSS), and suppositories (Anusol, etc).

11. CARDIOPULMONARY ARREST

Immediate Actions
   1. Assess responsiveness.
   2. If nonresponsive, follow algorithm in Figure I–4.

I. Problem. One week after above knee amputation, a patient is found unresponsive and pulseless in bed.

II. Immediate Questions
   A. Is the patient responsive? Basic cardiopulmonary resuscitation (CPR) begins with a vigorous attempt to arouse the patient. Call the patient and shake him or her by the shoulders.

   B. Is the airway obstructed? Finger sweep or suction out the patient's mouth. Listen for air movement.

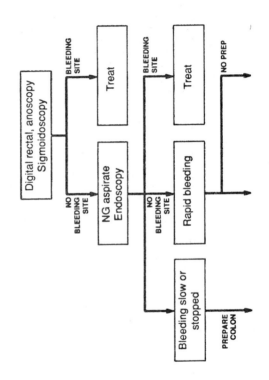

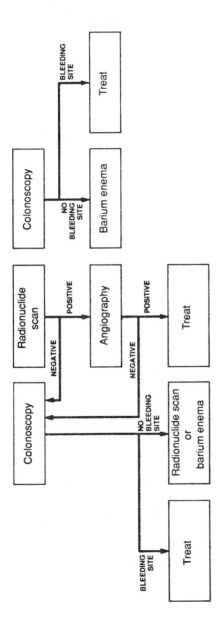

Figure I-3. Suggested scheme for the management of lower gastrointestinal hemorrhage. **NG** = nasogastric tube. *(Reproduced, with permission, from Schrock TR: Large intestine. In: Current Surgical Diagnosis & Treatment, 10/e. Way LW (editor). Appleton & Lange, 1994.)*

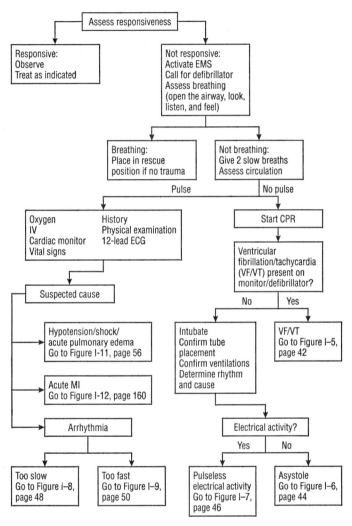

Figure I–4. Universal algorithm for adult emergency cardiac care (ECC). *(Reproduced, with permission, from Adult Advanced Cardiac Life Support. JAMA 1992;268, No. 16.)*

C. **Are there vital signs?** Check for carotid pulse and blood pressure.

After these basic questions are asked and maneuvers performed, begin mouth-to-mouth or, preferably, ventilation with 100% oxygen by bag and mask, and chest compressions. The following questions are then asked as ACLS is started.

D. **What medication is the patient taking?** Cardiac medications are particularly important, especially antiarrhythmics and digoxin. An adverse reaction to a recently administered medication may be determined.

E. **Are there any recent lab values, particularly potassium or hematocrit?** Hyperkalemia (usually > 7 mEq/L) or severe anemia, usually acute, may cause cardiac arrest.

F. **What are the patient's major medical problems?** Ask about coronary artery disease, previous myocardial infarction, hypertension, previous pulmonary embolus, and recent surgery.

III. **Differential Diagnosis.** Arrest rhythms include ventricular fibrillation and tachycardia, asystole, bradycardia, and electromechanical dissociation (EMD). Causes of cardiopulmonary arrest may include:

A. **Cardiac**
   1. Myocardial infarction.
   2. Congestive heart failure.
   3. Ventricular arrhythmias.
   4. Cardiac tamponade. Usually posttraumatic.

B. **Pulmonary**
   1. Pulmonary embolus.
   2. Acute respiratory failure.
   3. Aspiration.
   4. Tension pneumothorax.

C. **Hemorrhagic.** Undiagnosed severe bleeding can result in cardiac arrest, such as ruptured aortic aneurysm.

D. **Metabolic**
   1. **Hypokalemia, hyperkalemia.** These may induce arrhythmias.
   2. **Acidosis.** Severe acidosis may suppress myocardial function.
   3. **Warming from hypothermia.** Arrhythmias may be induced.

IV. **Database**

A. **Physical Exam Key Points.** As described, check responsiveness and vital signs. Resuscitation should always be initiated before a detailed physical exam is performed.
   1. Check ventilation and perform airway opening maneuvers (jaw thrust or chin lift) as needed.

    2. Look for tracheal deviation as evidence of a tension pneumothorax.

    3. Distended neck veins may indicate pericardial tamponade or pneumothorax.

B. Laboratory Data. These should be obtained as soon as possible, but should not delay the start of therapy.

    1. Arterial blood gas.

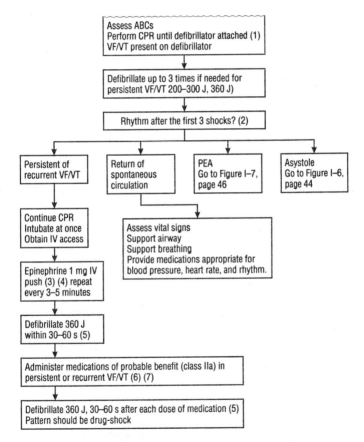

Figure I–5. Algorithm for ventricular fibrillation and pulseless ventricular tachycardia (VF/VT). *(Reproduced, with permission, from Adult Advanced Cardiac Life Support. JAMA 1992;268, No. 16.)*

    2. Serum electrolytes, with special attention to the potassium.
    3. CBC. Especially important is the hematocrit.

C. Radiologic and Other Studies
    1. Continuous cardiac monitoring, frequently checking lead placement.
    2. Other studies may be performed after the patient has been resuscitated.

V. Plan. Therapy for cardiac arrest is based on specific algorithms outlined by the American Heart Association (AHA). Specific AHA algorithms for ventricular fibrillation, ventricular tachycardia, bradycardia

Footnotes to Figure I–5
Class I: Definitely helpful.
Class IIa: Acceptable, probably helpful.
Class IIb: Acceptable, possibly helpful.
Class III: Not indicated, may be harmful.

(1) Precordial thump is a class IIb action in witnessed arrest, no pulse, and no defibrillator available.
(2) Hypothermic cardiac arrest is treated differently after this point. See section on hypothermia.
(3) The recommended dose of epinephrine is 1 mg IV push every 3–5 min. If this approach fails, several class IIb dosing regimens can be considered:
    Intermediate: epinephrine 2–5 mg IV push, every 3–5 min.
    Escalating: epinephrine 1 mg–3 mg–5 mg IV push (3 min apart).
    High: epinephrine 0.1 mg/kg IV push, every 3–5 min.
(4) Sodium bicarbonate (1 mEq/kg) is class I if patient has known preexisting hyperkalemia.
(5) Multiple sequenced shocks (200 J, 200–300 J, 360 J) are acceptable here (class I), especially when medications are delayed.
(6) Lidocaine 1.5 mg/kg IV push. Repeat in 3–5 min to total loading dose of 3 mg/kg; then use:
    Bretylium 5 mg/kg IV push. Repeat in 5 min at 10 mg/kg.
    Magnesium sulfate 1–2 g IV in torsades de pointes or suspected hypomagnesemic state or severe refractory VF.
    Procainamide 30 mg/min in refractory VF (maximum total 17 mg/kg).
(7) Sodium bicarbonate (1 mEq/kg IV):
    Class IIa
    If known preexisting bicarbonate-responsive acidosis.
    If overdose with tricyclic antidepressants.
    To alkalinize the urine in drug overdoses.
    Class IIb
    If intubated and continued long arrest interval.
    Upon return of spontaneous circulation after long arrest interval.
    Class III
    Hypoxic lactic acids.

Figure I–5. (*continued*)

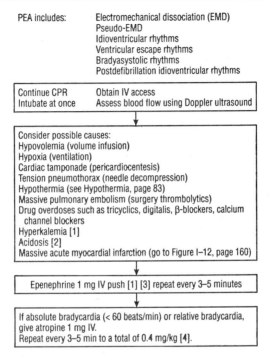

PEA includes: Electromechanical dissociation (EMD)
                       Pseudo-EMD
                       Idioventricular rhythms
                       Ventricular escape rhythms
                       Bradyasystolic rhythms
                       Postdefibrillation idioventricular rhythms

Continue CPR	Obtain IV access
Intubate at once	Assess blood flow using Doppler ultrasound

Consider possible causes:
Hypovolemia (volume infusion)
Hypoxia (ventilation)
Cardiac tamponade (pericardiocentesis)
Tension pneumothorax (needle decompression)
Hypothermia (see Hypothermia, page 83)
Massive pulmonary embolism (surgery thrombolytics)
Drug overdoses such as tricyclics, digitalis, β-blockers, calcium
   channel blockers
Hyperkalemia [1]
Acidosis [2]
Massive acute myocardial infarction (go to Figure I–12, page 160)

Epenephrine 1 mg IV push [1] [3] repeat every 3–5 minutes

If absolute bradycardia (< 60 beats/min) or relative bradycardia,
give atropine 1 mg IV.
Repeat every 3–5 min to a total of 0.4 mg/kg [4].

Figure I–6. Algorithm for pulseless electrical activity (PEA) (electromechanical dissociation [EMD]). *(Reproduced, with permission, from Adult Advanced Cardiac Life Support. JAMA 1992;268, No. 16.)*

asystole, and electromechanical dissociation are shown in Figures I–5 through I–9. Frequently used resuscitation medications are located inside the back cover. Every physician should have these memorized.

In addition, successful resuscitation is based on a team approach with one leader monitoring the rhythm and ordering therapy according to the appropriate algorithm. Everyone must remain calm and must be assigned to a specific job.

Resuscitation begins with the ABCs: **A**irway (intubate whenever possible), **B**reathing (ventilate), and **C**irculation (chest compression). For adults, the ratio of 5 compressions to 1 breath is used in two person CPR.

Footnotes to Figure I–6
Class I: Definitely helpful.
Class IIa: Acceptable, probably helpful.
Class IIb: Acceptable, possibly helpful.
Class III: Not indicated, may be harmful.

[1] Sodium bicarbonate 1 mEq/kg is class I if patient has known preexisting hyperkalemia.
[2] Sodium bicarbonate 1 mEq/kg:
   Class IIa
      If known preexisting bicarbonate-responsive acidosis.
      If overdose with tricyclic antidepressants.
      To alkalinize the urine in drug overdoses.
   Class IIb
      If intubated and continued long arrest interval.
      Upon return of spontaneous circulation after long arrest interval.
   Class III
      Hypoxic lactic acids.
[3] The recommended dose of epinephrine is 1 mg IV push every 3–5 min. If this approach fails, several class IIb dosing regimens can be considered:
      Intermediate: epinephrine 2–5 mg IV push, every 3–5 min.
      Escalating: epinephrine 1 mg–3 mg–5 mg IV push (3 min apart).
      High: epinephrine 0.1 mg/kg IV push, every 3–5 min.
[4] Shorter atropine dosing intervals are possibly helpful in cardiac arrest (class IIb).

Figure I–6. (*continued*)

A. **Ventricular Fibrillation and Pulseless Tachycardia.** See Figure I–5. Torsade de pointes, a rare ventricular arrhythmia, is treated with a temporary pacemaker, rarely bretylium, but never lidocaine. Most often congenital or drug induced, it is characterized by "twisting" or direction changes of the QRS complex around the isoelectric line.

B. **Electromechanical Dissociation.** See Figure I–6. In surgical patients, always consider pulmonary embolism, especially in high risk patients (obese, previous embolism, certain pelvic and orthopedic cases), and hypovolemia as causes of EMD. In trauma patients, consider tension pneumothorax and cardiac tamponade. Treat hypovolemia with aggressive fluid resuscitation, tension pneumothorax with tube thoracostomy, and pericardial tamponade with pericardiocentesis.

C. **Asystole.** See algorithm in Figure I–7. The prognosis is very poor in cases of asystole. Defibrillate if there is any question about the rhythm being fine ventricular tachycardia.

D. **Bradycardia.** See Figure I–8 and Problem 9, page 31.

E. Tachycardia. See Figure I–9 and Problem 67, page 215. Emergency cardioversion is reviewed in Figure I–10.

F. Hypotension, shock, and acute pulmonary edema. May arise independently or associated with a cardiac event. See Figure I–9 and Problem 47, page 159.

REFERENCE

Adult Advanced Cardiac Life Support. JAMA 1992;268:2199.

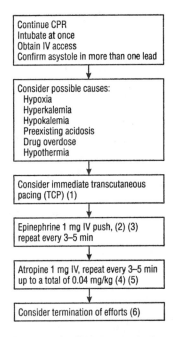

Figure I–7. Asystole treatment algorithm. *(Reproduced, with permission, from Adult Advanced Cardiac Life Support. JAMA 1992;268, No. 16.)*

12. CHEST PAIN

I. **Problem.** Four days following a radical nephrectomy a 62-year-old patient tells the nurse of an ongoing episode of chest pain that has lasted for ten minutes.

II. **Immediate Questions.** The conditions that lead a patient to complain of "chest pain" range from inconsequential to life-threatening. The purpose of the immediate questions is to determine the urgency of response and, in particular, to ascertain if ischemic heart disease is the cause of the pain.

 A. Does the patient have a history of coronary artery disease; if so, does the current pain resemble previous episodes of angina pectoris? In patients with documented cardiac disease, particularly if

Footnotes to Figure I–7
Class I: Definitely helpful.
Class IIa: Acceptable, probably helpful.
Class IIb: Acceptable, possibly helpful.
Class III: Not indicated, may be harmful.

(1) TCP is a class IIb intervention. Lack of success may be due to delays in pacing. To be effective TCP must be performed early, simultaneously with drugs. Evidence does not support routine use of TCP for asystole.
(2) The recommended dose of epinephrine is 1 mg IV push every 3–5 min. If this approach fails, several class IIb dosing regimens can be considered:
Intermediate: epinephrine 2–5 mg IV push, every 3–5 min.
Escalating: epinephrine 1 mg–3 mg–5 mg IV push (3 min apart).
High: epinephrine 0.1 mg/kg IV push, every 3–5 min.
(3) Sodium bicarbonate 1 mEq/kg is class I if patient has known preexisting hyperkalemia.
(4) Shorter atropine dosing intervals are class IIb in asystolic arrest.
(5) Sodium bicarbonate 1 mEq/kg IV:
Class IIa
If known preexisting bicarbonate-responsive acidosis.
If overdose with tricyclic antidepressants.
To alkalinize the urine in drug overdoses.
Class IIb
If intubated and continued long arrest interval.
Upon return of spontaneous circulation after long arrest interval.
Class III
Hypoxic lactic acids.
(6) If patient remains in asystole or other agonal rhythms after successful intubation and initial medications and no reversible causes are identified, consider termination of resuscitative efforts by a physician. Consider interval since arrest.

Figure I–7. (*continued*)

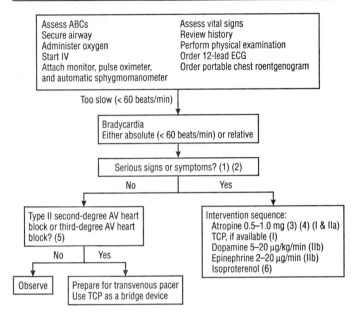

Assess ABCs   Assess vital signs
Secure airway   Review history
Administer oxygen   Perform physical examination
Start IV   Order 12-lead ECG
Attach monitor, pulse oximeter,   Order portable chest roentgenogram
and automatic sphygmomanometer

Too slow (< 60 beats/min)

Bradycardia
Either absolute (< 60 beats/min) or relative

Serious signs or symptoms? (1) (2)

No   Yes

Type II second-degree AV heart   Intervention sequence:
block or third-degree AV heart   Atropine 0.5–1.0 mg (3) (4) (I & IIa)
block? (5)   TCP, if available (I)
                                          Dopamine 5–20 µg/kg/min (IIb)
No   Yes   Epinephrine 2–20 µg/min (IIb)
                                          Isoproterenol (6)

Observe   Prepare for transvenous pacer
           Use TCP as a bridge device

Footnotes

(1) Serious signs or symptoms must be related to the slow rate.
    Clinical manifestations include:
      Symptoms (chest pain, shortness of breath, decreased level of consciousness) and
      signs (low BP, shock, pulmonary congestions, CHF, acute MI).
(2) Do not delay TCP while awaiting IV acess or for atropine to take effect if patient is
    symptomatic.
(3) Denervated transplanted hearts will not respond to atropine. Go at once to pacing,
    catecholamine infusion, or both.
(4) Atropine should be given in repeat doses in 3–5 min up to a total of 0.04 mg/kg.
    Consider shorter dosing intervals in severe clinical conditions. It has been suggested
    that atropine should be used with caution in atrioventricular (AV) block at the His-
    Purkinje level (type II AV block and new third degree block with wide QRS complexes)
    (class IIb).
(5) Never treat third-degree heart block plus ventricular escape beats with Lidocaine.
(6) Isoproterenol should be used, if at all, with extreme caution. At low doses it is class IIb
    (possibly helpful); at higher doses it is class III (harmful).
(7) Verify patient tolerance and mechanical capture. Use analgesia and sedation as needed.

Figure I–8. Bradycardia algorithm (patient not in cardiac arrest). *(Reproduced,
with permission, from Adult Advanced Cardiac Life Support. JAMA 1992;268, No. 16.)*

the current episode resembles previous known anginal attacks, the pain should be treated as myocardial ischemia with sublingual nitroglycerin (0.4 mg typical initial dose) without delay.

B. What is the location, nature, and severity of the pain? Location of the pain (substernal, epigastric), radiation of the pain to other areas (jaw, arms, flank, abdomen), nature of the pain (burning, crushing, tearing, stabbing), and the severity of the pain (mild, moderate, severe) can help define patterns of chest pain that fit certain diagnostic categories. However, chest pain cannot be defined by clinical criteria alone because there is considerable overlap in pain from varied causes as the thoracic viscera share common neural pathways. Classic angina is retrosternal and may radiate to the jaw or left arm. Thoracic aortic dissection is usually described as tearing or ripping and peptic ulcer is often burning or gnawing.

C. What was the patient doing when the pain began? The inciting activity (or factors that alleviate pain) at the onset of an episode of chest pain is helpful in defining the diagnosis. Classic angina is brought on by exertion, pleuritic pain is exacerbated by coughing, and esophagitis is often exacerbated by recumbency.

D. Are there any symptoms associated with the episode of chest pain? Inquire specifically about nausea, dyspnea, diaphoresis, dizziness, syncope, abdominal pain, pleuritic pain, palpitations, and presence of acid taste in the mouth.

III. Differential Diagnosis. The differential diagnosis of chest pain is one of the classic points of discussions in medical school clerkships because of the frequency of the complaint, the range of diagnostic possibilities, and the importance of making the correct diagnosis.

A. Cardiac/Vascular
   1. **Acute myocardial infarction.** Crushing retrosternal chest pain lasting longer than 1 hour and unrelieved by nitroglycerin.
   2. **Angina pectoris.** The pain of angina is typically described as crushing, substernal, often with radiation to the arms or jaw. There is often associated nausea, diaphoresis, dyspnea, or palpitations and usually relieved by nitroglycerin.
      a. Coronary artery disease
      b. Coronary artery spasm (Prinzmetal's angina). Variant angina, usually occurs at rest.
      c. Aortic regurgitation or mitral valve prolapse. Heart murmur will usually be present.
   3. **Aortic dissection.** The pain is tearing in nature and radiates to the back and is usually associated with a history of hypertension.

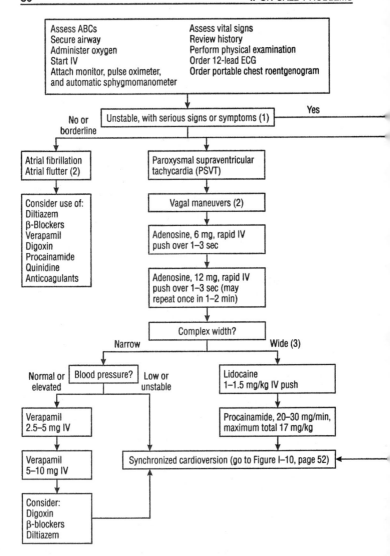

Figure I–9. Tachycardia algorithm. *(Reproduced, with permission, from Adult Advanced Cardiac Life Support. JAMA 1992;268, No. 16.)*

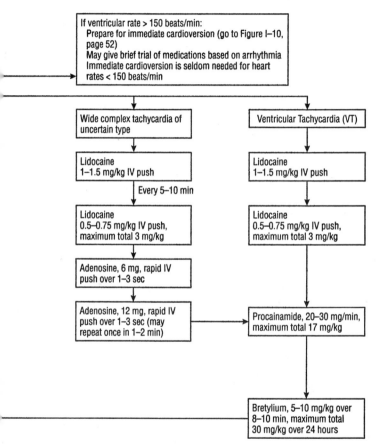

If ventricular rate > 150 beats/min:
Prepare for immediate cardioversion (go to Figure I–10, page 52)
May give brief trial of medications based on arrhythmia
Immediate cardioversion is seldom needed for heart rates < 150 beats/min

Wide complex tachycardia of uncertain type

Lidocaine 1–1.5 mg/kg IV push

Every 5–10 min

Lidocaine 0.5–0.75 mg/kg IV push, maximum total 3 mg/kg

Adenosine, 6 mg, rapid IV push over 1–3 sec

Adenosine, 12 mg, rapid IV push over 1–3 sec (may repeat once in 1–2 min)

Ventricular Tachycardia (VT)

Lidocaine 1–1.5 mg/kg IV push

Lidocaine 0.5–0.75 mg/kg IV push, maximum total 3 mg/kg

Procainamide, 20–30 mg/min, maximum total 17 mg/kg

Bretylium, 5–10 mg/kg over 8–10 min, maximum total 30 mg/kg over 24 hours

Footnotes

(1) Unstable condition must be related to the tachycardia. Signs and symptoms may include chest pain, shortness of breath, decreased level of consciousness, low blood pressure (BP), shock, pulmonary congestion, congestive heart failure, acute myocardial infarction.
(2) Carotid sinus pressure is contraindicated in patients with carotid bruits; avoid ice water immersion in patients with ischemic heart disease.
(3) If the wide-complex tachycardia is known with certainty to be PSVT, and BP is normal/elevated, sequence can include verapamil.

Figure I–9. (*continued*)

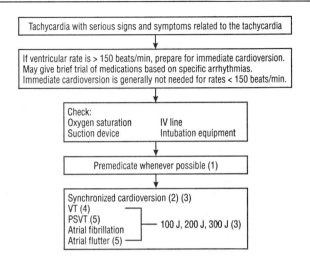

Tachycardia with serious signs and symptoms related to the tachycardia

↓

If ventricular rate is > 150 beats/min, prepare for immediate cardioversion.
May give brief trial of medications based on specific arrhythmias.
Immediate cardioversion is generally not needed for rates < 150 beats/min.

↓

Check:
Oxygen saturation   IV line
Suction device   Intubation equipment

↓

Premedicate whenever possible (1)

↓

Synchronized cardioversion (2) (3)
VT (4)
PSVT (5)   ┐
Atrial fibrillation   ├── 100 J, 200 J, 300 J (3)
Atrial flutter (5)   ┘

Footnotes
(1) Effective regimens have included a sedative (eg, diazepam, midazolam,
    barbituates, etomidate, ketamine, methohexital) with or without an analgesic
    agent (eg, fentanyl, morphine, meperidine).
    Many experts recommend anesthesia if service is readily available.
(2) Note possible need to resynchronize after each cardioversion.
(3) If delays in synchronization occur and clinical conditions are critical, go to
    immediate unsynchronized shocks.
(4) Treat polymorphic VT (irregular form and rate) like VF:
    200 J, 200–300 J, 260 J.
(5) PSVT and atrial flutter often respond to lower energy levels (start with 50 J).

Figure I–10. Electrical cardioversion algorithm (patient not in cardiac arrest).
(Reproduced, with permission, from Adult Advanced Cardiac Life Support. JAMA 1992;268, No. 16.)

4. **Acute pericarditis.** A friction rub may be present and an effusion typically seen on echocardiogram.
   a. **Infectious:** Most commonly viral or tuberculosis.
   b. **Myocardial infarction (MI):** There can be early pericarditis
      in the first few days or pericarditis 1–4 weeks post MI
      (Dressler's syndrome).
   c. **Uremia.**
   d. **Malignant neoplasm:** Most often breast or bronchogenic.
   e. **Connective tissue diseases.**
5. **Primary pulmonary hypertension.** The pain is mild, and dyspnea on exertion is a prominent symptom.

B. Pulmonary

1. **Pulmonary embolus/infarction.**
2. **Pneumothorax.** Acute onset, often with dyspnea; suspect in young patients or those with COPD.
3. **Pleurodynia.** Bornholm disease caused by coxsackie viral illnesses.
4. **Pneumonia/pleuritis.** This pain is typically pleuritic (made worse on deep inspiration).

C. Gastrointestinal

1. **Gastroesophageal reflux.** The patient often describes an acid taste in the mouth, associated with recumbency.
2. **Esophageal spasm.** Easily confused with angina pectoris as it may cause substernal pain relieved by nitrates.
3. **Gastritis.** Alcoholism or results from overuse of medications, such as NSAIDs.
4. **Peptic ulcer disease.** Typically epigastric pain and usually relieved by eating.
5. **Biliary colic.** Usually associated with eating, especially fatty foods, and located in the epigastrium or right upper quadrant.
6. **Pancreatitis**

D. Musculoskeletal. Pain is reproduced by palpation of the chest wall.

1. **Costochondritis.** Point tenderness over costochondral junction.
2. **Muscle strain/spasm.** There is often a history of exercise or exertion.
3. **Rib fractures after trauma.**

IV. Database

A. Physical Exam Key Points

1. **Vital signs.** Hypotension is an ominous sign and may represent cardiovascular collapse (extensive MI, dissecting aneurysm, pulmonary embolus, or tension pneumothorax). Hypertension in the face of a myocardial infarction or aortic dissection requires emergency therapy to reduce the pressure. Fever (usually low grade) may represent an embolus or other inflammatory process (eg, pneumonia, pleurisy, or pericarditis). Tachycardia may also require urgent cardioversion.
2. **HEENT.** Thrush (especially in immunosuppressed patients) may represent *Candida* esophagitis.
3. **Neck.** Venous distention with CHF or pneumothorax.
4. **Chest.** Chest wall tenderness or contusion with rib fracture; sternal instability after median sternotomy may indicate infection. Point costochondral tenderness with costochondritis.

5. **Lungs.** Rales with CHF, dullness to percussion with fluid or pneumonic consolidation, friction rub with pleural inflammation, decreased breath sounds with fluid or pneumothorax.
6. **Heart.** Murmur with valvular disease, friction rub with pericarditis (**Note:** a "normal finding" immediately after open heart surgery), and displaced PMI with CHF.
7. **Abdomen.** Determine presence or absence of bowel sounds, inflammation, or other evidence of intra-abdominal pathology.
8. **Neurologic.** Aortic dissection may cause a characteristic hemiplegia.
9. **Extremities.** Edema with CHF or asymmetric swelling with venous thrombosis.

B. **Laboratory Studies**
1. **Hemogram.** Leukocytosis in infectious illnesses, particularly lymphocytosis in viral conditions.
2. CPK with isoenzymes every 8 hours to evaluate myocardial injury.
3. ABG in most cases and always if there is any dyspnea.

C. **Radiologic and Other Studies**
1. **ECG.** Obtain a baseline study. Evaluate systematically and compare to prior ECGs. Document presence and degree of pain at the time of the ECG. ECG findings of an MI may include Q-waves, ST-wave changes (depression or elevation) or T-wave inversions. With a subendocardial infarction, the Q-wave may not be present. Arrhythmias may also be present.
2. **Chest x-ray.** If there is any possibility of myocardial ischemia obtain a portable chest x-ray so that the patient is not left unmonitored in the radiology department. Look for pneumothorax, effusions, infiltrates, globular heart shadow (pericardial effusion), and silhouette of the thoracic aorta and mediastinum (widened with aneurysm or dissection).
3. **Echocardiogram.** This evaluates the patient for pericardial effusion, cardiac wall motion, valvular disease, and aortic dissection.
4. **Aortogram/contrast CT scan.** To diagnose aortic dissection.
5. **Venogram/ventilation.** Perfusion scan/pulmonary angiogram to diagnose pulmonary emboli. A negative V/Q scan essentially rules out a PE. However, an equivocal scan or "probable" scan requires confirmation with pulmonary arteriography, or the patient should be treated based on clinical grounds.

V. Plan. The treatment plan is dictated by establishing the correct diagnosis. Of the conditions previously listed, myocardial ischemia, aortic dissection, tension pneumothorax, and pulmonary embolism are most immediately life threatening but treatable. If a reasonable suspicion of myocardial ischemia as the source of pain exists, do not hesitate to treat the patient accordingly. The most commonly confused diagnoses are esophageal spasm and musculoskeletal pain (see Figure I–11).

A. Emergency Management
1. Treat with oxygen therapy by mask or cannula.
2. Obtain an ECG and leave the leads in place to serve as a monitor and to repeat the ECG if pain recurs or increases.
3. Request an immediate portable chest x-ray and a room air blood gas.
4. If myocardial ischemia is a possibility, treat with sublingual nitroglycerin as a diagnostic and therapeutic trial.

B. Myocardial Ischemia
1. **Nitrates.** Sublingual nitroglycerin 0.4 mg (1/150 grain) is a typical starting dose. Monitor symptomatic relief and blood pressure. Repeat every 5–10 minutes up to three doses. If nitroglycerin is effective but pain recurs, establish a nitroglycerin drip at 10/20 μg/min and titrate to pain relief. Keep systolic BP above 90.
2. **Morphine.** If pain is not relieved by nitroglycerin or if the patient cannot tolerate nitrates, treat with 1–3 mg morphine IV.
3. Oxygen 4 liter by nasal prongs (approximately equal to 35% mask).
4. **Lidocaine.** If clear-cut infarction by ECG or if prominent ectopy, treat with 75–100 mg bolus IV, then begin a continuous IV infusion at 2 mg/min.
5. Continue monitoring and make arrangement to admit to CCU/ICU.
6. Coronary thrombolysis using streptokinase, urokinase, or tissue-plasminogen activator may be indicated and is coordinated by the cardiologist.

C. Aortic Dissection.
Initial treatment attempts to eliminate pain and reduce systolic blood pressure. Surgical correction is indicated for all symptomatic aneurysms.
1. **Nitroprusside (Nipride).** A continuous infusion of 0.5–1.0 μg/kg/min titrated up to control blood pressure.
2. **Propranolol.** Decreasing systolic blood pressure suddenly may cause a rebound increase in contractility and shear force; treat with propranolol 1–3 mg IV prior to Nipride.
3. **Morphine.** Use 1–3 mg IV prn to relieve pain.

D. Pulmonary Embolus
1. Check baseline coagulation parameters (PT/PTT).
2. Give heparin IV bolus of either 10,000 units or 100 U/kg, then begin a continuous IV infusion of 10 U/kg/hr. Check the PTT in 3–4 hours and adjust heparin to keep PTT approximately twice normal.
3. If anticoagulation is contraindicated, then place intracaval filter. Filters are also indicated in patients who present with recurrent emboli despite adequate anticoagulation.

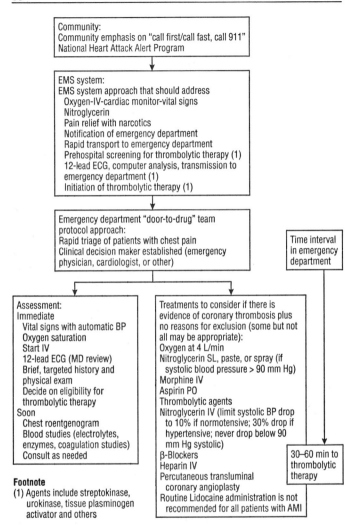

Figure I–11. Acute myocardial infarction (AMI) algorithm. Recommendations for early treatment of patients with chest pain and possible AMI. *(Reproduced, with permission, from Adult Advanced Cardiac Life Support. JAMA 1992;268, No. 16.)*

  E. Pneumothorax. Tube or emergency needle thoracostomy (page 305).
  F. Pericarditis
  a. Monitor for tamponade.
  b. Indomethacin or other anti-inflammatory agents.
  G. Gastritis/Esophagitis
  a. Antacids
  b. H^2-receptor blockers (cimetidine, ranitidine).
  H. Costochondritis. Treat with nonsteroidal anti-inflammatory drugs (ibuprofen, etc).

13. CHEST TUBE PROBLEMS

(Chest tube placement is discussed in Section III, Bedside Procedures)

Immediate Actions

Suspicion of a tension pneumothorax (based on tachycardia, hypotension, and absent or diminished breath sounds) in a patient with a chest tube in place necessitates immediate insertion of a large bore needle (14 gauge) at the anterior axillary line to allow egress of the air. Time must not be wasted obtaining a chest x-ray.

  I. Problem. The chest tube in a 20-year-old male admitted for spontaneous pneumothorax is malfunctioning.

 II. Immediate Questions

  A. What are the vital signs? Tachycardia, tachypnea, and hypotension may indicate a tension pneumothorax in a patient with a malfunctioning chest tube.
  B. What is the problem? Problems may include changes in drainage quality or quantity, persistent air leak, drainage around the tube dressing, increasing subcutaneous emphysema, or patients' complaints of discomfort.
  C. When and why was the tube inserted? The problem will be approached differently if the tube was put in during an operation, or emergently to drain an effusion, or to evacuate air from a spontaneous pneumothorax.
  D. When was the last x-ray obtained? If recently, immediately go check the film, if not, obtain a current one.

III. Differential Diagnosis

A. Faulty Drainage System. Collection containers may be full, tubing may be kinked, or the wall suction may not be adequate (usually 20-cm suction for most adult chest tubes).

B. Continuous Air Leak. Indicated by persistent bubbling in the air seal chamber of the chest tube drainage system.
  1. Cracked tube or other mechanical problem, ie, a loose connection.
  2. Last hole (hole closest to the drainage system) is outside the pleural space.
  3. Lung parenchymal injury with persistent leak (bronchopleural fistula). May be posttraumatic lung injury (penetrating injury) or iatrogenic during tube placement.

C. Bloody Drainage
  1. **Intercostal vessel injury.** Generally avoided because the tube is placed over the top of the rib.
  2. **Bloody effusion.** Malignant effusions are often bloody.
  3. **Pulmonary artery injury.** A rare problem.
  4. **Posttraumatic.** Most traumatic pneumothoraces are associated with some degree of bleeding.
  5. **Parenchymal lung injury.** Possibly at the time of tube placement.

D. Decreased Drainage
  1. Clotted tube.
  2. Resolution of the problem that led to tube placement.

E. Subcutaneous Emphysema
  1. Migration of the last hole outside the chest cavity.
  2. Improper placement (subcutaneous tube).
  3. Significant air leak requiring placement of a second chest tube.
  4. Tension pneumothorax.

IV. Database

A. Physical Exam Key Points
  1. **Vital signs.** Tachypnea may indicate a pneumothorax or respiratory compromise. Tension pneumothorax may decrease blood pressure.
  2. **Neck.** Tracheal deviation may indicate a tension pneumothorax. (Trachea deviates away from the side of the tension pneumothorax).
  3. **Lungs.** Check for symmetric breath sounds. Hyperresonance may signify a pneumothorax, whereas dullness may suggest an effusion or hemothorax.
  4. **Chest wall.** Determine if there is crepitance that signifies subcutaneous emphysema. Examine the insertion site for signs of tube migration, infection, or skin bleeding.

B. Laboratory Data
1. **Arterial blood gases.** Are indicated if patient is dyspneic.
2. Coagulation studies (PT/PTT/platelets) especially in cases of severe bleeding.

C. Radiologic and Other Studies
1. **Obtain a chest x-ray.** This is probably the most important diagnostic maneuver. Check tube position, see where the last hole of the tube is located, and note if there is any effusion (either new or recurrent) or any residual pneumothorax.

V. Plan. Note: In general, a chest tube should not be clamped because of the risk of a tension pneumothorax.

A. Air Leak
1. Be sure that the last hole is in the chest cavity (on x-ray). One may notice a rush of air at the site, which usually indicates that the last hole is outside the chest. If the last hole is outside the chest, replace the tube. Pushing the tube in is associated with a risk of empyema.
2. To differentiate tube problems from system problems, try clamping the tube **briefly** at the entry site. A persistent air leak indicates a problem in the drainage system, not the patient or tube.

B. Drainage Around the Tube. An enormous effusion is treated simply by reinforcing the dressing. Be sure the last hole is in the chest. Tight closure of skin around the tube at the entry site may cause subcutaneous dissection of fluid or air.

C. Change in Drainage Quality
1. The sudden appearance of bloody drainage after inserting a tube can indicate damage to intercostal vessels or, more significantly, may indicate damage to lung parenchyma. This may also represent minor bleeding after repeated attempts at placement of an ipsilateral subclavian line.
2. Intercostal vessel damage may stop on its own, but if persistent will require operative exposure and ligation.
3. Blood tingeing of a previously straw-colored effusion is usually of little significance.

D. Change in Drainage Quantity. A sudden increase in drainage is rare, unless the drainage becomes bloody and is related to a vascular mishap. This should be correlated with the recent x-ray. Is there a new effusion on that side? A sudden decrease in drainage with appearance of a new effusion usually warrants removal of the tube and/or placement of a new one.

E. Subcutaneous Emphysema. A pneumothorax is often associated with subcutaneous air, and there is often some air after placement of the tube. However, new subcutaneous emphysema, especially after a tube has been in for a while, may indicate migration

of the tube, such that the last hole is now out of the chest. This usually indicates a poorly functioning tube and necessitates replacement. The appearance of a great deal of subcutaneous air right after tube placement may be alleviated by enlarging the tube entrance site, to allow egress of the air rather than forcing the air (from a pneumothorax) to track subcutaneously. Large air leaks may require a second tube.

F. **Patient Discomfort.** There is always some pleuritic pain after placement of a tube, especially at the entrance site. Such pain must be differentiated from chest pain of other causes. Sudden onset of new pain must be investigated, looking at the position of the end of the tube, evidence of pneumothorax, and examining the entrance site. Treat with NSAIDs, eg, ibuprofen or Naprosyn; occasionally narcotics may be needed.

14. CHANGING NEUROLOGIC STATUS

I. **Problem.** You are called to evaluate a 34-year-old woman for somnolence two days after a right modified radical mastectomy.

II. **Immediate Questions**

A. **What are the vital signs?** Shock of any cause can result in poor cerebral perfusion and altered mental status. A changing respiratory pattern may indicate increased intracranial pressure, with an initial slowing followed by a rapid respiratory rate.

B. **Was the patient fully awake at any time since surgery?** Get an idea of the time course for the change in neurologic status.

C. **What medication is the patient taking?** Especially any sedatives (sleeping medications), as well as the amount of narcotics needed for pain control. Look at the medication records to see how much pain medicine and sedation the patient has received, not just how much has been ordered.

D. **Is the patient a diabetic?** Either hypoglycemia or hyperglycemia may cause altered mental status.

E. **Are there any intravenous fluids?** This can lead to metabolic causes of somnolence and coma. What is their composition?

F. **Was there a traumatic event?** For example, did the patient fall out of bed, or is the problem a result of a motor vehicle accident? Long bone fractures may cause fat embolism syndrome.

III. **Differential Diagnosis**

A. **Trauma**

1. **Subdural hematoma.** The most common intracranial mass lesion resulting from head injury.

2. **Epidural hematoma.** Usually associated with a skull fracture and a lacerated meningeal vessel.
3. **Concussion.** A clinical diagnosis of cerebral dysfunction that clears within 24 hours of the injury.
4. **Contusion.** Usually associated with neurologic deficits that persist for longer than 24 hours after injury and that demonstrate small hemorrhages in the cerebral parenchyma on CT scan.
5. **Fat embolus syndrome.** After long bone fracture.

B. **Metabolic Causes**
   1. **Exogenous.** Alcohol (including withdrawal "delirium tremens"), drugs (including drug withdrawal), narcotics, cimetidine, anesthetic agents (delayed clearance postop), poisoning.
   2. **Endogenous**
      a. **Endocrine**
         i. **Pancreas**–Insulin, hypo- and hyperglycemia
         ii. **Pituitary**–Hyper- and hypopituitarism
         iii. **Thyroid**–Hyper- and hypothyroid
         iv. Adrenal insufficiency
         v. Parathyroid
      b. **Fluids/electrolytes**
         i. **Sodium**–Hypo- and hypernatremia may cause confusion.
         ii. Hypo- and hyperkalemia
         iii. Hypo- and hypercalcemia
         iv. Hypo- and hypermagnesemia
         v. Acidosis (especially respiratory) or alkalosis
         vi. Osmolarity disturbances (hyperosmolar coma)
      c. **Organ Failure:** Including renal, hepatic, or pulmonary (hypoxia, hypercarbia, fat embolism syndrome [long bone fracture related]).

C. **Infection**
   1. Central nervous system infections (meningitis, encephalitis).
   2. Systemic sepsis.

D. **Tumors**
   1. Primary or metastatic to CNS.
   2. Paraneoplastic syndromes.

E. **Psychiatric Causes.** In psychogenic coma, the neurologic and laboratory profile is completely normal. Depression may also cause dementia especially in the elderly. ICU psychosis, and post-cardiotomy delirium are occasionally seen. ICU psychosis is seen frequently in the elderly patient and can be brought on by sleep deprivation or medications.

F. **Miscellaneous**
   1. **Seizures.** Including postictal states.
   2. **Cerebrovascular disease.** Infarction or hemorrhage, arteriovenous malformation (AVM), hypertensive encephalopathy.

3. **Syncope** (see Problem 66, page 212).
4. **Decreased cardiac output** (shock).
5. **Other CNS diseases.** These are usually more chronic: Alzheimer's, normal pressure hydrocephalus, Wernicke's encephalopathy (thiamine deficiency).

IV. **Database.** If the event occurs during the postop period, determine the nature, onset, and duration of event. Furthermore, ascertain anesthetic used, medications given, and IV fluids administered.

A. **Physical Exam Key Points**
  1. **Vital signs.** Hyper- or hypotension, tachy- or bradycardia, and respiratory rate may give a clue to the diagnosis.
  2. **HEENT.** Papilledema (increased intracranial pressure from a mass or hypertensive encephalopathy), meningeal signs such as nuchal rigidity (meningitis), pupillary reaction (pinpoint with narcotic, unilateral fixed and dilated, suggest herniation, dilated and fixed (anoxia). Conjunctival and fundal petechiae suggest fat embolism. Fruity breath is associated with ketoacidosis. Bruits may indicate a stroke.
  3. **Skin.** Jaundice, spider angiomata, palmar erythema with liver disease. Petechiae in neck and upper chest.
  4. **Neurologic exam.** (See Appendix for Glasgow Coma Scale.) Evaluate patient for spontaneous movements, response to pain, cranial nerve function.

B. **Laboratory Data**
  1. **CBC, platelet count.** To evaluate for infection or anemia.
  2. **Complete blood chemistry.** Includes electrolytes, BUN, creatinine, calcium, magnesium, osmolality; glucose can be rapidly checked with a "finger-stick" glucometer available on most nursing units.
  3. **Arterial blood gases.** A respiratory or metabolic cause may be found. Hypoxia may also cause delirium.
  4. **Serum ammonia.** Elevation indicative of hepatic failure.
  5. Urine and serum toxicology screening if indicated.
  6. Cultures for sepsis, if indicated.

C. **Radiologic and Other Studies**
  1. **Chest x-ray.** Especially if infectious or pulmonary source possible.
  2. **CT of the head.** If there is any indication of a CNS cause of coma—especially focal neurologic signs or presence of papilledema.
  3. **Lumbar puncture** (see page 317).
  4. **Electrocardiogram.** Myocardial infarction or atrial fibrillation (mural thrombi with emboli).
  5. **Electroencephalogram.**

V. Plan. While the therapy of changing neurologic status must be directed at the underlying cause, certain initial steps should be taken immediately. Ensure adequate airway, breathing, and circulation. Intubation may be necessary to protect the airway.

   A. Metabolic Causes. Treat the defect shown on lab studies. Refer to specific abnormality in the index. A single ampule of 50% dextrose can be given IV if there is any suspicion of hypoglycemia. The effect on a patient in diabetic ketoacidosis is minimal, so it is always safer to give the dextrose.

   B. Exogenous Causes. Any suspicion of narcotic-induced somnolence can be safely treated with naloxone, 0.4–0.8 mg IV push. Repeat dose may be necessary (up to 4–5 ampules are commonly given in this situation).

   C. Tumor. Somnolence in the presence of metastatic or primary CNS tumors is an emergency usually treated by radiotherapy. Give dexamethasone bolus 0.1–0.2 mg/kg.

   D. Infection. Treated with high dose antibiotics as appropriate to the Gram's stain organisms.

   E. Cardiac syncope or low cardiac output. Treated by approaching the underlying cardiac problem.

   F. Vascular. Intracranial bleeding is usually treated like other causes of increased intracranial pressure. Contact the neurosurgeon. Increased intracranial pressure should be emergently treated because herniation may occur. Intubation with hyperventilation, osmotic diuresis with mannitol (1–1.5 gm/kg over 20 minutes) and steroids (dexamethasone 10 mg IV) may acutely decrease intracranial pressure.

   G. ICU psychosis. This is a diagnosis of exclusion and based on clinical suspicion. Provide the patient with a companion and use restraints as a last resort. Occasionally haloperidol (Haldol) may be needed.

15. COAGULOPATHY

 I. Problem. Following placement of a LeVeen shunt, a patient has bleeding from both peritoneal and neck incisions as well as oozing from an intravenous site.

II. Immediate Questions

   A. What is the patient's blood pressure? Determine if the bleeding episode is extensive enough to cause hypovolemia and shock. Assess volume status by blood pressure, urine output, and central pressures if available. If central lines need to be placed, work up extent of coagulopathy before inserting needles into major vessels.

B. **How much external bleeding is there?** One of the most frequent calls on a surgical service is that a wound is bleeding or the blood stain on a dressing is increasing. One way to separate the clinically significant bleeding episodes from the insignificant ones is to quantitate the bleeding. Look at the wound to see if there is active bleeding, and ask to have any old dressings saved so that you can see the amount and the nature of the wound drainage.

C. **Do factors exist which increase the likelihood of generalized bleeding?** In the example previously given the patient could be expected to have problems with disseminated intravascular coagulation. In general, when confronted with a bleeding or oozing wound, ask the patient about liver disease, relatives with bleeding disorders, and use of medications such as aspirin, NSAIDs, or anticoagulants. Look for easy bruising or petechia.

D. **Could bleeding into the wound cause mechanical problems with a hematoma?** This question is pertinent to neck wounds where a wound hematoma can compress the trachea, and mediastinal wounds where undrained bleeding could cause pericardial tamponade. In both cases be prepared to open the wound quickly if emergent problems develop.

III. Differential Diagnosis

A. **Inadequate Surgical Hemostasis.** The most common cause of localized bleeding in the postoperative patient. In most cases, the bleeding is minor.

B. **Platelet Disorders**
   1. **Thrombocytopenia**
      a. **Decreased production:** Often secondary to chemotherapy or bone marrow replacement by fibrosis or neoplasia.
      b. **Sequestration:** Caused by splenic enlargement due to portal hypertension, neoplasia, or storage diseases.
      c. **Destruction:** Idiopathic thrombocytopenic purpura, thrombotic thrombocytopenic purpura (TTP), and drug reactions (eg, heparin) can cause platelet destruction.
   2. **Qualitative platelet disorders**
      a. **von Willebrand's disease:** An autosomal dominant disease with decreased platelet adhesion.
      b. **Platelet release defects:** Due to interference with cyclooxygenase metabolism by aspirin and NSAID.
      c. **Glanzmann's disease.**
      d. **Bernard-Soulier syndrome.**

C. Coagulation Defects
  1. **Congenital**
     a. **Hemophilia A:** A factor VII deficiency, X-linked, with an incidence of 1/10,000 male births.
     b. **Hemophilia B:** A factor IX deficiency, X-linked, with an incidence of 1/100,000 male births.
  2. **Acquired**
     a. **Disseminated intravascular coagulation (DIC):** Associated with sepsis, trauma, burns, disseminated malignancy, obstetric catastrophes, and following peritoneovenous (LeVeen) shunt (due to proteinaceous material entering the venous system).
     b. **Vitamin K deficiency:** Vitamin K is needed for synthesis of coagulation factors II, VII, IX, and X.
     c. **Hepatic failure:** Not only vitamin K-dependent factors but also I, V, and XI are synthesized by the liver.

IV. Database.
The keystone in diagnosing a coagulopathy is understanding and using the appropriate laboratory tests. It is important to draw blood for needed tests before instituting therapy or transfusions.

A. Physical Exam Key Points
  1. **Vital signs.** Tachycardia, orthostatic hypotension, and other signs of hypovolemia signify a major loss of blood.
  2. **Skin.** Petechia, purpura, easy bruising, and oozing from IV sites suggest a systemic rather than a local cause.
  3. **Incision.** Examine the incision for hematoma or active bleeding.
  4. **Abdomen.** Splenomegaly, hepatomegaly, or ascites may suggest a diagnosis.
  5. **Extremity.** Hemarthrosis may be seen with hemophilia.
  6. **Neurologic exam.** Needed as a baseline and to assess CNS bleeding if present.

B. Laboratory Data
  1. **Hemogram.** Follow serial hematocrits in ongoing bleeding.
  2. **Platelet count.** Adequate numbers do not imply adequate function of platelets.
  3. **PT and PTT.** The PT is elevated if there is a deficiency of factors I, II, V, VII, or X. The PTT assesses all coagulation proteins except factor VII and XIII. Factor VII has the shortest half-life and is the usual cause in generalized problems, such as liver disease. In lupus erythematosus there is a circulating anticoagulant that elevates the PT/PTT but does not cause a bleeding diathesis.
  4. **Thrombin time.** Assays functional fibrinogen level and can assay for heparin effect.

5. **Fibrinogen and fibrin split products (FSP).** In DIC fibrinogen is decreased and FSP are increased.
6. **Bleeding time.** Evaluates platelet function. Uremia, liver disease, and aspirin therapy within a week may adversely effect function.
7. **Peripheral blood smears.** May reveal fragments and helmet cells in DIC and TTP.
8. Type and crossmatch to the blood bank if needed.
9. Save one or two tubes of blood prior to therapy to assay for any coagulation factors that may be needed.

C. **Radiologic and Other Studies**
   1. **Chest x-ray.** If there are indications of intrathoracic bleeding.
   2. **Bone marrow biopsy.** May be performed at some point to assess platelet production.

V. **Plan.** Assess the rate of bleeding and differentiate between mechanical bleeding and true coagulopathy. Almost all external bleeding that is mechanical can be controlled by applying direct pressure and elevation. Treatment of a medical coagulopathy requires the laboratory results previously discussed to make the correct diagnosis and institute treatment. In the acute setting, assess all cases for the amount of blood loss and the volume status and treat with intravenous fluids.

A. **Thrombocytopenia**
   1. Use random donor platelet transfusion usually 5–10 units at a time for a platelet count < 10,000 or with a lesser degree of thrombocytopenia if there is ongoing bleeding. Patients receiving multiple platelet transfusions will develop antibodies and do better with HLA-matched single donor platelets. Immunocompromised patients should receive irradiated platelets to avoid a graft-vs-host reaction.
   2. **Drug reaction.** Discontinue the drug and transfuse platelets if necessary. Penicillins (infrequently) and chronic subcutaneous heparin can cause thrombocytopenia.
   3. **ITP.** No treatment is usually needed until the platelet count is < 10,000. Chronic ITP is treated with prednisone, cyclophosphamide (Cytoxan), azathioprine, or danazol. The best long-term results are with splenectomy. Platelet transfusions before splenectomy in these patients will be very short-lived.
   4. Document functional defect with bleeding time.

B. **von Willebrand's Disease**
   1. **Cryoprecipitate** (see Section V, page 341).
   2. **DDAVP.** A vasopressin analog that increases von Willebrand factor levels (see Section VII, page 366).

C. **Hemophilia A.** The half-life of factor VIII is about 12 hours. One unit per kg of factor VIII transfused raises the body activity about

2%. Load a patient with 50 U/kg IV, then give 25 U/kg every 12 hours. Cryoprecipitate contains a 20-fold increase in factor VII activity compared to FFP. There is also factor VIII concentrate.

D. Hemophilia B. FFP or plasma enriched in prothrombin complex is frequently used.

E. DIC. Treat the underlying cause. Support the bleeding patient with FFP, platelet transfusions, and blood transfusions.

F. Vitamin K Deficiency/Liver Disease. If immediate treatment is needed transfuse with 2–4 units of FFP and follow the PT/PTT. In all cases begin treatment with vitamin K 10 mg SQ every day for 3 days in a row.

16. COLOSTOMY PROBLEMS

I. Problem. A 68-year-old patient 6 days after abdominoperineal resection has problems with the function of his colostomy.

II. Immediate Questions

A. How old is the colostomy, and what type of colostomy is it? A new colostomy can retract into the wound, whereas obstruction tends to be a problem with an older colostomy. Loop or "double barrel" colostomies are temporary and usually are decompressive, whereas "end" colostomies are usually permanent.

B. What kind of appliance is on the colostomy? Poorly fitting appliances can cause leakage and skin irritation.

C. What color is the mucosa? Mucosal ischemia can occur in the immediate postoperative period.

D. What is the volume and nature of the output? A colostomy that has been working and suddenly stops can be approached differently than one that has never worked. The majority of colostomies are left-sided, end, descending colostomies. In the first few postoperative days, the output is scant and usually blood-tinged. When peristalsis resumes, the appliance will usually become filled with gas before the discharge of liquid feces, usually around the third or fourth postoperative day. Is output liquid and frequent? High output stomas are usually related to outlet stenosis, intra-abdominal infection, recurrence of disease, or resection of an excessive length of bowel.

III. Differential Diagnosis. There are a variety of potential problems with stomas that are discussed in two groups: new stomas and existing stomas. Problems with new stomas are likely to arise in the first few days after surgery.

A. New Stoma Problems
   1. **Stomal retraction/prolapse.** A surgical emergency because if the stoma retracts into the peritoneal cavity, it can lead to fecal spillage. Usually requires immediate operative intervention.
   2. **Stomal necrosis.** The outcome of a necrotic stoma depends on how much necrosis is present. The cause is usually compromised blood supply when the stoma was made. This can lead to a superficial slough of the mucosa or progress to complete full-thickness necrosis necessitating reoperation.
   3. **Stomal bleeding.** Can be from inadequate hemostasis at operation, peristomal bleeding due to intra-abdominal hemorrhage, skin bleeding, intraluminal bleeding, or mucosal irritation.

B. Existing Stoma Problems
   1. **Impaction/obstruction.** Obvious from history and examination of the stoma with a gloved finger.
   2. **Bleeding.** See Problem 10, page 34.
   3. Mucosal slough.
   4. Poor fitting appliance/skin irritation.
   5. Paracolostomy hernia.
   6. **Stenosis.** Often associated with high output of liquid and detected by examination with a gloved, well-lubricated finger. Can be at skin level or at the fascia.

IV. Database
   A. Physical Exam Key Points
      1. Examine at the stoma for ischemia, retraction, and carefully evaluate color. Most often, this can be accomplished by pressing the transparent colostomy bag gently against the stoma and using a penlight. A key point is that a viable stoma will transilluminate and a nonviable stoma will often not transilluminate. After a few postoperative days, the stoma normally will appear edematous with a dull pink-brown color. A pale tan color usually signifies ischemia. Black mucosa with a faint greenish tint signifies necrosis, and no mucosa visible signifies retraction. If the mucosa or surrounding site is bloody, quantitate and look for a local source.
      2. Examine the abdomen for signs of peritonitis, distention, or evidence of parastomal herniation.
   B. Laboratory Data. These are usually only helpful if excessive bleeding is a problem. (Clotting studies [PT/PTT] and hemogram).
   C. Radiologic and Other Studies
      1. **Abdominal films.** Look for obstructive pattern of bowel either at the level of the stoma or proximally (air-fluid levels, etc).
      2. Gastrografin enema through colostomy to evaluate obstructing

lesions. Gastrografin is also a cathartic. Barium or dilute barium will be used less frequently.

V. Plan. The treatment of stomal problems, of course, depends on the nature of the problem and its etiology. While some problems with stomas are purely cosmetic, there are a few that require rapid evaluation and treatment for optimal results.

A. Stomal Ischemia. A truly ischemic new stoma requires careful evaluation and then reoperation to revise the stoma correcting any technical or mechanical problems that led to ischemia (tight fascia, kinked mesentery).

B. Stomal Retraction. If the stoma retracts fully into the abdominal cavity, immediate operation is required.

C. Fecal Impaction. Usually caused by dehydration, narcotics, or lack of bulk in the diet. It is usually managed by warm colostomy irrigation, gentle cathartics, and it is prevented long term by stool softeners, bulk laxatives, and adequate fluid intake.

D. Bleeding. If a site of bleeding in the skin or on the mucosa is clearly visible, it can often be corrected with a bedside cautery, silver nitrate, or a suture. Use caution with cautery because colonic gas may be flammable. If the bleeding is resulting from any of the causes of gastrointestinal bleeding, a full evaluation is indicated (see Problem 10, page 34).

E. Appliance Problems. Consultation with an enterostomal care specialist can often be helpful to select the best appliance for the patient. Protective paste or Stomahesive (TM) may be applied to protect skin.

F. Stenosis. Usually responds to early digital dilatation, and reoperation sometimes is needed only if the stenotic area is at the level of the fascia.

G. Continuous Colostomy Drainage. Many patients are unhappy with the continuous discharge of fecal contents into the end-descending colostomy. Often the colon can be "trained" to evacuate only after colostomy irrigation. Transverse colonic "loop" colostomies are more difficult to manage because the output is usually a continuous liquid that is almost impossible to regulate.

H. Obstruction. Fecal impaction may be cleared as previously discussed. More serious causes may represent recurrent tumor.

17. COMA AND ACUTE MENTAL STATUS CHANGES

(See also Problem 14, page 60)

I. Problem. The night nurse wants an order to sedate an elderly patient who is agitated, uncooperative, and confused.

II. Immediate Questions

A. **What is the patient's baseline mental status?** If this behavior deviates from the patient's normal level of function, it indicates another underlying cause.

B. **What medication is the patient taking?** Many medications have a primary affect on the CNS (eg, pain medications and sedatives) or can affect neurologic changes as a side effect or following overdosage or an adverse drug reaction.

C. **Does the patient have a history of alcohol, narcotic, or prescription drug abuse?** Surreptitious use while in the hospital or withdrawal symptoms can occur.

D. **Has the patient suffered any recent trauma, especially head injury?** This may suggest the cause.

E. **Are there any other associated symptoms?** Such as wheezing, tachypnea, chest pain, paresthesias, or bleeding.

F. **What is the patient's state of consciousness?** Coma is unresponsiveness to external stimuli, while stupor and lethargy represent states of gradually less impairment. Delirium is acute confusion and decreased alertness—commonly with agitation and hallucinations. Dementia is a chronic condition of mental deterioration with loss of memory and cognitive functions.

III. Differential Diagnosis

A. **Traumatic**
  1. Subdural or epidural hematoma.
  2. Contusion.
  3. Concussion.

B. **Cerebrovascular**
  1. Subarachnoid hemorrhage.
  2. Intracerebral hemorrhage.
  3. Hypertensive encephalopathy.
  4. Eclampsia.

C. **Metabolic**
  1. **Exogenous**
    a. Narcotic or alcohol abuse
    b. Medication overdose
    c. Poisoning
  2. **Endogenous**
    a. **Endocrine:** Hypoglycemia, DKA, hypo- and hyper- (pituitary, thyroid, parathyroid, and adrenal).
    b. **Organ failure:** Hepatic, renal, respiratory, and cardiac.
    c. **Vitamin deficiency:** Thiamine, B_{12}
    d. **Acid-base, fluid and electrolyte disorders:** Hypo- and hyper- (kalemia, natremia, calcemia, magnesemia, and osmolarity).

   D. Infectious. Meningitis, encephalitis, abscess.

   E. Neoplasm. Space occupying lesion or hydrocephalus.

   F. Syncope or Postictal State.

   G. Psychiatric. Depression, Alzheimer's disease.

IV. Database

   A. Physical Exam Key Points
   1. **Vital signs.** Fever suggests infection, brady- or tachyarrhythmia, hypotension in shock or intoxication, respiratory rate and pattern (Cheyne-Stokes in transtentorial herniation, ataxic with medullary lesion).
   2. **HEENT.** Especially pupils for reactivity, shape, size (pinpoint with narcotics), and fundi for papilledema or retinopathy. Cranial nerves. Odor of breath (alcohol, uremia, fruity with DKA).
   3. **Skin.** Cyanosis, turgor, bruising and bleeding.
   4. **Chest.** Breath sounds, cardiac murmurs
   5. **Neurologic.** Include observations on posturing, level of consciousness, cranial and peripheral nerve function, reflexes, and motor function.

   B. Laboratory Data
   1. Serum glucose-glucose is the primary brain substrate. Short periods of hypoglycemia can result in permanent brain damage.
   2. **Serum electrolytes.** To evaluate obvious metabolic causes.
   3. **Drug screen.** Barbiturates, narcotics, and alcohol.
   4. **Arterial blood gas.** Acidosis, hypoxia, and hyperpnea are correctable.
   5. **PT/PTT and platelet count.** For coagulation study
   6. **Hemogram.** Leukocytosis in infection, assess anemia.

   C. Radiologic and Other Studies
   1. **Chest x-ray.** Pneumothorax, pleural effusion.
   2. **ECG.** To diagnose MI or arrhythmia.
   3. **Head CT.** To evaluate stroke, mass lesion, edema, shift.
   4. **Lumbar puncture.** Hemorrhage or infection.
   5. **EEG.** Seizure activity, cerebral cortical function.

V. Plan. As diagnostic information is being collected, therapy should be provided simultaneously, correcting obvious abnormalities. History should be obtained from family, friends, or caregiver with particular attention to head trauma, especially a lucid interval following initial loss of consciousness, illicit drug usage, poison ingestion, seizure, respiratory distress, history of diabetes, heart, lung or kidney disease.

Patients with changes in mental status on the wards should be moved to a unit for closer monitoring. Resuscitation should follow general guidelines.

A. Ventilatory Support. Supplemental oxygen, positioning, intubation and mechanical ventilation if necessary. (Airway, Breathing).

B. Circulatory Support. IV access and fluid administration if appropriate. Any source of bleeding should be identified and controlled, and blood products given as needed.

C. Dextrose. 50 ml of 50% solution IV if serum glucose is unknown or < 50 mg/dL.

D. Thiamine. 10 mg IV initially and 100 mg IM for 3 days if alcoholism is suspected.

E. Naloxone. 0.4–0.8 mg IV for unknown cause of coma or opiate intoxication. Repeat dosage may be necessary.

F. Flumazenil (Romazicon). 0.2 mg IV over 60 seconds, repeat as needed up to 3–5 mg for suspected benzodiazepine overdose. **Caution:** Can precipitate seizures in patients with history of seizures.

G. Supportive Care. Including nutrition, hydration and joint ROM. Prophylaxis for stress ulcers (H_2-receptor blockers, antacids), pressure sores (turn every 2 hours, air mattress, heal pads) and corneal abrasions (tape eyes shut).

18. CONSTIPATION

I. Problem. A 75-year-old bedridden woman from a nursing home has not had a bowel movement in 7 days.

II. Immediate Questions

A. What are the patient's vital signs? Fever, tachycardia, and hypotension may indicate infection or sepsis.

B. Is the patient's abdomen tense, tender, or distended, and is the patient passing flatus? Bowel obstruction with or without perforation or infarction is a life-threatening emergency. Obstipation (failure to pass flatus and stool) is often a more ominous problem.

C. What is the patient's bowel history? Nursing home patients are often laxative dependent. Surgical history may suggest obstruction from tumor or adhesions.

D. What medication is the patient taking? Narcotics and anticholinergics use can reduce bowel motility.

III. Differential Diagnosis

A. Mechanical Obstruction

1. **Mild constipation.** Can also be caused by painful perianal disease (eg, hemorrhoids) causing spasm.
2. **Fecal impaction.** Common in the elderly and related to dehydration, poor diet, and inactivity.
3. Obstruction due to a mass (inflammatory or neoplastic), volvulus, or adhesions from prior surgery.

B. Pharmacologic.
Medications that commonly cause constipation include narcotics and iron supplements. Low residue diets can also cause constipation.

C. Neurologic.
Pelvic or spinal trauma can result in anal sphincter dysfunction. Neoplastic involvement of pelvic nerve roots can result in colonic dysmotility (Ogilvie's syndrome or pseudoobstruction of the colon).

D. Other Causes.
Inactivity, poor fluid intake, and laxative abuse predispose to constipation. Electrolyte disturbances rarely may cause dysmotility (hypokalemia).

IV. Database

A. Physical Exam Key Points

1. **Vital signs.** Fever suggests an infectious cause.
2. **Abdominal exam.** Determine presence or absence as well as quality of bowel sounds. Look for distention, palpate for masses. Determine if pain is present at rest or with palpation.
3. **Rectal exam.** Hard stool in rectum, presence of blood, mass are sought.
4. **Neurologic exam.** Examine for evidence of previous stroke or other neurologic disease.

B. Laboratory Data

1. **Fecal occult blood.** Suggests mass or ischemia.
2. **Serum electrolytes.** Hypokalemia is an infrequent cause of bowel dysmotility.
3. **Hemogram.** Leukocytosis may indicate infection. Anemia may indicate GI bleed, which could suggest obstructing neoplasm.
4. **Arterial blood gas.** Indicated if obstruction and bowel infarction are suspected (hallmark is refractory metabolic acidosis).

C. Radiologic and Other Studies

1. Mild constipation and impaction usually need no further studies.
2. Abdominal films especially if obstruction is suspected (see Problem 1, page 1).
3. **Contrast studies and abdominal CT scan.** These are usually needed if there is evidence of chronic constipation or if there is evidence of blood in the stool (see Problem 10, page 34).

V. Plan. Medications that predispose patients to constipation (narcotics, anticholinergics) should be stopped whenever possible. Correct existing electrolyte abnormalities with specific attention paid to hypokalemia.

   A. Prevention. Postoperative and bedridden patients benefit from stool softeners (sodium docusate), fiber rich diet (fruits, vegetables, or bran or supplemented with agents such as psyllium) and adequate fluid intake.

   B. Laxatives and Enemas. Mild constipation can be treated in a variety of ways depending on physician preference: motility stimulant (bisacodyl), laxative (milk of magnesia), or gentle enemas (tap water, soap suds). Lactulose syrup is an excellent laxative for chronic constipation. Doses can be found in Section VII, Commonly Used Medications. In general, laxatives are **contraindicated** in the presence of obstruction.

   C. Disimpaction. Gentle digital disimpaction (well-lubricated, gloved finger) is required when hard stool in rectum cannot be passed. This procedure can then be followed up with careful retention enemas (soap suds or mineral oil may be used) and then with stool softeners to prevent recurrence.

   D. Other. Perforation, acute obstruction, and sepsis require emergency operation. If partial obstruction (no obstipation) is present, gentle clearing with enemas followed by contrast studies or colonoscopy is indicated.

19. COUGH

I. Problem. A patient being treated with IV antibiotics for cellulitis complains of a cough.

II. Immediate Questions

   A. Is the patient bringing up sputum with the cough? What are the characteristics of the sputum? A productive cough is more suggestive of significant infection than a nonproductive one, particularly if the sputum appears purulent. The presence of blood in the sputum raises a host of other issues (see Problem 36, page 125).

   B. Is the patient tachypneic or dyspneic? Usually a cough does not require emergent or urgent action. One exception is the patient with chronic pulmonary or cardiac disease who may suffer respiratory compromise with a new acute pulmonary event.

   C. Is the cough acute or chronic? In patients with a chronic cough, the key question is whether the nature or characteristic of the cough has changed. In the absence of other respiratory complaints, a new cough in a smoker may represent cancer.

D. **Is the patient immunocompromised?** Ask specifically about medications (steroids, chemotherapeutics) or secondary conditions (diabetes, AIDS, cancer) that predispose to serious pulmonary infections.

E. **Is the cough associated with any activity?** A cough that occurs with recumbency may signify pulmonary edema. A coughing spasm during sleep may be aspiration pneumonitis. A cough following eating or drinking could be a tracheoesophageal fistula or neurologic disorder.

III. **Differential Diagnosis.** The differential diagnosis for a cough can be structured by the causative agent stimulating the cough reflex.

A. **Inflammatory**
1. **Acute.** Bacterial, viral, fungal, and acid-fast organisms are causative agents. Associated systemic signs of infection such as leukocytosis, fever, viral exanthem, and purulent sputum. Certain sputums are characteristic such as rust-colored for pneumococci, currant-jelly for *Klebsiella,* and foul-smelling for anaerobic organisms.
2. **Chronic.** Chronic bronchitis occurs almost exclusively in smokers and is defined as a chronic productive cough for at least 3 months a year for 2 years.

B. **Mechanical.** Mechanical stimulation of the cough reflex can occur via inhalation or intrinsic or extrinsic mechanical stimuli.
1. **Inhalation**
   a. **Foreign body aspiration:** Localized wheezing with risk factors of depressed level of consciousness.
   b. Particulate aerosols.
   c. **Aspiration of gastrointestinal secretions:** Nighttime or early morning coughing spells are characteristic.
   d. Allergens in sensitive persons.
2. **Intrinsic**
   a. **Pulmonary edema:** Can be cardiogenic or noncardiogenic. Typical symptoms include acute dyspnea and copious frothy sputum.
   b. **Interstitial lung disease:** Restrictive disease by PFTs and diffuse interstitial changes of fibrosis on chest x-ray.
   c. **Bronchogenic carcinoma:** Risk factors of smoking, asbestos exposure, and systemic signs of weight loss and possible hemoptysis.
   d. **Bronchial adenoma:** Usually no systemic symptoms and possible hemoptysis.
3. **Extrinsic**
   a. **Thoracic aneurysm:** Can cause bronchial or tracheal compression.
   b. **Lymphadenopathy:** Secondary to sarcoidosis, chronic in-

fection, lymphoma, or cancer. There are often associated systemic symptoms (fever, fatigue, etc).

C. Chemical. These cause topical irritation.
   1. Smoke inhalation.
   2. Toxic fumes.

IV. Database

A. Physical Exam Key Points

   1. Vital signs. Temperature and respiratory rate are useful. Use of accessory respiratory muscles and nasal flaring suggest severe distress.

   2. Pulmonary
   a. Stridor: Represents upper airway obstruction or epiglottitis.
   b. Rhonchi: Seen with bronchitis and inhalation injuries.
   c. Signs of consolidation such as bronchial breath sounds, egobronchophony, and tactile fremitus in pneumonia.
   d. Rales: These are the hallmarks of pulmonary edema.
   e. Localized wheezing/rhonchi: May signify foreign body or obstructing neoplasm.

   3. Cardiac. Signs of cardiac failure (cardiomegaly, S3 gallop).

   4. Skin/extremities. Cyanosis and clubbing are typical in chronic obstructive respiratory disease (COPD). Rash can be seen in some viral illnesses.

B. Laboratory Data

   1. Hemogram. Leukocytosis and left shift in infectious diseases.

   2. Calcium. Hypercalcemia is a paraneoplastic syndrome in some bronchogenic carcinomas.

   3. Arterial blood gas. If indicated by dyspnea or cyanosis.

   4. Arterial carboxyhemoglobin. In cases of smoke and carbon monoxide inhalation.

C. Radiologic and Other Studies

   1. Chest x-ray. Evidence of pulmonary edema, neoplasm, pneumonia, interstitial lung disease, hilar lymphadenopathy, and in some cases, an aspirated foreign body (eg, teeth, coins). Acute aspiration may not be apparent on an initial x-ray.

   2. Sputum. Look at gross appearance noting color, viscosity, odor, and amount. Gram's stain, acid-fast stain, fungal stains, and appropriate cultures are essential. Obtain sputum cytology if pulmonary neoplasm is a possibility.

   3. PPD skin test. If tuberculosis is possible.

   4. Pulmonary function tests (PFT). A restrictive pattern (decreased total lung capacity and vital capacity) in interstitial lung disease.

5. **Bronchoscopy.** To evaluate and biopsy neoplasm, obtain brushings and biopsies for culture. Obtain postbronchoscopy sputum cultures. May be therapeutic for foreign body aspiration.

V. Plan. Attempt to obtain a sputum sample even if told initially that cough is nonproductive and order a chest x-ray. If patient is dyspneic, obtain a room air ABG and begin oxygen therapy.

A. Infectious Conditions. (See Section IX for drug dosages).
1. **Unknown community acquired pneumonia.** Penicillin G (useful in treating pneumococcal infections) or erythromycin (useful in treating mycoplasma or pneumococcal infections).
2. **Community acquired/compromised host (COPD/Alcoholic).** Cephalosporin or tetracycline.
3. **Hospital acquired.** Aminoglycoside and nafcillin or aminoglycoside and cephalosporin.
   a. **Anaerobic:** Penicillin G or clindamycin.
   b. **Mycoplasma:** Erythromycin or tetracycline.
   c. **Tuberculosis.** Isoniazid and rifampin.
   d. **Immunosuppressed patient:** (eg, after transplant).
      i. Requires coverage for *Legionella* (erythromycin) plus an aminoglycoside plus PCN/or a cephalosporin.
      ii. When a specific organism is identified by Gram's stain and culture, antibiotic therapy is adjusted appropriately.
      iii. *Pneumocystis carinii* pneumonia is particularly prevalent in AIDS patients and treated with trimethoprim/sulfamethoxazole or pentamidine.

B. Pulmonary Edema
1. Oxygen.
2. Upright posture.
3. **Diuretics.** Usual choice is furosemide 20–40 mg IV. If patient is on a chronic oral Furosemide (Lasix) dose, give 1–2 times normal dose intravenously. Follow for hypokalemia.

C. Nonproductive Cough. Either associated with viral upper respiratory infection or tracheal irritation.
1. **Cough suppressant**
   a. Codeine/hydrocodone preparation most effective.
   b. **Dextromethorphan:** A codeine derivative that acts centrally.
   c. Avoid cough suppressants in patients with a productive cough.
2. **Expectorants.** There is no clear evidence to be of value. Best established is guaifenesin (Robitussin etc). A multitude of preparations often combining a cough suppressant, expectorant, and an antihistamine are available.

20. CENTRAL VENOUS LINE PROBLEMS

(Central venous catheterization techniques are discussed in Section III, page 295.)

I. **Problem.** The central venous pressure (CVP) catheter placed in a patient to undergo total hip replacement in the morning is not functioning.

II. **Immediate Questions**

A. **What is the appearance of the tracing?** A CVP should have a slowly undulating waveform, which varies with the patient's respirations if properly positioned in the chest. Absence of a waveform may indicate that the catheter is clotted. In the absence of a transducer, the column of fluid in the manometer should fluctuate with respirations.

B. **Can blood be aspirated from the line?** Inability to aspirate blood doesn't imply a nonfunctioning catheter that can't be used for fluid infusions. It may mean the tip is against the vessel, but also may indicate a kinked or clotted line.

C. **How long has the line been in place?** The longer a line is in place, the higher the incidence of infection.

D. **Is the line in correct position?** This must be evaluated on a chest x-ray. The tip should be in the superior vena cava. If there is any question, get a new film and compare it to the post-placement x-ray.

E. **Is there bleeding from the site?** This may represent a local problem or a diffuse coagulopathy.

III. **Differential Diagnosis**

A. **Clotted Catheter.** This happens more frequently with slowly running lines.

B. **Catheter in Incorrect Position.** Evaluated by chest x-ray. Subclavian lines occasionally go up into the neck and will not fluctuate with respiration.

C. **Kinked Catheter.** These include kinking of the line at the skin entry site or kinking under the clavicle because of the angle of placement to enter the vein. This can usually be seen as an acute bend on x-ray.

D. **Other Mechanical Problems.** Cracking of the catheter at the hub or a loose connection.

E. **Flush Line or Transducer Malfunction.** Easily ruled out by checking the system, the nursing staff can be very helpful in evaluating this.

F. **Infected Catheter.** Any question of sepsis originating in a central venous line requires expeditious evaluation. The best technique involves drawing cultures through the catheter, removing the line, and culturing the tip.

IV. Database

A. Physical Exam Key Points

1. **Vital signs.** Fever signifies infection, whereas tachycardia and hypotension may represent excessive bleeding, tension pneumothorax, or hemothorax.

2. **HEENT.** Tracheal deviation may indicate an expanding hematoma or tension pneumothorax, especially immediately after CVP line placement.

3. **Lung.** Diminished breath sounds may indicate a pneumothorax, hemothorax, or hydrothorax.

4. **Check line site.** Inspect for evidence of cellulitis, bleeding, catheter kinking, or leakage from a cracked hub. Check the transducer and flush line.

B. Laboratory Data

1. Draw blood cultures such as Dupont Isolator® if sepsis must be evaluated. Obtain cultures from both the catheter and peripherally (see V-E below).

2. CBC or coagulation profile if bleeding is present.

V. Plan.

In general, replacing the line will usually solve problems associated with the line itself. Unless the line is infected, it can be changed over a guidewire. Be sure to carefully suture it in place to avoid kinking at the hub. All line manipulations should be performed using sterile technique and with the patient in the Trendelenburg (head down) position to prevent air embolus.

A. **Clotted Catheter.** A new line thought to be clotted can often be declotted safely with a syringe. The decision to attempt to declot a catheter should be approached cautiously because the clot may act as an embolus. The catheter can be gently aspirated or flushed with a 1 mL tuberculin syringe. The smaller diameter of this syringe matches the diameter of the catheter more closely and transmits more pressure than a larger syringe. Use heparin flush solution (100 U/mL). One can also use streptokinase to declot a line (See Section VII, page 366 for dose), but side effects can limit its use.

B. **Kinked Catheter.** Inspection of the site may reveal a kinked catheter that can be easily corrected by repositioning the skin sutures using sterile technique. A subclavian catheter that is kinked at the entry to the vein under the clavicle must be replaced. Subclavian lines are the easiest to affix to the skin and prevent kinking, whereas internal jugular are the most difficult.

C. Misdirected Catheter. Usually requires removal and replacement, often to another site. Rarely, fluoroscopy may be needed to direct a difficult catheter.

D. Bleeding. Site bleeding can usually be controlled with direct pressure.

E. Workup of the Infected Catheter. Draw one blood culture from the line, one from a peripheral site, and evaluate the colony counts at 24 hours as described by Mosca. If the colony count from the culture is 5 or more times greater than the peripherally drawn culture, the line is implicated as the culprit and must be replaced at another site.

F. Hints for Catheter Insertion. (See Section III, page 295). There are many "tricks" to inserting a central venous catheter, most of which are personal preferences rather than proven helpful tools.

    1. The most common locations are subclavian and internal jugular (IJ). The problem with IJ lines is fixing them to the patient for long periods of time. Subclavian lines are easier to fix to the skin. Femoral lines are acceptable when there is no upper body alternative and when rapid access is needed during CPR.

    2. Most commonly for subclavian lines, the patient is placed with a roll between the scapulae, in the Trendelenburg position. This presumably makes the vein more prominent and simplifies puncture. Recent evidence in the literature, however, contradicts this commonly held view. The needle is passed below the clavicle and aimed toward the sternal notch. After obtaining a good blood return (make sure it is venous), the syringe is removed, carefully holding the needle still. Watch for spontaneous blood return. The guidewire is passed through the needle and the needle removed. The guidewire should pass easily. Remember that if the guidewire goes to the right ventricle, arrhythmias may be induced. The skin is nicked with a scalpel, and the catheter passed over the guidewire. After removing the guidewire, it should be nearly straight. Affix the catheter at the hub to the skin.

    3. The internal jugular vein is approached with the patient turning his or her head away from the side approached. The needle is inserted two fingerbreadths above the clavicle, in the V shaped area between the two heads of the sternocleidomastoid muscle. Aim for the ipsilateral nipple. Identifying the vein with a small needle (eg, 20 gauge) before using the large needle to pass the guidewire is highly recommended.

    4. In placing a central venous line there are four signs of successful placement:

        a. Easy aspiration of blood through the syringe.

      b. Easy passing of the guidewire.

      c. After removal, the guidewire should be nearly straight.

      d. Blood should aspirate easily through the catheter after placement.

21. DEATH

I. Problem. On a cold night a homeless man is brought to the emergency room unresponsive and pulseless after being found on a park bench.

II. Immediate Questions

    A. Is the patient responsive? See Problem 11, page 37 and Problem 17, page 69.

    B. Is the patient cold from exposure? If the core body temperature is less than 32.2°C, the patient is hypothermic and must be warmed. Warm air ventilation, warming blanket, warm bladder and gastric lavage, and warm intravenous fluids are all effective. The most effective warming is done on cardiac bypass.

    C. What medications or drugs has the patient taken? Narcotics, alcohol, and overdosage may cause coma and cardiac arrhythmias.

    D. Does the patient have a declaration of agreement regarding organ donation? If unavailable, the next of kin can allow procurement if the patient is an acceptable candidate. Respiration and cardiac function must be supported until procurement.

    E. Are the family or close friends available? Family should be notified when a patient's hospital course changes markedly. In the acute setting, many health care workers suggest that families **not** be informed of the patient's unexpected death over the phone, but be asked to come to the hospital immediately. For chronically ill patients, it may be appropriate to inform the family of the patient's death by telephone.

    F. Is rigor mortis present? Resuscitation is not appropriate in this patient.

III. Differential Diagnosis. History from family, witnesses, and EMS personnel may assist in diagnosis.

    A. See Problem 11, page 37 and Problem 17, page 69 for a complete list of acute causes.

    B. Intoxications and metabolic disorders are common causes of coma and cardiopulmonary arrest that can be reversible if corrected in time. CPR must continue (according to ACLS protocol) unsuccessfully for 20 minutes before pronouncing the patient dead.

C. Hypothermia. Core temperature below 32°C is protective against hypoxic neurologic damage. Death cannot be pronounced until the patient has been warmed to at least 32.2°C and a full 20 minutes of ACLS protocol CPR given (see page 37).

IV. Database

A. Physical Exam Key Points

1. **Vital signs.** Temperature must be documented to be above 32.2°C. Lack of spontaneous respiration must be documented (following ventilation with 100% O_2, withdraw support and observe for 10 min to allow CO_2 to > 60 mm Hg). Absence of pulse or functional cardiac rhythm should be documented.

2. **CNS test for cranial nerve and reflex function.** For brain death, patients must be comatose with no spontaneous motion or response to stimulation, pupils dilated and unresponsive to light, and corneal, oculocephalic, oculovestibular, and oropharyngeal reflexes must be absent.

3. **Chest.** Confirm absence of apical pulse and spontaneous respirations.

4. **Skin.** Any patient arriving at the emergency department with livor or rigor mortis is considered dead and CPR does not need to be initiated. (Same for injuries obviously incompatible with life, eg, decapitation).

B. Laboratory Data. As needed in diagnosis of inciting cause of death.

1. **Hemogram.** Sepsis, anemia.

2. **Serum electrolytes.** Arrhythmogenic abnormalities, uremia, glucose.

3. **Drug screen.** Alcohol, barbiturates, opiates, or benzodiazepines.

4. **Arterial and venous blood gases.** Acid-base abnormalities.

C. Radiologic and Other Studies. As needed in the diagnosis of inciting cause of death.

1. **Chest x-ray.** Pneumothorax, hemothorax, etc.

2. **Head CT.** For all comatose patients.

3. **ECG.** Arrhythmia, EMD.

4. **EEG,** blood flow study, brain scintigraphy, or cerebral angiography to document brain death.

V. Plan

A. Resuscitation. See Problem 17, page 69 and Problem 11, page 37.

Following full resuscitation and thorough investigation of possible causes and their treatment, if the patient has no response to CPR for 20 min of ACLS protocol, they can be pronounced dead. Make sure temperature, intoxicant and brain death criteria are met, if applicable. Do not electrically cardiovert a hypothermic patient. Hypothermia causes refractory ventricular fibrillation that is reversible with warming. Allow a longer period of observation in traumatic injury in children as they are more resilient to hypoxic injury than adults.

B. Pronouncing Death. Confirm death and note time.

C. Maintain support of ventilation and circulation if patient is a potential organ donor.

D. Notification
1. Attending physician, chief of service or appropriate contact
2. **Next of kin.** It is appropriate to have a family designate contact remaining family members once the designate has been notified. Inquire regarding autopsy or organ donation.
3. **Transplant coordinator.** If appropriate, they usually should be made aware of a potential donor before the declaration of death. The coordinator generally makes arrangements to approach the family regarding organ procurement to eliminate burden on the caregiver and the possible appearance of conflict of interest to the family.
4. **Morgue.** The transfer usually is arranged by nursing staff. Allow time for family of the deceased to view the body in the patient's room before transfer to the morgue.
5. **Coroner.** Laws regarding definition of coroner's cases differ among states. The medical examiner will usually investigate all traumatic, perioperative, and suspicious deaths.

E. Preparation. Most institutions have standard "mortuary packs" containing a plastic shroud and state death certificate. All IV lines, chest and endotracheal tubes, and other invasive devices are left in place. ETT is disconnected, IV lines are tied off or capped. The nursing staff usually complete this task for you.

F. Documentation
1. **Discharge summary.** The patient needs to be formally discharged.
2. **Death certificate.** Do **not** list cardiopulmonary arrest as the cause of death—this is how everyone dies. Give the main reason for hospitalization as the primary cause of death, eg, adenocarcinoma of the lung. Other events contributing to death can be listed secondarily, eg, pneumonia, acute renal failure.

G. Reflection. If you felt particularly close to the patient, do not forget that you are allowed to grieve as well. Families will appreciate a kind word and communicating with them provides a sense of closure. Consider the patient's history and course and what measures could have been effective in preventing death. This is usually done formally at morbidity and mortality hospital review conferences.

22. DIARRHEA

I. Problem. A 56-year-old man develops diarrhea 2 days after an aortobifemoral vascular graft is placed.

II. Immediate Questions

A. What are the patient's vital signs? Tachycardia may indicate volume depletion. Hypotension and fever may indicate sepsis. Tachypnea can be found in sepsis and is a response to significant metabolic acidosis as may be found in ischemic injuries such as bowel infarction.

B. What are the characteristics of the stool? Is the diarrhea bloody? Bloody diarrhea may be seen after ischemic injury to the bowel, with colonic neoplasms (carcinoma and villous adenoma), and infection (*Shigella*) and other inflammatory states.

C. Is this an acute or chronic problem? Acute diarrhea is usually infectious in origin, medication induced, or from mesenteric ischemia. Chronic diarrhea usually does not require urgent treatment.

D. What medication is the patient taking? Many medicines cause diarrhea. Antibiotics can cause diarrhea by altering colonic flora leading to malabsorption or *Clostridium difficile* overgrowth and pseudomembranous colitis, a toxin-induced diarrhea.

E. Is there a history of pelvic radiation therapy? Radiation therapy for malignancies (cervix, prostate, rectal) can cause chronic diarrhea.

III. Differential Diagnosis

A. Acute Diarrhea

1. Infectious. Rare causes of acute diarrhea in the surgical patient include viral and bacterial infections and parasitic infestations (*Salmonella, Shigella, Campylobacter, Yersinia*).

2. Ischemic. A catastrophic cause of diarrhea, mesenteric ischemia is a surgical emergency. Abdominal distention and severe pain, loss of bowel sounds, and bloody diarrhea in the critically ill, hypotensive patient or the vascular surgery patient after aortic crossclamping and ligation of the inferior mesenteric artery are suspicious for mesenteric ischemia and bowel necrosis.

3. Gastrointestinal hemorrhage. Blood acts as a cathartic agent (see Problem 10, page 34).

    4. Drug induced.
- a. Quinidine, digoxin, colchicine, antacids (magnesium based), chemotherapeutic agents (methotrexate, adriamycin) and laxatives. Opioid withdrawal.
- b. Antibiotics cause diarrhea by altering normal flora and causing malabsorption, or by inducing *C difficile* overgrowth and toxin production (pseudomembranous enterocolitis). Many antibiotics may cause pseudomembranous colitis—most frequently implicated include clindamycin, cephalosporins, and ampicillin parenteral aminoglycosides.

B. Chronic Diarrhea
1. **Inflammatory.** Regional enteritis and ulcerative colitis cause diarrhea as can radiation injury of the bowel.
2. **Neoplastic.** Colon cancer can cause diarrhea. Classically, villous adenoma causes copious watery diarrhea.
3. **Endocrine.** Diarrhea can be found with carcinoid syndrome, hyperthyroidism, and in the islet-cell tumors (gastrinoma, Zollinger-Ellison syndrome and VIPoma [Vasoactive-Intestinal Polypeptide hormone secreting tumors]).
4. **Postoperative.** Diarrhea can be seen after gastrectomy (dumping), significant small and large bowel resections, and pancreatic resection.
5. **Pancreatic.** Exocrine pancreatic dysfunction results in steatorrhea and malabsorption.
6. **Paradoxic.** Fecal impaction may result in diarrhea as only liquid stool can be expelled past the point of impaction.
7. **Other.** Psychogenic, irritable bowel syndrome, lactose intolerance, radiation induced.

IV. Database

A. History.
Diarrheal episodes, quality and quantity of loose stools, associated abdominal pain, and use of medicines and laxatives may aid in the diagnosis.

B. Physical Exam Key Points
1. **Vital signs.** Irregular pulse may indicate atrial fibrillation, a possible source of embolus and mesenteric ischemia.
2. **Abdominal exam.** Pain is rarely seen with diarrhea. When present, bacterial infections, such as *Shigella* and *Yersinia,* and mesenteric ischemia must be considered. Distention is seen with bowel ischemia. Bowel sounds vary, but absent sounds may indicate ischemic injury.
3. **Rectal exam.** Must always be performed to rule out neoplasm and impaction and to check for occult blood.
4. **Skin.** Jaundice, spider angiomata, palmar erythema should be looked for to determine possible liver and, secondarily, pancreatic disease from alcohol abuse.

C. Laboratory Data
   1. Stool for occult blood using a Hemoccult or other test kit. Serial exams increase sensitivity.
   2. Stool culture for enteric pathogens, examine for ova and parasites, fecal leukocytes (see page 285), *C difficile* toxin assay.
   3. **Hemogram.** Monitor hematocrit, especially if there is evidence of gastrointestinal bleeding. Look for leukocytosis as evidence of infection or perforation.
   4. **Electrolytes.** Severe diarrhea may derange serum electrolytes. Hypokalemia and bicarbonate loss may lead to metabolic acidosis with a normal anion gap (see page 250).
   5. **Arterial blood gas.** To assess metabolic acidosis, especially if mesenteric ischemia is suspected.
   6. **Stool electrolytes.** Potassium, sodium, and bicarbonate determinations make fluid replacement more physiologic in severe cases. See Section IV, page 337 to guide replacement.

D. Radiologic and Other Studies
   1. **Sigmoidoscopy.** This should be performed in patients suspected of having pseudomembranous colitis and severe diarrhea. Classic findings are whitish green plaques or confluent pseudomembrane. Patients with a mass on rectal exam should undergo sigmoidoscopy and biopsy of the suspicious area. In addition, ischemic injury in the left colon can often be seen through a sigmoidoscope.
   2. **Nasogastric aspiration.** An NG tube should be placed to rule out upper GI bleeding if diarrhea is grossly bloody or melanotic.
   3. **Abdominal and chest radiographs.** Look for evidence of obstruction or ileus (dilated loops and air-fluid levels) or perforation (free air, best appreciated on an upright chest film), air in the portal system (ischemic bowel necrosis), pancreatic calcifications.
   4. **Paracentesis.** If ischemia and gangrene are suspected, peritoneal tap should be performed and culture, Gram's stain, white blood cell count, and amylase determined on the aspirated fluid. If the fluid is cloudy, bloody, or malodorous, bowel gangrene is probably present. See Section III, page 295.
   5. **Arteriography.** This should be conducted when ischemic bowel injury is first considered.
   6. **Barium or Gastrografin enema.** Should be performed when inflammatory bowel disease or neoplasm suspected.
   7. **Colonoscopy.** Is sometimes indicated.
   8. **ECG.** Rarely, mesenteric embolization can occur from atrial thrombus in atrial fibrillation or after myocardial infarction.

V. Plan

A. Fluid and Electrolytes
   1. Significant dehydration can occur with acute diarrhea; shock requires careful, yet aggressive, rehydration with the help of a

central venous catheter and, rarely, with a pulmonary artery catheter. Alpha-adrenergic agents used to support blood pressure will worsen mesenteric ischemia, but may be unavoidable in severe cases.

2. Frequent loose stools of toxic or endocrine origin (carcinoid) often require fluid replacement with additives, such as bicarbonate to duplicate the electrolyte makeup of the stools. See Section IV, page 337.

B. Stop Possible Causative Medications and Antibiotics

C. Control Agents. (Medication doses can be found in Section VIII, page 376).

1. **Narcotics.** Tincture of opium, diphenoxylate with atropine (Lomotil), loperamide, codeine, and paregoric can be used carefully to control diarrhea. These agents rarely prolong infection diarrhea making the illness worse. Additionally, they should not be used in cases of impaction or low lying neoplasms.

2. **Bismuth subsalicylate (Pepto-Bismol).** Shown to control some types of diarrhea, in part by inhibiting prostaglandin synthesis.

3. Kaolin and pectin do not work in most cases.

4. Cholestyramine is a useful adjunct to vancomycin in treating pseudomembranous colitis.

5. Dietary changes.
   a. Avoid lactose containing foods.
   b. Clear liquid diet for 24–48 hours.
   c. Advance diet slowly.

D. Antibiotics

1. **Bacterial diarrhea.** Trimethoprim-sulfamethoxazole covers most infections, but therapy should be based on bacteriologic results. In most cases, with the exception of shigellosis, however, antibiotics are not necessary and are indicted in the immunocompromised patient only.

2. **Pseudomembranous colitis.** Can be treated with vancomycin 125 mg PO every 6 hours or metronidazole 500 mg PO every 6 hours, usually for 7 days. Cholestyramine can be added 4 times a day as an adjunct. If pseudomembranous colitis is strongly suspected, empiric therapy can be initiated prior to the results of the clostridium toxin assay.

E. Operation. Embolectomy, bowel resection, mesenteric artery bypass for mesenteric ischemia. Resection is required for colonic malignancies, villous adenoma, and some complicated cases of inflammatory bowel disease. When possible, tumor localization and resection should be performed for carcinoid and islet-cell tumors.

F. Other

1. **Control GI bleeding.** See Problems 10 and 34, pages 34 and 118.

2. **Disimpaction.** Manual with a gloved finger and adequate lubrication.
3. **Pancreatic insufficiency.** Give high doses of replacement enzymes (pancrease, Viokase, etc).
4. **Control thyrotoxicosis.** PTU or methimazole, iodide, β-blockers, dexamethasone.
5. Steroids or sulfasalazine if inflammatory bowel disease.
6. High dose cimetidine for diarrhea caused by gastrinoma.

23. DRAIN OUTPUT—CHANGING AMOUNT

I. **Problem.** You are notified that a patient, 2 days following a hepatic lobectomy, has a three-fold increase in the volume from a Jackson-Pratt drain over the prior eight hours.

II. **Immediate Questions**

A. **Exactly where is the drain and what operative procedure was done?** To begin to manage problems with drains, one must know the basic facts. For example, a drain in the gallbladder bed following a cholecystectomy (low drainage expected) is very different from a T-tube following a common duct exploration (much higher drainage than from the gallbladder bed).

B. **What is the nature of the drain fluid?** There is a limited number of body fluids that can account for an increase in drain output. The list includes serous/serosanguineous fluids, blood, pus, lymph (chyle), bile, pancreatic juice, intestinal contents, urine, or CSF. Some of these fluids can be identified by gross visual inspection and others by laboratory analysis.

C. **Are there any new symptoms concurrent with the change in drain output?** Ask specifically about pain, signs of infection, hypotension, and abdominal distention.

D. **What is the pattern of postoperative drainage?** Variations in drain output may reflect variability in the ability of the drains to function rather than actual increased fluid production. For example, if in the time period before increased drainage the output was unexpectedly low, the increased output may reflect a sudden outflow of accumulated fluids. Also, check for more than one drain in the same area and look at the total output for all drains.

E. **Has there been any change in the patient's activities coincident with changing drain output?** A patient started on oral intake would be expected to have increased drainage of pancreatic secretions, thoracic duct flow, or T-tube output. Also, if a patient has increased physical activity such as ambulation or physical therapy then drains in extremity/lymph node dissection area may increase.

III. Differential Diagnosis. Drains may be categorized by the location and type of drain. The list below contains the more commonly used surgical drains, states the purpose of the drain, and points out specific problems to be expected in terms of changing output. Drain management is neither mysterious nor complicated, but rather is a simple plumbing matter with a finite number of possible explanations for a given situation.

A. Extremity/lymph node dissection (axillary, inguinal) drains.
1. The purpose is to prevent the accumulation of lymph and serous fluid so that wound healing is facilitated.
2. Increased output is usually lymph and is often associated with increased motion of the area of the wound. Treatment is to immobilize the affected area.

B. Mediastinal tubes. Placed during open heart surgery.
1. Function is to identify excessive bleeding and prevent cardiac tamponade.
2. Increased output is usually bloody and may be due to a specific bleeding point.
3. A sudden decrease in output may be due to an obstructed tube and may precede tamponade.

C. Chest Tubes (pleural). (See also Problem 13, page 57.)
1. Functions to drain blood, pus, air, or fluid from pleural cavities.
2. One specific case of increased drainage associated with oral intake may indicate fluid from injured thoracic duct.

D. Hepatic/Biliary Tube
1. **Hepatectomy**
   a. Drains lymph, bile, and blood from cut surface of the liver, as well as any bile leak from the ligated hepatic duct.
   b. **Examine for bile:** Often multiple drains are present so be aware of total output.
2. **Cholecystectomy** (often not drained).
   a. Drain identifying leak from ligated cystic duct or excessive bleeding.
   b. Examine drain output for bile.
3. **Common duct exploration.**
   a. T-tube stents the choledochotomy, prevents bile leaks, and provides a path for further diagnostic or therapeutic inquiries (cholangiogram or extraction of retained stones).
   b. Increased output may signify distal obstruction from a retained stone, edema, or the start of oral intake.

E. Pancreatic Procedures
1. Used when pancreatic parenchyma is violated (islet-cell tumor resection, trauma) or when ductal system is opened (external drainage of pseudocyst) to prevent the accumulation of pancreatic fluid.

    2. Drain output increases with feeding or with distal duct obstruction.

F. Esophageal Procedures
1. Function to identify leaks and evacuate potentially irritative/infectious fluid.
2. **Output increased with leak.** Examine for appearance of saliva or refluxed gastrointestinal contents.

G. Urinary Tract Procedures
1. Usually after radical cystectomy and urinary diversion, radical prostatectomy or other procedures where the collecting system or bladder had been opened. Prevents urinoma formation and in the case of a concomitant node dissection, lymphocele formation.
2. Increase may represent increased lymph leakage or urinary leakage from an anastomotic site.

IV. Database

A. Physical Exam Key Points
1. Examine drainage fluid for color and characteristics looking for blood, pus, and bile. Also look at the tube for clots or other obstructing material.
2. **Lungs.** Changes or absent breath sounds in chest tube.
3. **Cardiac.** Physical signs of tamponade such as increased jugular venous pressure, pulsus paradoxus, or quiet heart sounds.
4. **Abdomen.** Pain, abdominal distention, or a fluid wave may be present with accumulating fluid.
5. **Extremities.** Examine for collections of undrained fluid under surgical site.

B. Laboratory Data
1. **Hemogram.** Especially if infection or excess bleeding may be present.
2. **Hematocrit of drainage fluid.** Often grossly bloody fluid is still mostly serum or lymph. Compare the drainage hematocrit to the blood hematocrit.
3. **Gram's stain.** Culture of drainage if any question of infection.
4. **Chemistries.** These can be performed on material from the drain to help identify specific types of fluids being drained.
   a. **Amylase:** Markedly elevated in pancreatic secretions, also present in saliva.
   b. **Triglycerides:** Elevated in thoracic duct lymph.
   c. **Creatinine:** If it is possible that the drained fluid is urine, creatine in the fluid will be markedly elevated.
   d. **pH:** Pleural fluid pH < 7.2 may be associated with an empyema.
   e. **LDH and protein:** See Section III for a discussion of ascitic fluid (paracentesis) and pleural fluid (thoracentesis).

C. Radiologic and Other Studies
1. **Chest x-ray.** Especially if changing amount in pleural or mediastinal tube to determine if there is an increasing fluid collection.
2. **Plain films.** Most drains are marked with a radiopaque stripe so that drain position can be verified with plain films.
3. **Contrast studies.** Routine with T-tube following common duct exploration. Contrast studies can identify fistulas, leaks, or cavities of accumulated fluid.

V. Plan. Identify type of drain, location, and type of fluid draining; formulate ideas about the likely source of fluid.

A. Emergency Management. Usually drain management does not require emergent or urgent action with the exception of mediastinal tubes on the cardiac surgery service.
1. **Increased output.** Almost always blood. Document rate of bleeding by accurately noting output every 30–60 minutes and following serial hematocrits. Measure coagulation parameters and correct as necessary with FFP and platelets. Notify senior staff and operating team about rate of bleeding when possibility of returning to the operating room exists.
2. **Decreased output.** A sudden decrease in output may be a result of a clot in the tube and may lead to an episode of cardiac tamponade. If blood pressure decreases, be prepared to open the lower portion of the wound and evacuate blood and clot gently from the retrosternal space.

B. Routine Management
1. Record accurately the amount, characteristics, and lab analysis of increased drain output.
2. Replace high output with appropriate fluids
    a. **Pancreatic, biliary & small bowel:** See Section IV.
    b. **Mediastinal bloody drainage:** Use blood.
3. Occasionally, suction on a drain will encourage persistent drainage. It is sometimes appropriate to put drains on "passive" (gravity) drainage to decrease the volume.
4. Remember that drain management is an area where individual idiosyncrasies abound. Never pull a drain unless you believe it is appropriate and the surgeon in charge wants it pulled.

24. DRAIN OUTPUT—CHANGING CHARACTER

I. Problem. A 45-year-old male, 2 days after cholecystectomy, now has bilious drainage from a right flank Penrose drain.

II. Immediate Questions

A. What are the characteristics of the drainage? Bloody, bilious, serous, serosanguineous, urine-like may be used to describe the nature of the drainage.

B. What kind of drainage was there previously? A drain that had serous drainage and is now draining blood is an obvious cause for concern. Similarly, a previously serous fluid that now looks like urine may indicate a new fistula.

C. What volume of drainage is present? This is important to evaluate because this volume often must be replaced and is addressed in Problem 23, page 88.

D. What was the operation and where was the drain placed? These questions must be answered to assess the nature of new drainage.

III. Differential Diagnosis. Clearly, the differential diagnosis depends on the characteristics of the drainage and the location of the drain. For a further discussion of drainage, see Problem 23, page 88.

A. Bloody Drainage. Of obvious concern after any surgical procedure. Read the operative note to see if there is any mention of a "generalized ooze" of blood at the end of the procedure.

B. Serous Drainage. Usually of no concern a few days after surgery. An increased volume of drainage may be a result of irritation from the drain.

C. Purulent Drainage. Indicates infection.

D. Bilious Drainage. Rarely placed after cholecystectomy but may be a leak from the ducts of Luschka after cholecystectomy, but can be from an injured common duct as well.

E. Intestinal Drainage. Of obvious concern after any operation. May be a fistula to the skin wound.

F. Urine Drainage. A fistula may have developed; for example, perineal urinary drainage after an abdominoperineal resection indicates a bladder fistula.

G. Chylous Drainage. Indicates injury to the thoracic duct.

IV. Database

A. Physical Exam Key Points

1. **Vital signs.** Signs of infection (tachycardia, fever) and volume loss.
2. **Abdomen.** Check for signs of peritonitis.
3. **Wound.** Examine for signs of infection or fluid collection.

   B. **Laboratory Data**
      1. **Hemogram.** Check white blood cell count and hematocrit. **Note:** While counts may be elevated up to 24 hours after surgery, they may not represent an infection.
      2. **Coagulation profile.** PT/PTT platelets, fibrin split products if bleeding is excessive.
      3. **Send drain fluid for chemistry as appropriate.** See Problem 23, page 88.

   C. **Radiologic and Other Studies**
      1. **Angiogram.** May help localize bleeding site if rate is at least 1 ml/min.
      2. **Fistulogram.** Useful to identify origin of cutaneous fistulae.
      3. **CT scans and ultrasound.** May localize undrained fluid collections.

V. **Plan**

   A. **Supportive care in patients who are bleeding.** Administer fluids or blood to maintain blood pressure. Determine the bleeding site and control by angiogram, reoperation, or correction of coagulopathy.

   B. Antibiotics are indicated in certain fistulae such as colovesical fistulae.

   C. Reoperation may be needed, as in the case of biliary drainage from an abdominal wound or drain, not present previously.

   D. Purulent drainage from within a body cavity always mandates continuous drainage until the abscess is cleared. Operative intervention may be needed but often percutaneously under CT or ultrasound guidance additional fluid can be removed.

   E. Replace fluids as needed (see Section VI, page 359).

25. DELIRIUM TREMENS (DTs)

I. **Problem.** A 55-year-old intoxicated man is admitted with abdominal pain and an elevated amylase. Narcotic analgesia is initiated. On the third hospital day, he is found talking to the walls and shaking violently.

II. **Immediate Questions**

   A. **What are the patient's vital signs?** Hypertension, tachycardia, and fever may represent signs of autonomic overactivity, common in delirium.

B. **What is the patient's mental status?** Altered levels of consciousness and impaired cognitive function define delirium. Hallucinations and confusion are important observations. These coupled with autonomic hyperactivity are typical of delirium. Delirium can also present as unresponsiveness, but disorientation and confusion are still prominent. As a general rule, visual hallucinations, "pink elephants," are more commonly associated with toxic psychosis (EtOH, etc), and auditory hallucinations are more commonly associated with psychiatric illness.

C. **What is the patient's airway status?** Any patient with an altered level of consciousness is at increased risk of aspiration.

D. **What medication is the patient taking?** With particular attention to addictive substances.

E. **Is there a history of drug or alcohol abuse?** This is central to the accurate diagnosis.

III. **Differential Diagnosis.** Delirium is a manifestation of diffuse cerebral dysfunction. Focal neurologic deficits point to a structural abnormality (stroke, brain tumor, etc). The differential diagnosis of delirium is more extensive than the following list indicates and includes any source of diffuse cerebral dysfunction (see also Problem 14, page 60). The patient presenting with delirium may be suffering from a very wide range of problems. The patient described may be delirious based on any of the following diagnoses.

A. **Withdrawal Syndromes**
  1. **Delirium tremens.** A potentially life-threatening form of alcohol withdrawal, DTs must be thought of in any patient known to be a heavy drinker who developed delirium 3–4 days after hospitalization. In the patient not known to be a drinker, other causes must be investigated.
  2. **Barbiturate withdrawal.** Indistinguishable from DTs clinically.
  3. **Opioid withdrawal.** Occurs up to 48 hours after cessation of agent (most rapid with heroin) and symptoms include restlessness, rhinorrhea, lacrimation, nausea, diarrhea, and hypertension.

B. **Metabolic Abnormalities**
  1. **Electrolyte abnormalities.** Chronic vomiting, pancreatitis, renal failure, and severe liver disease can all cause electrolyte and metabolic abnormalities, which can manifest as delirium.
  2. **Hypoxia.** Congestive heart failure can produce hypoxia and delirium in an indolent fashion.
  3. **Drug intoxication.**

C. **Endocrine Abnormalities.** Abnormal thyroid and adrenal cortical function can cause delirium. Hypoglycemia from an insulin secreting tumor or from intentional or accidental insulin overdose should be considered. Diabetic ketoacidosis and hyperosmolar coma should also be considered.

D. **CNS Infections.** Meningitis and encephalitis can cause delirium.

E. **Intensive Care Unit Psychosis.** A special, rather common form called "Post pump psychosis" or "Post pericardiotomy syndrome" or ICU psychosis is associated with patients having undergone coronary bypass procedures.

F. **Sepsis.** Any cause of sepsis can lead to altered mentation.

IV. Database

A. **Physical Exam Key Points**
1. **Vital signs.** Tachycardia is a common manifestation of withdrawal states.
2. **Neck.** Look for jugular venous distention, which suggests congestive heart failure (CHF) and thyroid masses (hyperthyroidism).
3. **Chest exam.** Signs of congestive heart failure and other causes of pulmonary edema and hypoxia should be sought.
4. **Abdomen.** Check for bladder distention, a common cause of agitation in the elderly patient.
5. **Skin.** Profuse sweating is typical of DTs.
6. **Neurologic exam.** Mental status changes define delirium. Hallucinations, confusion, and disorientation are typical. Reflexes will be exaggerated but symmetrical. Pupils are reactive. Any focal findings on motor, sensory, deep tendon, or cranial nerve examination point to a structural abnormality, either spinal or intracranial.

B. **Laboratory Data**
1. **Electrolytes and glucose.** Look especially for hyponatremia and hypoglycemia. These are potentially life threatening. Calcium abnormalities should also be ruled out.
2. **ABGs.** Obtain if hypoxemia is likely.

C. **Radiologic and Other Studies.** History, physical exam, and simple tests usually provide the diagnosis of delirium. A chest x-ray might show cardiomegaly and pulmonary edema. Evaluation of the CNS by head CT scan or lumbar puncture is occasionally necessary, especially in the septic patient or one with focal neurologic findings. Rarely is electroencephalography (EEG) useful.

V. Plan

   A. Prevention. The patient at risk for delirium tremens should be
      treated while hospitalized with around-the-clock benzodiazepines,
      most commonly oxazepam (15–30 mg PO every 4–6 hours) or
      chlordiazepoxide (25–50 mg PO every 6–8 hours).

   B. Delirium tremens. Alcohol abusers typically display other poten-
      tial causes of delirium, most notably electrolyte abnormalities
      (from vomiting) and hepatic encephalopathy.
      1. Benzodiazepines given intravenously initially (diazepam 5–
         10 mg IV every 4–6 hours) followed by oral treatment with
         diazepam, chlordiazepoxide, or oxazepam in the nonvomiting
         patient.
      2. Restraints to prevent injury may be needed, often in the prone
         position (decrease risk of aspiration).
      3. Intravenous fluid replacement for volume and electrolyte ab-
         normality correction are usually needed. Intravenous fluids are
         supplemented with thiamine (100 mg), multi-vitamins, magne-
         sium (1–2 g), and calcium (500 mg) to replete wasted stores in
         these often malnourished patients.
      4. Withdrawal seizures are treated with phenytoin or paraldehyde.

   C. Hypoxia
      1. **Oxygen therapy.** Supplemental mask.
      2. **Morphine sulfate and diuretics.** These are used in the setting
         of pulmonary edema.
      3. **Digoxin or dopamine and nitrates.** These are used in the set-
         ting of pulmonary edema caused by congestive heart failure.

   D. Other
      1. **Narcotics withdrawal.** This can be treated with relatively high
         doses of minor tranquilizers or with methadone (10–20 mg PO,
         q2–6H). Clonidine may be used as alternate therapy to combat
         autonomic symptoms of withdrawal.
      2. **Drug intoxication.** Usually, a safe and supportive environment
         suffices until the effects of the drug wears off. Minor or major
         tranquilizers can be used, especially in the violent patient.
      3. **Endocrine abnormalities.** These are treated appropriately.
      4. **CNS infections.** Appropriate antibiotics, with or without drain-
         age of abscess, are indicated.
      5. **ICU psychosis.** Make an attempt to keep the patient oriented.
         Attempt to reproduce day-night environment and adequate
         sleep. Agitation can be controlled with oral or parenteral
         haloperidol (Haldol). TV or radio programs or, optimally, a com-
         panion help to orient the patient.
      6. Thiamine prophylaxis should be given to patients with a pre-
         disposing history (EtOH abuse).
      7. **Sepsis.** Treat with appropriate antibiotics and fluid resuscita-
         tion.

26. DYSPNEA

I. Problem. A patient on the trauma service with a diagnosis of myocardial contusion complains of difficulty breathing.

II. Immediate Questions

A. **What was the patient doing when the dyspnea occurred?** Shortness of breath with exertional activity may indicate an underlying problem depending on the severity of the dyspnea. Dyspnea associated with a reclining position (ie, orthopnea) points to cardiac dysfunction.

B. **Did the dyspnea occur abruptly, or did it have a gradual onset?** The differential diagnosis for acute dyspnea differs from subacute or chronic dyspnea and points often to a specific event such as a pulmonary embolus, pneumothorax, or myocardial infarction.

C. **What is the baseline respiratory status of the patient?** A complaint of "not getting enough air" in a well-trained athlete indicates a more serious dysfunction than an equivalent complaint in a chronic smoker with emphysema. Inquire specifically about current work and recreational physical activities.

D. **Are there other symptoms such as chest pain coincident with the dyspnea?** A patient may focus on the shortness of breath and not disclose chest pain or pressure unless asked. However, dyspnea may be the sole presenting symptom of an acute myocardial infarction.

E. **Is there wheezing or stridor?** Both acute asthma attacks and anaphylactic reactions are readily treatable but must be identified and have appropriate therapy instituted quickly.

F. **Is there a history of asthma or other pulmonary condition?**

III. Differential Diagnosis. As previously mentioned, dyspnea may be classified as acute or subacute/chronic. Within each category the underlying mechanism is either predominantly pulmonary or cardiac.

A. **Acute**
   1. **Pulmonary**
      a. **Pneumothorax:** Can be caused by trauma—associated with rib fractures and may progress over hours and can be associated with a hemothorax. Spontaneous usually in males with tall thin body habitus.
      b. **Pulmonary embolus:** Maintain a high index of suspicion. Risk factors of immobilization, recent surgery, neoplastic disease, and estrogen use.

   c. **Asthma or allergic reactions:** Asthma clearly identified by wheezing. Anaphylactic reactions identified by stridor, atopic history, hives, and facial edema (see Problem 5, page 19).
   d. **Aspirated foreign body.** Usually obvious by history, but in young or mentally impaired need to rely on physical exam and radiologic studies.
   e. **Reflux with aspiration:** See Problem 8, page 28.
 2. **Acute myocardial infarction.** Especially if cardiac risk factors. Usually associated with chest pain or pressure but not always.
 3. **Anxiety attack.** Not a common cause of shortness of breath and often difficult to exclude organic causes. Further complicated by being frequently associated with chest pain. Often tachypnea cycles with period of normal breathing and tachypnea may resolve when patients are not aware of being observed.

B. **Subacute/Chronic**
 1. **Pulmonary**
    a. **COPD:** These patients usually have a smoking history with baseline dyspnea on exertion. In progression of baseline dyspnea look for evidence of infectious process.
    b. **Pneumonia:** Often associated with leukocytosis, fever, productive sputum, and chest x-ray changes (infiltrates).
    c. **Interstitial lung disease:** Chest x-ray and pulmonary function tests are diagnostic.
 2. **Cardiac**
    a. **Congestive heart failure:** Physical exam shows elevated jugular venous pressure, rales, peripheral edema, cardiac gallop, and displacement of left ventricular impulse. Dyspnea is associated with lying down.

IV. **Database**

A. **Physical Exam Key Points**
 1. **Vital signs.** Fever may signify infection, but may also be seen with a pulmonary embolus. Tachypnea may accompany hypoxia, embolus, or a pneumothorax.
 2. **Lung.** Observe respiratory rate, work of breathing, and use of accessory muscles. Listen for wheezes, stridor, rales, evidence of consolidation, and decreased breath sounds.
 3. **Cardiac.** Elevated jugular venous pressure, displacement of left ventricular impulse, new murmur of mitral regurgitation. Check for pulsus paradox.
 4. **Extremities.** Leg swelling as evidence for deep venous thrombosis. Evaluate for evidence of cyanosis.
 5. **Neurologic.** Confusion and drowsiness may signify severe hypoxia.

B. Laboratory Data
1. **Hemogram.** Leukocytosis may be present with infection.
2. **ABG.** Documents level of respiratory compromise and guides therapeutic decisions.
3. **Sputum Gram's stain/culture.** In patients with pneumonia or tracheobronchitis.
4. **Blood chemistries.** May reveal evidence of renal failure.

C. Radiologic and Other Studies
1. **Chest x-ray.** Of obvious importance. If patient is in distress obtain immediate portable chest x-ray.
2. **ECG.** Always obtain ECG if any question of cardiac cause.
3. **Pulmonary function tests.** Not applicable to acute situation but helpful in patients with obstructive or restrictive chronic lung disease.
4. **V/Q scan.** Ventilation/perfusion scan will evaluate for pulmonary embolism.
5. **Pulmonary angiogram.** Especially with an equivocal V/Q scan in the diagnosis of pulmonary embolus, angiography is the "gold standard" in the diagnosis of pulmonary emboli.
6. **Radionuclide angiogram.** This documents left ventricular ejection fraction and level of congestive heart failure.
7. **Exercise tolerance test.** Useful if episode of dyspnea related to ischemic heart disease.
8. **Echocardiography.** Evaluates for valvular disease, akinesis, failure, etc.

V. Plan

A. Emergent Therapy
1. **Oxygen supplementation.** If patient is short of breath, institute oxygen therapy. Acutely 100% may be used, with adjustments made to keep arterial oxygen at least 60–80 mm Hg or oxygen saturation > 90% based on blood gas measurements or pulse oximetry. Long term oxygen therapy at this level can cause toxicity. Do not worry about suppression of hypoxic drive (chronic lung disease) in the acute situation. Patients with a history of COPD and CO_2 retention may be at increased risk to lose their "hypoxic drive" to breathe, but it is impossible to predict which patients may be affected.
2. Stat portable chest x-ray, ECG, and blood gases are usually indicated if the cause is not immediately obvious.

B. Specific Urgent/Immediate Treatments
1. **Asthma.** In most cases, order an immediate treatment of Alupent nebulizer 0.3 ml in 2–3 ml normal saline by respiratory therapist. In younger patients in extreme distress, give 0.25 ml (or 0.01 ml/kg) 1:1000 subcutaneous epinephrine. If the patient is not on theophylline treatments, start loading doses of 5–6 mg/kg IV aminophylline over 20–30 minutes.

    2. Anaphylaxis. Refer to Problem 5, page 19.

    3. Myocardial ischemia. If immediate evaluation is consistent with myocardial ischemia, give sublingual nitroglycerin. Refer to Problem 12, page 47.

    4. Acute congestive heart failure. Treat with oxygen, diuretics (IV Lasix 10–40 mg dependent on prior exposure), sit the patient upright if blood pressure allows.

    5. Pneumonia. Treat with antibiotics and pulmonary toilet.

    6. Pneumothorax. Place a chest tube as outlined in Section III, page 295.

27. DYSURIA

  I. Problem. A patient complains of dysuria 4 days after an uncomplicated radical neck dissection.

  II. Immediate Questions

    A. How long has this symptom been present? Knowing the time course of any illness can provide clues to the cause. If the illness is more chronic, check on any previous urinalysis available.

    B. What is the patient's urologic history; specifically, is there any history of infections or stone disease? Some patients, especially females, are prone to recurrent urinary infections. Urethritis or prostatitis may be present in males.

    C. Are there any associated voiding symptoms? Fever, chills, and back pain are often signs of upper urinary tract infection (pyelonephritis). Frequency, urgency, and pain on urination suggest lower urinary tract infection (cystitis, prostatitis, urethritis).

    D. Has the patient recently had a Foley catheter removed? A catheter may result in an infection. Mild urethral irritation usually resolves shortly after the catheter is removed.

  III. Differential Diagnosis

    A. Urinary Tract Infection

      1. Upper. Pyelonephritis may occasionally cause dysuria, although this is infrequent.

      2. Lower. Cystitis is often associated with urgency and frequency. Urethritis may be gonococcal or nongonococcal, often caused by *Chlamydia*. Prostatitis may be acute (associated with fever, chills and signs of sepsis) or chronic (associated with voiding symptoms or recurrent urinary tract infections).

B. Vaginitis. Can present with initial complaints of dysuria. Can be due to *Candida, Trichomonas, Gardnerella* organisms. Atrophic vaginitis in postmenopausal women.

C. Genital Infections. Such as herpes or due to condylomata.

D. Chemical Irritants. Allergic reaction to a variety of agents (deodorant, douches).

E. Postprocedure. A frequent complaint after bladder catheterization or cystoscopy, usually resolves spontaneously if no infection intervenes.

F. Urethral Syndrome. Frequent syndrome in women with dysuria and voiding complaints without evidence of urinary tract infection. Often worsened by certain foods.

G. Miscellaneous. Urethral stricture, bladder tumor, urolithiasis, and interstitial cystitis.

IV. Database

A. Physical Exam Key Points
1. **Abdominal exam.** Look for signs of suprapubic tenderness or costovertebral angle tenderness.
2. **Genitalia.** Including urethral meatus, urethra, testicles, and epididymis in men. Vaginal discharge suggests vaginitis. Females may require a formal pelvic exam if the cause is not readily obvious.
3. **Rectal exam.** Including prostate. Mandatory to evaluate prostatitis. Be aware that vigorous exam of an acutely inflamed prostate can induce bacteremia and may be contraindicated in the presence of high fever and chills.

B. Laboratory Data
1. **Urinalysis and culture.** Pyuria ($>$ 5 WBC/HPF), the presence of leukocyte esterase or nitrites and a positive culture suggest a urinary tract infection.
2. **Hemogram.** Leukocytosis and a left shift will be seen with acute pyelonephritis and acute prostatitis and not normally seen in urethritis, chronic prostatitis, or cystitis.
3. **Urethral discharge culture and Gram's stain.** Thayer-Martin media should be used if gonorrhea is suspected. *N gonorrhea* can be seen as gram-negative intracellular diplococci on Gram's stain.
4. **Urine cytology.** Dysuria may be a subtle manifestation of transitional cell carcinoma.

C. Radiologic and Other Studies.
Full urologic evaluation (excretory urography, cystoscopy, etc) may be required for definitive diagnosis, but is rarely performed acutely in this setting.

V. Plan

A. Positive Urinalysis. This is enough of a reason to start antibiotic therapy. If the patient is otherwise healthy and not systemically septic, then oral antibiotics (such as trimethoprim/sulfa or quinolone) may be started.

B. Systemic Sepsis. A patient with signs of fever, chills, nausea, malaise, or hypotension (often associated with acute pyelonephritis or prostatitis) should be evaluated with appropriate cultures (blood and urine). Start systemic antibiotics. A third generation cephalosporin (cefoperazone, ceftazidime, etc), or ampicillin with an aminoglycoside are good choices until culture and sensitivities are available.

C. Chronic Prostatitis. May have a positive urine culture with findings of prostatitis, but are not septic. Treatment is a 3 week course of trimethoprim/sulfa or quinolone.

D. Vaginitis. Should be treated appropriately; nystatin vaginal cream or suppositories for *Candida,* oral metronidazole for *Trichomonas,* dienestrol (AVC) cream for atrophic vaginitis.

E. Other Infections. Treated with appropriate antibiotics.
  1. **Gonococcal urethritis.** Many regimens are available (procaine penicillin G 4.8 million units IM plus probenecid 1 gm PO, ceftriaxone 250 mg IM, ampicillin 3 gm PO) followed by a 7-day course of tetracycline.
  2. **Nongonococcal urethritis (NGU)** *(Chlamydia).* Doxycycline 100 mg PO bid tetracycline 500 mg PO qid for 7–10 days.

F. Symptomatic Relief. Symptomatic relief of dysuria can usually be achieved using phenazopyridine (Pyridium) 100–200 mg PO tid (turns urine orange) while workup or treatment is in progress. A small subset of patients with dysuria are sensitive to excessively alkaline or acidic urine that may vary with diet.

28. EPISTAXIS

I. Problem. A 45-year-old hypertensive patient, 1 day after a laparoscopic cholecystectomy, complains of a nosebleed that has lasted for 2 hours.

II. Immediate Questions

A. What are the patient's vital signs? Hypertension is usually a response to epistaxis rather than a cause. Tachycardia usually represents agitation of the patient, but rarely indicates significant blood loss in this setting. Each patient should, therefore be checked for orthostatic hypotension.

B. Is there a history of nosebleed or any recent trauma? New onset of epistaxis should alert the evaluating physician to intranasal pathology. Recurrent epistaxis is usually traumatic, especially in the younger patient.

III. Differential Diagnosis. Epistaxis has multiple causes. Obscure causes, such as hematologic malignancies and coagulation disorders, will not be discussed in detail. Ninety percent of epistaxis has its origin in the anterior portion of the nasopharynx.

   A. Trauma. Injuries of the nose, caused by blunt trauma, often cause epistaxis that ceases spontaneously. Digital trauma (nose-picking) is a major cause of epistaxis. The source is almost always an anterior site called the Kiesselbach's triangle, a submucosal mat of blood vessels located on the anterior-most aspect of the nasal septum.

   B. Hypertension. Hypertension may make control of bleeding more difficult, and is rarely, if ever, a cause of bleeding in itself.

   C. Intranasal Pathology. The adult patient that presents with new epistaxis in the absence of trauma may have an intranasal lesion. These include polyps and benign and malignant tumors. Typically, no anterior source of bleeding is apparent. Local infections may also be an underlying condition.

   D. Systemic Illnesses and Medications. Patients who take anticoagulants, such as warfarin, can develop epistaxis when the prothrombin time is overly prolonged. Aspirin interferes with platelet function. Obscure causes of epistaxis include leukemia, hemophilia, and chemotherapy-induced thrombocytopenia. Arteriosclerosis commonly predisposes to posterior epistaxis in the elderly.

IV. Database

   A. Physical Exam Key Points

      1. Vital signs. Hypertension often improves as the patient relaxes. The chronically hypertensive patient can be treated. Orthostatic hypotension can be found after significant nasal hemorrhage.

      2. Skin. Look for petechiae and ecchymoses to suggest a systemic problem.

      3. Nose. Examination of the nasal cavity should be performed with a headlamp or mirror and a nasal speculum. Examine as much of the mucosa as possible for a possible bleeding site. Briefly examine the contralateral nasal cavity. Topical cocaine controls bleeding in the majority of cases if examination is difficult.

B. **Laboratory Data**
   1. **Coagulation studies.** These are occasionally useful but may reveal over-anticoagulation of a patient taking warfarin (Coumadin).
   2. **Hemogram.** The hematocrit will not accurately reflect blood loss in the acute period. Look for unsuspected thrombocytopenia.

V. Plan

A. **Initial Control of Bleeding.** A quiet atmosphere, bilateral alar pressure, and 5% cocaine applied locally constitute initial attempts to control bleeding. Cocaine acts as both a vasoconstrictor and anesthetic.

B. **Cauterization and Anterior Packing**
   1. **Silver nitrate sticks.** If examination reveals a likely bleeding source after initial control is achieved, silver nitrate sticks cauterize the site.
   2. **Anterior nasal packing.** An anterior pack can be placed if cauterization is not successful and is often placed anyway as reinforcement. A piece of Gelfoam can be placed over the bleeding site, and then bacitracin impregnated Nu-Gauz is layered into the nose. Tape a drip pad to the nose. Packing can usually be removed in 2–4 days. Patients who have packing should be started on antibiotics (ampicillin or erythromycin) to prevent sinusitis.

C. **Posterior Packing.** Persistent bleeding with no localized anterior site requires posterior packing and admission to the otolaryngology service. In addition to admission, these patients require antibiotics (as above), oxygen, and analgesia, usually with narcotic. Three methods are used commonly to place posterior packs.
   1. A 14 Fr Foley catheter can be passed into the nasopharynx, inflated with saline, and gently drawn into choani.
   2. Specialized nasal balloons are available (Nasal-Stat).
   3. A pack made of 4 × 4 cotton gauze can be placed. This method is more complicated. Three 4 × 4 gauze sponges are rolled and tied with 3 large silk ties. A rubber catheter is passed into the nose and pulled out the mouth with a clamp. Two sutures from the pack are tied to the catheter and then pulled up into the nasal pharynx, guided with a finger. An anterior pack is then placed and the posterior pack sutures tied. The remaining pack suture comes out the mouth and is taped to the face. This allows removal of the pack in 4–5 days.

D. **Recurrent bleeding.** Recurrent bleeding after removal of a posterior pack is an indication for angiography and either ligation or embolization of the causative vessel.

29. EPIDURAL CATHETER PROBLEMS

I. Problem. A nurse reports the inadvertent dislodgement of an epidural catheter in a patient 1 day after a radical nephrectomy.

II. Immediate Questions. Lumbar epidural catheters, usually placed for intraoperative anesthesia, are used for postoperative analgesia by the injection of narcotics or local anesthetics into the extradural space via a soft catheter.

   A. When was the last dose of epidural narcotic? Long-acting narcotics injected into the extradural space can provide reliable analgesia for 12–18 hours after each dose.

   B. Is the patient in pain? If yes, then supplemental intravenous or intramuscular narcotics will be required.

   C. Is the patient otherwise stable? Delayed respiratory depression can occur from systemic absorption of the narcotic.

   D. Is the catheter tip intact? A retained epidural catheter tip can lead to infectious complications, such as epidural abscess. The tip of the catheter is marked by a black dot.

III. Database

   A. Physical Exam Key Points

      1. Vital signs. Hypotension and respiratory depression can occur with unintentional intravascular injection even up to several hours later. Cardiopulmonary collapse occurs if epidural doses of narcotics or anesthetics are given into the subarachnoid space, usually 15–30 minutes following injection.

      2. Chest. Check breath sounds for depth and rate.

      3. Neurologic. Check mental status, determine level of anesthesia, if still present, as well as motor and sensory function. The patient should be able to move their feet and feel you touch them! Rarely, epidural hematomas can occur causing symptoms of an epidural mass, requiring immediate neurosurgical decompression.

      4. Catheter exit site. Examine for bleeding and signs of infection.

      5. Catheter tip. Examine the tip to make sure the entire catheter has been removed.

   B. Laboratory Data. Generally of little value unless coagulopathy or cardiopulmonary complications arise.

   C. Radiologic and Other Studies. Usually not needed.

IV. Plan

    A. Insure that no complications of epidural anesthesia have occurred.

        1. Overmedication. Contact anesthesia staff, provide adequate monitoring and support for the patient. Overmedication is the primary reason why patients receiving epidural anesthesia should remain in a monitored setting.

        2. Hematoma. Diagnose and correct any coagulopathy and contact neurosurgical service immediately.

        3. Inadvertent subarachnoid puncture. Causes a severe headache that persists past 2 days and does not respond to recumbency. CSF leak can be sealed with a "blood patch" procedure; contact anesthesia staff.

        4. Urinary retention. Infrequently seen with epidural anesthesia; use an indwelling catheter to drain the bladder.

        5. Itching. Commonly seen. Benadryl 25–50 mg IM or PO.

    B. Analgesia. Supplement pain relief with additional IV, IM, or PO analgesics. Make sure you know the last dose given through the catheter to avoid overmedication.

    C. Wound care. Cover site with a sterile, dry dressing and inspect daily for signs of infection.

    D. Positioning. Patients should remain recumbent for a few hours after catheter removal to decrease "spinal headache."

30. FALL FROM BED

  I. Problem. The day after an open reduction and internal fixation of a humeral fracture, a 60-year-old man fell from bed while trying to go to the bathroom. He has a laceration on his forehead.

  II. Immediate Questions. Most falls from bed are not associated with serious injury. However, they are extremely upsetting to the patient and the patient's family. Every fall from bed warrants a complete evaluation, documentation of the incident, and thorough search for injury.

    A. Is the patient able to speak? Quickly assess the airway and mental status by having the patient answer the question "What happened?"

    B. Is the patient back in bed? To avoid further injury, leg roll patient onto a back board, use in-line-traction or cervical immobilization before placing patient back in bed.

    C. Is the patient in pain? Pain will guide you to the obvious injuries.

III. Differential Diagnosis. History obtained from the patient, visitors, and staff may be helpful in determining the underlying reason for the fall. Specific injuries incurred from the fall will not be covered here. Head injury, skeletal fractures and dislocations lead the list.

   A. Delirium. See Problem 25, page 93 for a complete list.

   B. Dementia. Preexisting risk factor for falling and should be recognized for prevention.

   C. Acute Change in Neurologic Status. See Problem 14, page 60 and Problem 17, page 69.

   D. Delayed recovery from anesthesia.

   E. Musculoskeletal weakness in postoperative period.

IV. Database

   A. Physical Exam Key Points

   1. **Vital signs.** Fever can cloud the sensorium, hypotension a factor for septic or cardiogenic shock, arrhythmias, respiratory rate and pattern.

   2. **HEENT.** Closely examine scalp and face for signs of head injury, cranial nerve exam, examine teeth.

   3. **Neck.** JVD, C-spine tenderness, nuchal rigidity.

   4. **Chest.** Bilateral breath sounds, wheezing, consolidation, cardiac murmurs, palpate ribs.

   5. **Abdomen.** Tenderness, bowel sounds to screen for abdominal injury.

   6. **Skin.** Bruising, lacerations.

   7. **Extremities.** Tenderness, obvious fractures, check IV lines.

   B. Laboratory Data

   1. **Hemogram.** Anemia, infection.

   2. **Serum electrolytes.** Hypo- and hyperglycemia, kalemia, calcemia, natremia, and magnesemia; uremia, ammonia.

   3. **Cardiac enzymes.** If MI suspected.

   4. **Toxic drug screen.** If clinically indicated.

   5. **Arterial and venous blood gases.** Acid-base disorders, hypoxia.

   6. **Cultures.** Blood, urine, sputum, if infection suspected.

   C. Radiologic and Other Studies

   1. **ECG.** If MI suspected or arrhythmia noted.

   2. **Chest x-ray.** If respiratory or infectious source likely and to check for fractures. Rib detail films may be needed to evaluate for fractures.

   3. **Head CT.** For change in mental status.

4. **Plain x-rays.** Tender extremities and joints to check for fracture or dislocation.
5. **Lumbar puncture.** If indicated.
6. **EEG.** If indicated.
7. **Pulse oximetry.** Noninvasive means of checking hypoxia.

V. Plan. Overall, an underlying cause for the fall must be sought and treated. See Problem 17, page 69 and Problem 14, page 60 for specific treatment plans.

   A. Fractures and dislocations should be splinted and the orthopedic service contacted for definitive care and follow-up.

   B. Lacerations should be cleaned and sutured. Local wound care for abrasions.

   C. If C-spine injury suspected, immobilize neck and keep patient flat until the spine can be evaluated radiographically.

   D. Prevention of Further Injury. Mild sedation if warranted. Make sure side rails of bed are up and that the patient is properly oriented to and can reach the nurse call button. Restraints if necessary. A bedside commode may be useful for the weak or elderly as well as physical therapy for reconditioning.

   E. Incident Report. Risk management includes completion of the report and documentation of the incident in the chart.

31. FEVER

I. Problem. You are notified that a patient on another service who had a gastrectomy for cancer has a fever of 38.9°C.

II. Immediate Questions

   A. How many days postop is the patient? Most medical students know the mnemonic: "The Five W's: wind, water, walk, wound, wonder drugs" for postoperative fever. The time since operation helps to focus one's attention on the likely diagnosis. These five causes, in order from the mnemonic, are pneumonia, urinary tract, thrombophlebitis, wound infection, and drug reaction.

   B. What is the fever pattern? Check the chart for the previous 2–3 days to see any emerging or changing fever patterns. Spiking fevers are often associated with infections in a closed space (ie, abscesses). Continual fevers are often found in cases of vascular involvement such as infected prosthetic grafts or septic phlebitis.

   C. Does the patient have chills/rigors with the fever? Often rigors are associated with more serious fevers and indicate an episode of bacteremia. Fevers associated with drug reactions or atelectasis usually do not have associated rigors.

D. Did the patient have fevers before the operation? A patient may suffer from a chronic disease associated with fever (lymphoma, etc). Even if the patient does not have one of these diagnoses, keep them in mind when no other source of fever is identifiable.

E. Has the patient recently stopped taking an antipyretic agent? Occasionally a new fever is the realization of a suppressed fever in patients taking aspirin, acetaminophen, or NSAID. Noting this may be of importance in diagnosing fever in certain cases.

F. Has the patient recently been taking antibiotics? Find out why, which drug, and the time of the last dose.

G. Are there any associated complaints such as cough, dysuria, diarrhea, abdominal pain, or pain around any IV sites or incisions? May point to the cause of the fever.

III. Differential Diagnosis. Usually the febrile patient seen in an emergency room or outpatient setting has an acute infection readily diagnosed from associated complaints. This type of febrile patient will not be discussed. The common febrile patient on a surgical service is one with a postoperative fever. However, other patients (postoperative or otherwise) may have a fever of unknown origin defined as a temperature of at least 38.5°C daily for at least 3 weeks and no diagnosis after 1 week of inhospital investigation. The differential diagnosis of postoperative fevers and fever of unknown origin is given below.

A. Postoperative Fever

1. **Atelectasis.** The fever is usually < 39°C and occurs in first 12–48 hours postop.
2. **Urinary tract infection.** Typically occurs 3–5 days postop in the hospitalized patient and usually follows urinary tract manipulation such as a Foley catheter.
3. **IV catheter infection.** The longer a catheter is left in, the higher the risk of infection.
   a. **Peripheral:** The site will often appear infected.
   b. **Central:** Diagnosed on high degree of clinical suspicion and usually by positive blood cultures drawn through the line.
4. **Deep venous thrombosis.** The fever is usually low grade (37.5–38.5°C). Pulmonary embolus may also have an associated low grade fever.
5. **Wound infection**
   a. **Early:** Organisms are often *Clostridium* or *Streptococcus,* in first 12–36 hours postop.
   b. **Late:** More common 5–8 days postop, commonly because of *Staphylococcus, Pseudomonas,* etc.

6. **Drug reaction.** Most commonly antibiotics (penicillins, cephalosporins).
7. **CNS origin.** Central fever in trauma patient with head injuries or meningitis in spinal anesthetic complication.
8. **Thyroid storm.** Following thyroidectomy for Grave's disease.
9. **Blood transfusion.** See Problem 68, page 217.
10. **Postpericardiotomy syndrome.** Usually seen 5–7 days postop.
11. **Anastomotic bowel leak.** Usually seen 7–10 days postop and usually associated with peritoneal irritation.
12. **Otitis, sialadenitis, sinusitis.** Especially in patients with long-term nasogastric tubes.
13. **Addisonian crisis.**
14. **Acalculous cholecystitis.** May be seen with prolonged periods of being NPO, associated with trauma and other severe illnesses.
15. **Pancreatitis.**
16. *Clostridium difficile* **enterocolitis.** Typically diffuse green, watery, foul-smelling, or bloody diarrhea.

B. Fever of Unknown Origin
   ### 1. Infections
   a. **Granulomatous:** Caused by *Mycobacterium* or fungal agents.
   b. **Endocarditis:** Especially with valvular heart disease.
   c. **Abscess:** Hepatic, subphrenic renal or pelvic.
   ### 2. Neoplastic. Fevers can be a part of "paraneoplastic syndromes."
   a. Lymphoma.
   b. Renal cell carcinoma.
   c. Hepatic metastatic disease.
   ### 3. Connective tissue disease
   a. Systemic lupus erythematosus.
   b. Rheumatoid arthritis (usually juvenile).
   c. Polymyalgia rheumatica.
   ### 4. Miscellaneous
   a. Drug reaction.
   b. Recurrent pulmonary emboli.
   c. Inflammatory bowel disease.

IV. Database

A. Physical Exam Key Points
   1. **Vital signs.** Document all fevers rectally. Check orthostatic vital signs.
   2. **Skin.** Examine wound and all past and current IV sites.
   3. **HEENT.** Check for sialadenitis, otitis, and pharyngitis.
   4. **Pulmonary.** Listen for rhonchi, evidence of consolidation.

     5. Abdomen. Right upper quadrant tenderness, peritoneal signs.

     6. Trunk. Costovertebral angle tenderness.

     7. Extremities. Evidence for deep venous thrombosis (pain, swelling, etc).

     8. Wound. Check the wound for erythema, fluid collection, subcutaneous air, crepitation, and tenderness. If the wound is relatively recent, remember to use strict aseptic technique.

     9. Pelvic examination. To look for evidence of pelvic source.

B. Laboratory Data

     1. Hemogram. Leukocytosis, left shift with infection. Anemia may be seen with endocarditis.

     2. Electrolytes. Hyponatremia and hyperkalemia in addisonian crisis.

     3. Thyroid hormone levels, T_3 and T_4.

     4. Urinalysis, Gram's stain and culture.

     5. Throat culture if indicated.

     6. Wound culture if indicated.

     7. Blood cultures, at least two peripheral. Drawback cultures from central line if present. Also culture central line. Line exit site cultures are minimally helpful. Multiple cultures on different days may be best for endocarditis.

     8. Sputum Gram's stain and culture if indicated.

     9. Stool for fecal leukocytes and *C difficile* toxin assay.

C. Radiologic and Other Studies

     1. Chest x-ray. Linear densities with atelectasis; infiltrates with pneumonia; occasional wedge-shaped infarction with pulmonary emboli.

     2. ECG. ST elevations in postpericardiotomy syndrome.

     3. Venous Dopplers/venogram. If deep venous thrombosis suspected.

     4. Abdominal CT. For evaluation of intra-abdominal abscess. Ultrasound is good for hepatic or subphrenic abscesses but CT scan is procedure of choice if available.

     5. Abdominal Ultrasound. In acalculous cholecystitis can demonstrate sludge, pericholecystic fluid and may demonstrate abscesses.

     6. HIDA scan. Useful in acute acalculous cholecystitis.

     7. Gallium scan. Using labeled WBCs may help identify an otherwise elusive abscess.

V. Plan. The primary goal is to diagnose and treat the underlying cause. A second goal is to treat the fever. Antipyretics can be given with caution after cultures are obtained. Finally, some preventive measures for postoperative fever are discussed.

A. Treatment of Specific Causes

     1. Atelectasis and pneumonia

        a. Incentive spirometry, ambulation and coughing are general

measures to both treat and help prevent atelectasis and pneumonia.
   b. For pneumonia, antibiotics are empirically started, based on results of the Gram's stain, and finally based on culture results. The antibiotic susceptibility patterns of the particular hospital should be known because these are usually nosocomial organisms.
2. **Urinary tract infection.** See Problem 27, page 100.
3. **IV catheter sepsis**
   a. **Peripheral:** Remove all suspicious catheters and apply local heat to area. Use cefazolin or dicloxacillin as antibiotic if required. Observe for suppurative phlebitis, which usually requires vein excision.
   b. **Central:** Optimally remove line, treat with antibiotics (cephalosporin or vancomycin) for 1–2 days prior to a wire (see Problem 20, page 78). Using peripheral cultures as well as cultures drawn through the line, obtained in Isolator (Dupont) tubes, one can compare the number of colonies. If the number of colonies in the line culture is less than five times that in the peripherally obtained culture, the line is not the source of sepsis.
4. **Thyroid storm.** Treat with propylthiouracil (PTU) 400 mg q6H, sodium iodide 250 mg PO/IV q6H, propranolol 1 mg/min IV for 2.8 minutes, and hydrocortisone 100 mg IV.
5. **Postpericardiotomy.** Indomethacin 25–50 mg tid with food or antacids.
6. **Addisonian crisis.** 100 mg hydrocortisone IV q8H.
7. **Wound infection.** Open wound carefully, culture drainage, and pack with saline moistened gauze. Dress with dry gauze and secure to patient. Change three times daily.
8. *C difficile volitis* (see page 84).

B. **Treatment of Fever**
   1. **Antipyretics.** Acetaminophen 650 mg PO/pr q4–6H is preferred because aspirin inhibits platelet action.
   2. **Maintain adequate hydration.** Fever increases baseline fluid requirements 500 ml/24 hr/each degree centigrade above 38.3°C (101°F).
   3. **Cooling blanket.** Useful in lowering the body temperature.

C. **Preventive Measures**
   1. **Atelectasis.** Have smokers quit for a few weeks before an elective operation. Teach all patients incentive spirometry preoperatively.
   2. **Intravenous catheters.** Change peripheral IVs routinely every 2–3 days or sooner if needed.
   3. Deep venous thrombosis
      a. Early ambulation should be encouraged.
      b. For high risk patients (obesity, prior DVT, neoplasia) consider subcutaneous heparin.

c. Many surgeons routinely utilize sequential compression stockings in any patient undergoing a procedure that requires general or regional anesthesia. These are used postoperatively until the patient is ambulatory.

4. **Blood transfusion.** Acetaminophen 650 mg and diphenhydramine (Benadryl) 25–50 mg IM/PO about 30 minutes before transfusion in patients with a history of transfusion reaction may blunt the febrile response.

5. **Thyroid storm.** Use SSKI (saturated solution of potassium iodide) [KI] two drops tid and propranolol 20–40 mg PO qid for 7–10 days before surgery.

32. FOLEY CATHETER PROBLEMS

(Bladder catheterization is discussed in Section III, Bedside Procedures.)

I. **Problem.** The Foley catheter in a patient 2 days after sigmoid colon resection is not draining.

II. **Immediate Questions**

A. **What has the urine output been?** If the urine output has slowly tapered off, then the problem may be oliguria rather than a nonfunctioning Foley catheter. A Foley catheter that has never put out urine may not be in the bladder.

B. **Is the urine grossly bloody; are there any clots in the tubing or collection bag?** Clots or tissue fragments, such as those present after a prostate or bladder resection, can obstruct the flow of urine in a Foley catheter. Similarly, intraoperative bladder trauma in an abdominal case can lead to bleeding.

C. **Is the patient complaining of any pain?** Bladder distention often causes severe lower abdominal pain; bladder spasms are painful and may cause urine to leak out around the catheter rather than through the catheter.

D. **Was any difficulty encountered in catheter insertion?** Problematic urethral catheterization should raise the possibility that the catheter is not in the bladder.

III. **Differential Diagnosis**

A. **Low Urine Output.** It may be a result of dehydration, hemorrhage, acute renal failure, as well as a host of other causes (see Problem 56, page 187).

B. **Obstructed Foley Catheter**
1. Kinking of catheter or tubing.
2. **Clots, tissue fragments.** Most common after transurethral re-

section of the prostate or bladder. Grossly bloody urine suggests a clot has formed. "Tea" colored or "rusty" urine suggests an organized clot may be present even though the urine is no longer grossly bloody. Bleeding will often accompany "accidental" catheter removal with the balloon still inflated and with any coagulopathy.

3. **Sediment/stones.** Chronically indwelling catheters (usually > 1 month) can become encrusted and obstructed. Calculi can lodge in the catheter.

C. **Improperly Positioned Foley Catheter.** These problems are much more common in males. In traumatic urethral disruption associated with a pelvic fracture, the catheter can pass into the periurethral tissues. Strictures or prostatic hypertrophy may cause the end of the catheter to be positioned in the urethra and not the bladder.

D. **Bladder Spasms.** The patient may complain of severe suprapubic pain or pain radiating to the end of the penis. With a spasm, urine may leak around the sides of the catheter. Spasms are common after bladder or prostate surgery or surgery around the bladder. Spasms may be the only catheter complaint or may be so severe as to obstruct the flow of urine.

E. **Bladder Disruption.** Resulting from blunt abdominal trauma, operative complication, or caused by severe distention secondary to a blocked catheter.

F. **Inability to Deflate Foley Balloon.** Rare with modern catheters. All catheters should be tested before use.

IV. **Database**

A. **Physical Exam Key Points**
   1. **Vital signs.** Check for tachycardia or hypotension, which is characteristic of hypovolemia.
   2. **Abdominal exam.** Determine if the bladder is distended (suprapubic dullness to percussion with or without tenderness); may be indicative of an obstructed Foley catheter. Percuss the bladder to help identify distention.
   3. **Genital exam.** Bleeding at the meatus suggests urethral trauma or partial removal of the catheter with the balloon inflated.
   4. **Rectal exam.** A "floating prostate" suggests urethral disruption.
   5. **General.** Look for signs of hypovolemia causing low urine output such as skin turgor, mucous membrane appearance, etc.

B. **Laboratory Data.** Most problems are usually mechanical in nature so that laboratory data is somewhat limited in this setting.
   1. **BUN, serum creatinine.** Elevations may be seen with cases of renal insufficiency.

      2. Coagulation studies. Especially if there is severe bleeding present.

  C. Radiologic and Other Studies. In the acute setting of a Foley catheter problem, usually not needed. Ultrasound may demonstrate hydronephrosis in cases of obstructive uropathy.

V. Plan

  A. First, be sure the catheter is functioning. A rule of thumb is a catheter that will not irrigate is in the urethra and not in the bladder. Start by gently irrigating the catheter with aseptic technique using a catheter tipped 60 ml syringe and sterile normal saline. This may dislodge any clots obstructing the catheter. If sterile saline cannot be satisfactorily instilled and aspirated, the catheter should be replaced. Catheter irrigation or change in any patient who has undergone bladder or prostate surgery must be done with extreme care.

  B. If the catheter irrigates freely, workup the patient for anuria. See Problem 56, page 187.

  C. Bladder spasms can be treated with oxybutynin (Ditropan), propantheline (Pro-Banthine) or belladonna and opium (B&O) suppositories. (See dosage in Section IX, page 388). Be **sure** to discontinue these medications before removing the catheter to allow normal bladder function.

  D. Techniques to deflate a balloon that will not empty include:

      1. Injection of 5–10 mL mineral oil into the inflation port will cause balloon rupture in latex catheters in 5–10 minutes. Follow-up cystoscopy is recommended to make sure there are no retained fragments.

      2. Threading a 16 Fr central venous catheter or 0.38 guidewire into the inflation channel (after the valve is removed) may bypass the obstruction.

      3. As a last resort, ultrasound directed transvesical needle puncture of the balloon may be needed.

33. HEADACHE

I. Problem. A 42-year-old man complaining of a headache presents to the in clinic 4 days after inguinal hernia repair under spinal anesthesia.

II. Immediate Questions

  A. What does the headache feel like? Is it similar to previous headaches? A patient complaining worst headache of his life associated with vomiting and stiff neck may have a subarachnoid bleed or meningitis. Most other causes of headache require less immediate attention.

B. What makes the headache better or worse? Spinal headaches typically become worse as the patient sits up and get better when the patient lies flat.

III. Differential Diagnosis

A. Spinal Headache. Relatively common after spinal anesthesia or lumbar puncture because of a slow leak of CSF. The use of smaller spinal needles has reduced the incidence of such headaches.

B. Sinusitis. Often associated with specific areas of facial pain.

C. Vascular
  1. Cluster headaches and migraine headaches. Careful history usually reveals the presence of these prior to this current episode.
  2. Subarachnoid hemorrhage. Often leads to severe headache and nuchal rigidity.
  3. Others. Giant cell arteritis, and sub- or epidural hematoma may cause headaches.

D. Tension. This is by far the most common cause of headache in any patient population. Usually a constant, band-like pressure, often occipital and frequently associated with muscular tension in the neck.

E. Neoplastic. Rarely does neoplasm result in headache in the absence of other neurologic abnormalities.

F. Meningitis. Nausea, vomiting, headache, and stiff neck are hallmarks of this disease.

G. Other. Fever, hypertension, and systemic viral illnesses can cause headache.

IV. Database

A. History. Determine if the patient had recent operation under spinal anesthesia. Determine history of similar headache and associated symptoms such as scotomata or nausea and vomiting.

B. Physical Exam
  1. Vital signs. Check temperature and blood pressure.
  2. Head and neck
    a. Nuchal rigidity may indicate subarachnoid irritation or meningitis.

  b. Injected conjunctiva and excessive tearing are common with migraine.

  c. Percuss sinuses looking for tenderness.

  d. Tenderness in the temporal area, especially over the temporal artery is associated with temporal arteritis.

  e. Papilledema suggests increased intracranial pressure or space occupying lesion.

C. Laboratory Data

 1. Hemogram. An elevated white count may indicate infection.

 2. Erythrocyte sedimentation rate (ESR). A nonspecific test, but often elevated in temporal arteritis.

D. Radiologic and Other Studies

 1. Sinus radiographs. These should be performed if sinusitis is suspected clinically.

 2. Head CT scan. A scan of the head can be performed if subarachnoid hemorrhage is suspected or in new onset severe headache to rule-out intracranial mass. It should also be performed if neurologic exam reveals focal findings.

V. Plan. Careful exam and history reveal benign nature of headache in most cases. Most should be treated with acetaminophen or aspirin as needed.

A. Spinal headaches. After lumbar puncture, like for spinal anesthesia, headaches should not be overlooked in the postoperative patient. They can be very persistent and often require rest in supine position, analgesics, and IV hydration. Refractory spinal headaches can be treated by injecting autologous blood "patch" into the epidural space to seal the dural leak.

B. Migraine

 1. Acute therapy, mild-moderate migraine. Standard analgesics are usually effective. Agents such as NSAIDs, Fiorinal, Midrin, butorphanol nasal spray (once in each nostril, repeat in 3–5 hours).

 2. Acute therapy severe migraine. Sumatriptan (Imitrex) 6 mg SQ or dihydroergotamine (DHE 45) 1 mg IM, repeat two times at 1 hour intervals if needed.

 3. Some migraine patients require chronic prophylaxis with β-blockers, tricyclic antidepressants (amitriptyline), or methysergide.

C. Intracranial Tumor or Subarachnoid Hemorrhage. Require neurosurgical intervention.

D. Infections. For example, acute sinusitis and meningitis require urgent treatment with high dose antibiotics. Frontal sinusitis often needs to be drained.

34. HEMATEMESIS

Immediate Actions

1. Assess Airway, Breathing, and Circulation.
2. Obtain vital signs.
3. Intubate, if necessary.
4. Assure large bore IV access and begin lactated Ringer's (LR) 500 mL bolus.
5. Obtain blood for transfusion.
6. Place NG tube.

I. **Problem.** A patient admitted for an elective Le Veen shunt suddenly begins vomiting blood.

II. **Immediate Questions**

A. **What are the blood pressure and orthostatic signs?** The initial management focuses on maintaining intravascular volume and perfusion pressure. Blood pressure/orthostatic hypotension is the best on-the-ward estimate of the volume loss.

B. **Any bleeding tendencies?** Review available history, physical exam, and lab data regarding any correctable coagulation deficit.

C. **Any stigmata of alcohol abuse?** Of the major causes of upper GI bleeding, only esophageal varices is associated with any physical signs. Obtain history and physical signs for cirrhosis and portal hypertension, but keep in mind that a diagnosis of cirrhosis does not equate with a diagnosis of variceal bleed.

D. **Did the patient retch or vomit nonbloody material before hematemesis?** A Mallory-Weiss tear is the fourth most common cause of hematemesis in most series, and the patient, nurses, or any observer should be carefully asked about the episode. "Coffee ground" emesis indicates that the blood has been in the stomach long enough to be converted by gastric acid from hemoglobin to methemoglobin.

E. **Does the patient have any history of aortic disease or a prior aortic vascular procedure?** Although low in the list of causes of hematemesis, aortoduodenal fistula should always be included in the initial differential diagnosis of upper GI bleed. The phenomenon of a sentinel bleed allows some of these patients to be salvaged, but only if the diagnosis is made quickly.

III. **Differential Diagnosis.** Hematemesis is virtually always associated with bleeding proximal to the ligament of Treitz. The converse, however, is certainly not true (see Problem 10, page 34). In the most recent series, ulcer disease, gastritis, esophageal varices, and Mallory-Weiss tears account for 90–95% of episodes of hematemesis.

A. Esophagus

1. **Esophageal varices.** Associated with cirrhosis and portal hypertension.
2. **Mallory-Weiss tear.** Usually a mucosal tear at the gastroesophageal junction associated with severe retching with or without vomiting.
3. **Esophagitis.** Classic history of heartburn, "water brash" (regurgitation of gastric contents), and worsening of symptoms with recumbency.
4. **Esophageal tumors.** Benign squamous or adenocarcinomas.

B. Stomach

1. **Gastritis.** Significant hematemesis usually indicates severe stress gastritis, most often alcohol related.
2. **Gastric ulcer.** Pain typically exacerbated by eating, but may also be relieved with eating. Up to 42% associated with duodenal ulcer.
3. Gastric tumors.
4. Gastric varices.

C. Duodenum

1. Duodenal ulcer
2. **Aortoduodenal fistula.** Almost exclusively in cases of aortic reconstruction.

D. Hemobilia. Usually secondary to trauma, infection, stone disease, or iatrogenic causes.

E. Systemic Causes

1. **Coagulopathy** (DIC, leukemia, etc).
2. **Osler-Weber-Rendu.** Associated with multiple telangiectases.
3. **Peutz-Jeghers.** Associated with multiple hamartomas.

F. Non-GI source. Nasopharyngeal bleeding (see Problem 28, page 102).

IV. Database

A. Physical Exam Key Points

1. **Vital signs.** Orthostatic blood pressure measurements. Determine the pulse and blood pressure with the patient in the supine position for 5 minutes. Have the patient stand or dangle legs off the side of the bed. At 1 minute, determine BP and pulse. A drop in BP of > 10–20 or an increase in pulse of > 10 suggests volume depletion.
2. **Skin.** Cool, moist, pale skin indicates volume loss. Evidence of alcohol abuse as spider angiomata or palmar erythema. Signs

of systemic disease as multiple bruises, telangiectases, or hamartomas of lips, oral mucosa.

3. **HEENT.** Evidence of epistaxis or other nasopharyngeal source.
4. **Abdomen.** Scars from prior ulcer, vascular, or other procedure. Pain or evidence of peritoneal signs. Signs of portal hypertension as splenomegaly, caput medusa, or ascites.
5. **Rectal.** Check for gross blood or melena.
6. **Genitourinary.** Testicular atrophy and gynecomastia as evidence for alcohol abuse.

B. **Laboratory Data**
1. **Hemogram.** Obtain serial hematocrits and document time drawn and relation to transfusions.
2. **Platelet count.** Verify there are adequate numbers.
3. **PT/PTT.** Helps identify potentially correctable deficit in the coagulation cascade.
4. **Renal function.** Should be determined as a baseline.
5. **Liver function tests.** To document liver disease.
6. **Blood bank specimen.** Remember with the initial blood draw to type and crossmatch for up to 6–10 U of blood.

C. **Radiologic and Other Studies**
1. **Chest x-ray.** This will document aspiration.
2. **Upper endoscopy.** In most hospitals, the diagnostic procedure of choice (and sometimes therapeutic).
3. **UGI series.** May be used if endoscopy is unavailable and if bleeding has stopped. It interferes with endoscopy and angiography so not usually a first line study.
4. **Angiogram.** Rarely used unless endoscopy does not identify source.

V. **Plan.** Bleeding can be excessive, and as an example, up to 50% of patients with massive UGI bleeding from varices will die. Treat volume loss, establish diagnosis, and implement specific therapies. Continued bleeding in any of these conditions requires the appropriate surgical intervention. However, about 85% of cases of UGI bleeding resolve without operative intervention.

A. **Initial Management**
1. Large bore IVs (18 gauge or larger) and begin crystalloid.
2. Type and crossmatch for packed red blood cells (6 units minimum).
3. **Place NG tube.** This documents ongoing bleeding and clears the stomach for endoscopy. An Ewald tube may be needed to evacuate large volumes of clot.
4. **Monitor volume replacement**
   a. Always chart serial hematocrits, timing, and amount of transfusions because this measures the rate of bleeding,

which is the major criteria to decide if surgery is needed in many instances.
  b. Foley catheter
  c. Central line if needed especially in patients with cardiac/respiratory disease.
  5. Correct coagulopathy with platelets or FFP.
  6. Insert NG tube and irrigate with saline until clear. The temperature of the irrigant is not important. What matters is clearing the material from the stomach.
  7. Consider intubation to protect the airway from aspiration.
B. Specific Treatment. After acute bleed stabilized.
  1. Ulcer
    a. Antacids via NG tube q 1–2 hour.
    b. H$_2$-receptor blockers (cimetidine, ranitidine). May prevent rebleeding but probably does not stop ongoing bleeding. May be used with antibiotics.
    c. Laser endoscopy. Promising but unproven.
  2. Stress gastritis
    a. Antacids.
    b. H$_2$-receptor blockers have no effect in active bleeding.
  3. Esophageal varices
    a. Injection sclerotherapy by endoscopy.
    b. Vasopressin 0.4–0.6 U/min by peripheral IV for 1 hour. Repeat every 3 hours if successful.
    c. Balloon tamponade (Sengstaken-Blakemore Tube). Attempt only if experienced as complications of aspiration, respiratory arrest, and esophageal rupture are possible.
  4. Mallory-Weiss tear
    a. Vasopressin is of unclear effectiveness.
    b. Angiographic embolization.

35. HEMATURIA

I. Problem. A 51-year-old patient has blood in his urine 3 days after undergoing a vagotomy and pyloroplasty.

II. Immediate Questions

A. Is it gross or microscopic hematuria? Microscopic hematuria may have been present for a long time, without the patient being aware, suggesting a chronic process, while gross hematuria will not have gone unnoticed in the past.

B. Does the patient have a Foley catheter or stents in place? Irritation of bladder mucosa by a Foley catheter is a common cause of hematuria in the hospitalized patient; however, other causes should be investigated if the blood does not completely clear after the catheter is removed. Stents are often placed peri-operatively by cystoscopy for difficult pelvic cases and can cause minor bleeding.

C. Has the patient recently undergone abdominal surgery? Recent abdominal surgery (especially the night after surgery) may implicate a surgical problem such as ureteral, renal or bladder injury.

D. Does the patient have abdominal pain or fever? Abdominal pain may suggest an inflammatory or infectious process. Infection would often be accompanied by fever. Renal colic typically radiates from the flank into the groin and suggests a stone.

E. Has the urine output remained adequate? Urine output is the best indicator of adequate renal function and perfusion. A sudden decrease in urine output may be indicative of rapid changes in renal function or a mechanical blockage due to clots.

F. Does the patient have symptoms of urinary tract infection? Dysuria, frequency, and urgency are common symptoms associated with urinary tract infections.

G. What is the history? A history of recent TURP or resection of bladder tumor may explain the bleeding (microhematuria may persist 2–3 months after TURP). A remote history of bladder tumor may suggest a recurrent tumor. Chemotherapy with agents such as Cytoxan may cause acute hemorrhagic cystitis and cause bladder cancer many years later.

H. If female, when was the last period? Menses will often contaminate the urinalysis.

III. Differential Diagnosis

A. Foley Catheter Irritation/Trauma. This must be considered a diagnosis of exclusion in a patient with a Foley catheter. Be sure to complete the evaluation before attributing hematuria to this (see Problem 32, page 113.)

B. Stone. A calculus anywhere in the urinary tract from the kidney to the urethra can cause hematuria. It is usually associated with severe abdominal pain especially when the stone is in the ureter.

C. Infection. An infection in the urinary tract can cause hematuria. It is important to obtain a clean catch specimen for culture.

D. Tumor. Painless hematuria is the sine qua non of bladder tumors and can occur with renal cell carcinoma or prostatic carcinoma as well.

E. Trauma. Posttraumatic hematuria can be caused by a variety of lesions, such as renal parenchymal injury, or urethral injury secondary to pelvic fracture. A Foley catheter should **not** be inserted in any patient suspected of possible pelvic fracture until after a retrograde urethrogram has been performed to rule out urethral tear. Also consider an intraoperative complication if structures adjacent to the urinary tract were operated upon (colon, uterus).

F. **Excessive Anticoagulation.** A common cause of hematuria in anticoagulated patients and requires adjustment of drug dosage. Rarely this will unmask another problem, such as a neoplasm.

G. **Structural Abnormalities.** Polycystic kidney and medullary sponge kidney can cause hematuria. It is important to rule out other potential causes of hematuria in patients with known structural abnormalities.

H. **Prostatic Hypertrophy.** Benign prostatic hypertrophy can cause hematuria, but other causes must be ruled out as well. This is a common cause in older males.

I. **Glomerulonephritis.** Red cell casts are often seen on urinalysis.

J. **Enterovesical Fistula.** As with most fistulas to the urinary tract, hematuria usually will not be the first sign. Often, pneumaturia or an infection is the first sign.

K. **Vascular.** A variety of vascular lesions such as renal infarction, renal vein thrombosis, and A–V malformations cause hematuria.

L. **Renal Papillary Necrosis.** Predominantly a disease of diabetics.

M. **Drugs.** Especially cyclophosphamide, can cause hemorrhagic cystitis.

N. **Radiation Cystitis.** Patients with rectal or genitourinary malignancies are most frequent.

O. **Hemorrhagic Cystitis.** Usually a complication of chemotherapy with Cytoxan and may predispose to transitional cell carcinoma.

P. **Systemic Diseases.** Systemic lupus erythematosus, hemolytic-uremic syndrome, and Goodpasture's syndrome (see Problem 36, page 125).

Q. **Tuberculosis.** While the lung accounts for most tuberculosis in the United States, renal involvement does occur and can cause hematuria and is associated typically with sterile pyuria.

R. **Sickle-cell Anemia.** Black patients with hematuria and no other obvious cause should be evaluated for sickle-cell disease.

S. **Contamination.** Often caused by menstrual period or dysfunctional uterine bleeding. Check a catheterized specimen to exclude this cause.

T. **Benign Essential Hematuria.** A diagnosis of exclusion when no pathologic evidence of clinical bleeding can be found.

IV. Database

A. Physical Exam Key Points

1. **Abdominal.** Examine for palpable masses indicative of tumors or other masses and tenderness that may accompany infection, sickle cell disease, and inflammatory processes.

2. **Urethral meatus.** Look for gross blood at the meatus, especially in posttraumatic patients or in males with a pelvic fracture.

3. **Rectal exam.** Critical in the trauma patient. May reveal a "free floating prostate" that may signify urethral disruption. Prostatic carcinoma or prostatitis may also be detected.

4. **Pelvic exam.** For evidence of cervical bleeding.

B. Laboratory Data

1. **Urinalysis.** Red cell casts are associated with upper tract bleeding; myoglobinuria (from crush or electrical injury) may be confused with hematuria.

2. **Clotting studies.** To determine if anticoagulation is a cause of hematuria.

3. **Sickle-cell disease.** Screen in blacks suspected of sickle cell disease as a cause of hematuria.

4. **Hemogram.** Attention to hematocrit and platelet count.

5. **Urine cytology.** May diagnose transitional cell carcinoma, but not renal cell or prostate carcinoma. Many clinical labs offer "localization" studies whereby the site of bleeding can be identified as renal or postrenal based on the RBC morphology.

6. **Urine Culture.** To rule out bacterial infection. Acid-fast stain checked on several urine specimens will help rule out tuberculosis of the urinary tract.

7. **BUN and creatinine.** Baseline renal function should be determined.

C. Radiologic and Other Studies

1. **Abdominal plain x-ray, IVP.** A plain x-ray may show a urinary calculus (in 80% of cases).

2. **Excretory urography (IVP).** Usually the first diagnostic test performed after laboratory studies. All multiple trauma patients must have a "one shot" IVP, regardless of the presence of hematuria or not.

3. **Retrograde urethrogram/cystogram.** In cases of pelvic trauma or clinical suspicion of urethral disruption or bladder rupture.

4. Further studies that may be indicated include CT of the abdomen (especially in trauma patients), ultrasound, angiography and cystoscopy.

V. Plan.
The treatment depends on the cause, which could take several days to ascertain. The "standard workup" of hematuria in the adult is

physical exam, UA, urine culture, urine cytology, intravenous pyelogram, and cystoscopy. Hematuria is rarely a cause for significant acute blood loss, and as long as renal function and urine output are not impaired, the workup of hematuria is generally not an emergency.

A. Gross Hematuria with Clots. Most frequently arises from the bladder and usually requires placement of a large irrigating "three way" Foley catheter, (such as 24–26 Fr, 30 mL balloon). Irrigate out the clots with a 60 mL syringe because clots present in the bladder will perpetuate the bleeding. Irrigation with normal saline will often be necessary to keep the urine clear until the source of bleeding is corrected.

B. Specific Treatments

1. **Urinary tract infection.** Treated with appropriate antibiotics. Follow-up urinalysis is needed to document the resolution of hematuria.

2. **Urolithiasis.** If the stone is expected to pass spontaneously, (usually < 1 cm), expectant therapy with analgesics and hydration is customary.

3. **Tumors.** Requires complete evaluation usually with abdominal CT and other studies as indicated by urologic consultation.

4. **Tuberculosis.** Treated with antibiotics, long-term follow-up with IVPs is needed because strictures (often 5–10 years after treatment) can lead to loss of renal function.

5. **Collecting system abnormality.** Requires further workup, usually retrograde ureteropyelogram and cystoscopy and then management as indicated.

6. **Coagulopathy.** Adjust dose of anticoagulant or treat with fresh frozen plasma as indicated.

7. **Glomerulonephritis.** Medical management as indicated, usually requires a biopsy.

8. **Hemorrhagic cystitis.** Treated with saline irrigation and occasionally alum irrigation. Refractory, life-threatening cases may require formalin instillation in the operating room.

36. HEMOPTYSIS

I. Problem. A 50-year-old male smoker admitted for elective aortofemoral bypass shows you a specimen of bloody sputum he just coughed up.

II. Immediate Questions

A. What are the vital signs? Fever may signify pulmonary infection. Orthostasis signifies significant blood loss.

B. Has this happened before? Chronic hemoptysis, acute onset, amount of blood, history of epistaxis, and pain on coughing should all be sought.

C. **Is the patient a smoker?** Smoking history may suggest a neoplasm or chronic bronchitis.

D. **What volume of blood was coughed up?** Massive hemoptysis is defined as > 500 mL blood loss in a 24-hour period.

III. Differential Diagnosis

A. Pulmonary Sources

1. **Neoplastic**
   a. **Bronchial carcinoma:** Early, usually see streaked sputum only. Advanced cancer may erode into pulmonary vessels causing severe hemorrhage or exsanguination.
   b. **Bronchial adenoma:** These are uncommon, often highly vascular lesions.

2. **Infectious**
   a. Tuberculosis.
   b. Fungal infections.
   c. Bacterial pneumonia rarely results in more than blood-streaked sputum. Pneumonia caused by *Klebsiella* often results in bloody sputum. *Serratia marcescens* may produce a reddish sputum that is confused with blood.
   d. **Chronic bronchitis:** Usually associated with smokers.
   e. Bronchiectasis.

3. **Vascular**
   a. **Pulmonary infarction from emboli:** Hemoptysis in this setting is accompanied by dyspnea and pleuritic chest pain. Look carefully for deep venous thrombosis.
   b. **Vascular aneurysms:** Aortic aneurysms rarely erode into the bronchial tree resulting in rapid exsanguination.

4. **Trauma.** Pulmonary contusion after blunt trauma or vessel laceration after penetrating trauma can cause hemoptysis.

5. **Foreign body.**

6. **Mitral stenosis.** Rupture of pulmonary vessels due to elevated left atrial pressures.

B. Nonpulmonary Sources. Not strictly hemoptysis, some patients cannot differentiate pulmonary (ie, coughed) sources of blood from others such as gastrointestinal, oral, or nasal.

C. Systemic Causes. Rarely is hemoptysis the sole site of hemorrhage in a patient with a bleeding diathesis or systemic vasculitis, but problems to consider are the leukemias, idiopathic thrombocytopenic purpura (ITP), Henoch-Schönlein purpura (HSP), Goodpasture's syndrome, and lupus erythematosus.

IV. Database

A. Physical Exam Key Points

1. Vital signs including blood pressure, check for orthostasis, or presence of tachypnea.
2. **HEENT.** Look carefully for an oral and nasal source of bleeding.
3. **Chest.** Examine for decreased breath sounds, evidence of chest trauma, listen for pleural rub that may signify effusion or pulmonary infarction.
4. **Cardiac.** Irregular beats may signify atrial fibrillation and an atrial source of emboli. Mitral stenosis is heard as a low, rumbling diastolic murmur.
5. **Abdomen.** Look for tenderness that may be associated with peptic ulcer disease, a disease that can be confused with hemoptysis.
6. **Extremities.** Evidence of DVT or cyanosis may be present.

B. Laboratory Data

1. Hemogram with attention to hematocrit and platelet counts.
2. Coagulation studies.
3. Sputum examination.
   a. **Culture routinely and Gram's stain:** A properly collected specimen will have few epithelial cells. Large numbers of epithelial cells suggests more of a saliva collection than sputum.
   b. **AFB culture and stain**
   c. Cytology.
4. **Renal function.** Check BUN and creatinine, as renal dysfunction usually accompanies hemoptysis in Goodpasture's syndrome.

C. Radiologic and Other Studies

1. **Chest x-ray is mandatory.** It may reveal infiltrates, infarct, obstructing lesion, contusion and pneumothorax, rib fracture, or aortic aneurysm.
2. **Chest CT scan.** Will further define suspicious lesions seen on routine chest x-ray.
3. **Bronchoscopy.** Although not as readily available as a chest radiograph, bronchoscopy will often allow diagnosis of a pulmonary source of hemoptysis. This should be performed when the acute bleeding subsides, although rigid bronchoscopy may be helpful.
4. **Angiogram.** This may be needed to define a possible fistula between aneurysm (seen on x-ray or CT) and the bronchial tree or to visualize bleeding source not seen on bronchoscopy. Can also localize embolus leading to infarction. Pulmonary angiography provides the definitive diagnosis of pulmonary embolism.

5. **Electrocardiogram.** If irregular pulse felt and atrial fibrillation suspected.
6. PPD skin test to evaluate for TB infection.
7. **Nuclear ventilation/perfusion (V/Q) scan.** Indicated in the initial evaluation if pulmonary embolus is suspected.

V. Plan

A. **Immediate Management.** With significant hemorrhage, the patient should be monitored in the ICU.
1. Establish venous access with large bore (16 gauge or larger) IVs, begin volume replacement as for any patient with blood loss. Send specimens to blood bank for type and crossmatch.
2. Because these patients are at significant risk for asphyxia, the airway should be protected and endotracheal intubation considered.
3. Perform gastric lavage with a nasogastric tube if evaluation cannot differentiate between GI and pulmonary hemorrhage.

B. **Specific Plans**
1. **Neoplasm.** Pulmonary resection should be performed when feasible. This may be necessary on an emergent basis if there is massive bleeding.
2. **Infection.** Antibiotics should initially be started empirically. Subsequent antibiotics should be based on culture results.
3. **Vascular**
   a. Pulmonary infarction from embolization should be treated with heparin to prevent further clot propagation. Streptokinase or urokinase can be considered in the nonoperative patient, as can thoracotomy and embolectomy in the salvageable critically ill patient.
   b. **Aneurysm:** Sentinel bleeding from eroding aneurysms can precede exsanguinating hemorrhage. Resection should be attempted, with prosthetic replacement, when possible.
   c. Erosion into the innominate artery from a tracheostomy tube (usually heralded by minor sentinel bleeding episodes) is life-threatening. Carefully evaluate all tracheostomy patients who have even minor bleeding. Attempt to control bleeding in acute episode by digital pressure inside the anterior wall of the trachea or with the inflated balloon of an endotracheal tube.
4. **Trauma**
   a. Blunt flail chest with underlying pulmonary contusion leading to hemoptysis often results in severe respiratory decompensation. Mechanical ventilation with positive pressure and aggressive pulmonary toilet is the treatment for this condition.
   b. Penetrating trauma resulting in hemoptysis should be initially treated with tube thoracostomy; persistent bloody

drainage or hemoptysis mandates exploratory thoracotomy. Bronchial tree disruption can cause hemoptysis and requires thoracotomy.

5. Foreign body. Rigid bronchoscopy is usually successful in retrieving bronchial foreign bodies.

6. Massive hemoptysis

   a. Exploratory thoracotomy and resection are sometimes needed in cases of massive hemoptysis.

   b. Placement of double lumen endotracheal tubes allows for complete collapse of an affected lung, resulting in shunting of circulation away from this lung. This method of control also allows for localization of the bleeding site to the affected side.

37. HICCUPS (SINGULTUS)

I. Problem. A patient admitted for right upper quadrant pain with possible cholecystitis develops hiccups for 4 hours.

II. Immediate Questions

   A. Is there any new or increased abdominal pain? Hiccups may be associated with a variety of significant intra-abdominal diseases so a careful evaluation of associated abdominal symptoms is needed.

   B. Is there any shoulder pain or pain with respiration? A second major category of hiccup related disorders is diaphragmatic irritation. Both referred pain to the shoulder or pleuritic pain may point to a diaphragmatic process, such as subphrenic abscess.

   C. Does the patient have any cardiac history or symptoms? Although unusual, hiccups may be the presenting and sometimes only symptom of a transmural myocardial infarction. Always keep this in mind, especially if the patient looks ill with a complaint of hiccups.

   D. Are there any emotional problems with the patient? Hiccups related to anxiety or other psychogenic causes is very prevalent in women, but not in men. Inquire about previous problems with hiccups.

III. Differential Diagnosis. Hiccups are usually a short-term innocuous complaint, and they are often a result of aerophagia caused by rapid eating, drinking, or laughter. Even in chronic situations no organic cause may be found. The list below is some of the organic disorders in which hiccups may be present.

A. Diaphragmatic/Phrenic Nerve Irritation
   1. Subphrenic abscess
   2. Pneumonia/pleuritis
   3. Myocardial infarction
   4. Pericarditis
   5. Peritonitis
   6. Metastatic implants on the diaphragm
   7. Lung tumors
   8. Postoperative

B. Gastrointestinal Diseases
   1. Gastric dilatation
   2. Hiatal hernia
   3. Pancreatitis

C. Metabolic Diseases
   1. Uremia
   2. Diabetes
   3. Alcohol abuse

D. CNS Dysfunction. "Central hiccups" often caused by posterior fossa tumor or infarction or encephalitis. In neonates, may indicate a seizure.

E. Psychogenic. The hallmark is that these stop when the patient is asleep.

IV. Database

A. Physical Exam Key Points
   1. **Vital signs.** Spiking temperatures may indicate an abscess.
   2. **Pulmonary.** Evidence for decreased diaphragmatic excursion that may accompany diaphragmatic irritation or evidence for an infiltrate or effusion.
   3. **Cardiac.** Listen for pericardial friction rub.
   4. **Abdomen.** Distention (either ascites or gaseous), pain, peritoneal signs, hepatosplenomegaly, tympany, especially over the gastric area may suggest a diagnosis. "Punch tenderness" over the lower ribs may suggest diaphragmatic inflammation.

B. Laboratory Data
   1. **Hemogram** especially with infection.
   2. **Renal function tests.** Increased BUN and creatinine with uremia.
   3. **Glucose.** Glucose tolerance test may be needed at some point to diagnose diabetes.
   4. **Amylase.** Elevated in pancreatic disease.

C. Radiologic and Other Studies
   1. **Chest x-ray.** Elevation of diaphragm, effusion, infiltrate, or tumor.

    2. Abdominal x-rays. Gastric dilatation may be seen on this study or on chest x-ray as well.

    3. ECG. To rule out ischemic changes if clinically indicated.

    4. Ultrasound/CT abdomen. May reveal subphrenic fluid collections or other pathology.

    5. CT chest. Chest tumors may irritate the phrenic nerve.

V. Plan. Any significant associated condition (myocardial infarction, gastric dilatation, subphrenic abscess) should be treated in the appropriate manner. There are a variety of individual or "home remedies" to treat hiccups. Those listed below are found to have withstood at least some objective scrutiny.

  A Mechanisms to Interfere with Respiration. Low P_{CO_2} accentuates hiccups while high P_{CO_2} inhibits them. Maneuvers to increase P_{CO_2}:

    1. Breathholding.

    2. Drinking water rapidly.

    3. Rebreathing from a paper bag.

  B. Mechanisms to Alter Afferent Pathways

    1. Stimulate nasopharynx with cotton swab.

    2. Swallow a teaspoon of dry granulated sugar.

  C. Pharmacologic Management

    1. Chlorpromazine. 25–50 mg PO/IM q6H.

    2. Perphenazine. 4–8 mg PO or 5 mg IM q8H.

    3. Metoclopramide. 10 mg PO q6H for several days.

38. HYPERCALCEMIA

I. Problem. The clinical chemistry laboratory calls to tell you that one of your patients, a 45-year-old male scheduled for surgery in the morning, has a serum calcium of 12.5 mg/dL (normal 8.5–10.5 mg/dL).

II. Immediate Questions

  A. Is the patient symptomatic? Delirium, confusion, stupor and emotional lability, polydipsia, polyuria, anorexia, and nausea and vomiting are often seen with critical levels of hypercalcemia.

  B. Has the patient recently had surgery? In particular, adrenal surgery (hypoadrenalism) or long-term immobilization, which can cause excessive bone resorption and hypercalcemia.

  C. What IV fluids and medications are currently being given? There may be medications causing increased calcium levels (thiazide diuretics, vitamin D) or the administration of exogenous calcium.

   D. **Is there any history of cancer or parathyroid disease?**
      Hypercalcemia can be caused by a paraneoplastic syndrome as-
      sociated with cancer.

III. **Differential Diagnosis.** (See also Section II, page 245)

   A. **Hyperparathyroidism (HPT).** About 20% of patients with hyper-
      calcemia will have associated hyperparathyroidism. Primary HPT
      is usually diagnosed with elevated calcium, low phosphate, and el-
      evated parathyroid hormone.

   B. **Malignant Neoplasm.** This can be caused by bone metastasis or
      by factors secreted by the tumors (multiple myeloma, lung, breast,
      kidney) and is the most frequent cause.

   C. **Thiazide Diuretics.** Agents such as hydrochlorothiazide cause in-
      creased renal resorption of calcium.

   D. **Sarcoidosis.** The granulomatous tissue may produce a vitamin D
      metabolite.

   E. **Vitamin D Intoxication.** This history will usually reveal chronic in-
      gestion.

   F. **Milk-alkali syndrome.** Excessive alkali and calcium in the treat-
      ment of peptic ulcer disease (less frequent today with use of
      magnesium-containing antacids).

   G. Hyperthyroidism.

   H. Adrenal Insufficiency.

   I. **Paget's disease.** Usually with secondary hyperparathyroidism.

   J. Acute tubular necrosis (diuretic phase).

   K. Acromegaly.

   L. Excessive calcium administration.

   M. Long-term immobilization.

IV. **Database.** The classic history is "stones, bones, moans, and abdom-
    inal groans," and weight loss.

   A. **Physical Exam Key Points**
      1. **Vital signs.** Hypertension may accompany hypercalcemia.
      2. **Cardiac.** Arrhythmias may include bradycardia, tachycardia.
      3. **Chest.** Breast carcinoma may be suggested by a mass lesion
         or prior mastectomy.
      4. **Abdomen.** Check for masses.
      5. **Bones.** Tenderness to percussion that may indicate metastatic
         disease.
      6. **Nodes.** Lymphadenopathy with cancer or sarcoidosis.

    7. Neurologic weakness, hyperactive reflexes, impaired mentation (stupor, delirium).

    8. Skin. Evidence of pruritus.

B. Laboratory Data

    1. Serum calcium and albumin. Confirm elevation on a repeat determination. **Caution:** The units of calcium measurement may differ in different institutions (mg/dL vs mEq/dL). If the albumin is not normal, a corrected calcium level must be determined (see page 259). Symptoms usually appear at levels of 13 mg/dL.

    2. Phosphorous. Usually low in hyperparathyroidism except if renal failure present.

    3. Potassium, magnesium. Decreases may be associated with high serum calcium level.

    4. Arterial blood gases. Acidosis with hyperchlorhydria.

    5. Alkaline phosphatase. Elevated in hyperparathyroidism with bone disease.

    6. Renal function. Renal insufficiency will exacerbate hypercalcemia.

    7. Parathyroid hormone (PTH) level. Increased in primary or secondary hyperparathyroidism, often decreased in hypercalcemia not caused by hyperparathyroidism.

C. Radiologic and Other Studies

    1. Chest x-ray. May show hilar adenopathy with sarcoidosis or lymphoma.

    2. Abdomen x-rays. May show renal stones with hyperparathyroidism.

    3. Skull. Typical punched out lesions of multiple myeloma.

    4. Bones. May show osteolytic lesions of metastatic cancer.

    5. IVP. Will often reveal renal stones with hyperparathyroidism and, occasionally, renal cell carcinoma, which may have associated hypercalcemia.

    6. Barium swallow. The esophagus can be displaced with parathyroid adenoma.

    7. ECG. Hypercalcemia is associated with a shortened QT interval and prolonged PR interval.

    8. Cortisone suppression test. No response in hyperparathyroidism, but metastatic cancer, myeloma, sarcoid, vitamin D intoxication, milk-alkali syndrome, and adrenal insufficiency usually respond with a decrease in calcium.

V. Plan

    A. Initial Management. First, lower the serum calcium (if necessary), then control the underlying cause.

        1. Levels < 12 mg/dL. Usually directed only at the underlying cause.

   2. **Moderate elevation (12–15 mg/dL).** Treat with hydration and
      loop diuretics initially (see below).
   3. **Severe hypercalcemia (> 15 mg/dL or any symptomatic
      patient regardless of level).** A life-threatening emergency re-
      quiring more rigorous therapy.
B. **Specific Plans**
   1. Restrict calcium intake, encourage mobilization, and treat un-
      derlying disorder in all cases. Calcium-containing and calcium-
      increasing medications include calcium carbonate antacids
      (Tums), vitamins A and D, thiazide diuretics (hydrochlorothia-
      zide).
   2. **Saline diuresis.** To restore volume and produce at least
      1500–2000 ml/d of urine. Sodium increases calcium excretion
      by competing for resorption in distal tubule. In the presence of
      renal or cardiac failure, this must be done with caution. Monitor
      serum calcium, phosphate, potassium, magnesium, and BUN.
   3. Furosemide can be given 20–40 mg IV q2–4h to bring Ca be-
      low 12 mg/dL after hydration. Carefully monitor serum potas-
      sium during diuresis and replace as necessary.
   4. Mithramycin 15–25 µg/kg in 1 L saline over 3–6 hours. Used
      most often for PTH producing malignancies, osteolytic malig-
      nancies, vitamin D intoxication, and nonPTH producing tumors
      such as myeloma.
   5. Magnesium sulfate 2 mEq/kg IV over 8–12 hours (lg 20% solu-
      tion = 8 mEq/ml) to correct hypomagnesemia.
   6. **Corticosteroids.** Ineffective against primary HPT and may
      take 1–2 weeks to see effect, used with malignancies. Pred-
      nisone 5–15 mg PO daily is fairly typical dosing.
   7. **Dialysis.** As a last resort if extremely high levels cannot be
      treated.
   8. **Other agents.** Include etidronate, pamidronate, gallium nitrate,
      calcitonin, indomethacin, and phosphate.

39. HYPERGLYCEMIA

I. **Problem.** An elderly woman who has just undergone hemicolectomy
   is spilling sugar in her urine. A stat serum glucose is 185 mg/dL (normal fasting 70–105 mg/dL).

II. **Immediate Questions**
   A. **Is there a history of diabetes?** Diabetic patients who usually
      take insulin will need a portion of their usual daily dose even while
      taking nothing by mouth, usually 50% of their morning dose.
      Surgical stress may temporarily create insulin requirements in the
      non-insulin-dependent diabetic. Lastly, no history of diabetes must

suggests other problems: overalimentation, sepsis, side effects of glucocorticoid use, etc.

B. What are the vital signs? Fever may represent a septic episode, which can cause glucose intolerance. New onset hyperglycemia or a sudden increase in serum glucose in a diabetic can be the first sign of sepsis.

III. Differential Diagnosis. (See also Section II, page 245).

A. Diabetes

1. **Insulin-dependent (type I) (formerly called juvenile diabetes).** Insulin-dependent diabetics require insulin even when taking nothing by mouth.

2. **Non-insulin-dependent** (type II) (formerly called Adult Onset Diabetes or AODM). Surgical stress often aggravates diabetes. Thus, patients controlled with diet or oral hypoglycemic agents may develop a worsening of their diabetes.

B. Sepsis. Glucose intolerance is often an early sign of sepsis in the critically ill patient.

C. Hyperalimentation. Typical central parenteral nutrition solutions contain up to 35% glucose solution. If these are advanced too quickly or the patient receives amounts above nutritional requirements, hyperglycemia can develop.

D. Gestational Diabetes. Some women develop hyperglycemia during pregnancy.

E. Other Causes

1. **Medication.** Steroid use causes insulin resistance in many patients, other agents include oral contraceptives.

2. Cushing's syndrome.

3. Pancreatic disease or resection.

IV. Database

A. Physical Exam Key Points

1. **Vital signs.** Fever and tachycardia suggest infection, and hypotension suggests sepsis. Kussmaul respiration (deep, rapid respiratory pattern) may be seen with severe ketoacidosis.

2. **HEENT.** Fruity odor on the breath may signify ketoacidosis.

3. **Lungs.** Listen for evidence of pneumonia.

4. **Abdomen.** Exclude intra-abdominal causes of sepsis.

5. **Neurologic.** Obtundation may indicate deterioration of a diabetic condition and the development of ketoacidosis.

B. Laboratory Data. Significantly elevated chemsticks should be confirmed with a serum glucose determination.

1. **Serum electrolytes.** Potassium and phosphorus must be monitored closely in diabetic ketoacidosis (DKA).

2. Arterial blood gas. Any suspicion of sepsis or DKA should be followed-up with a determination of serum pH and Po_2.

3. Lactic acid measurements may be useful in DKA.

4. Hemogram. Elevated leukocyte count may indicate infection.

5. Cultures of blood, urine, central lines, etc, should be done if infection is suspected.

6. Urine glucose. Thresholds for spilling glucose in the urine can vary widely; confirm with a serum glucose if any doubt exists.

C. Radiologic and Other Studies. These studies should be selected based on clinical impression. For example, infection in the postoperative hyperglycemic patient may be evaluated with a chest x-ray if a pulmonary source is suspected, or an abdominal CT scan if an intra-abdominal abscess is considered.

V. Plan

A. Initial Management. Controlling serum glucose quickly and safely and treating predisposing infection appropriately.

B. Specific Plans

1. Sliding scale insulin. Small doses of subcutaneous regular insulin can be given every 6 hours based on rapid, automated evaluation of blood sugars using chemsticks. Typically, serum glucose of < 200 mg% is considered adequate control. A typical sliding scale will give no insulin with serum glucose determinations under 180 mg%, 3–5 U from 180–240 mg%, 6–10 U from 240–400 mg%, and 9–15 U for > 400 mg%. Any chemstick > 400 mg% should be confirmed with a stat serum measurement from the lab. Patients who have not been on insulin previously will need smaller doses until their own response to insulin is assessed.

2. Diet. Modification is needed in diabetic patients, with caloric restriction in the obese patient being important.

3. Oral hypoglycemic agents. Many type II diabetics admitted on these medications may require insulin supplements after an operation, but are usually discharged on the same agent.

4. Severe glucose intolerance owing to sepsis and DKA. These require aggressive therapy, usually in an ICU setting. DKA is usually manifest as tachypnea, dehydration, ketones on the breath, abdominal pain, with hyperglycemia, hyperketonemia, and metabolic acidosis.

a. Precipitating factors: In the surgical patient, infection precipitates severe glucose intolerance. It should be appropriately treated.

b. Dehydration: Typically, patients become volume depleted, often because of severe glycosuria. Rehydrate the patient initially with dextrose free saline. Increased urine output in these patients may be a result of osmotic diuresis and not a reflection of the true volume status. Volume status must be assessed by other means, such as a central venous pressure line.

c. **Potassium:** Potassium levels will go down as DKA improves. The potassium ions become intracellular, thus decreasing serum levels. However, the patient actually is total body potassium depleted.

d. **Bicarbonate:** Correction of severe acidosis with bicarbonate is sometimes needed. Insulin must be continued until the bicarbonate normalizes. This may mean using both insulin and glucose intravenously.

e. **Insulin:** Start with a 10–20 U IV bolus and follow this with a continuous drip. Infusion rate will vary, but should be approximately 2–5 U/hr initially and adjusted as needed.

f. **Dextrose:** IV fluids should be changed to those containing 5% dextrose when serum glucose levels decrease to 300 mg/dL.

g. **Maintenance insulin:** Once IV therapy has controlled severe hyperglycemia, maintenance insulin will be needed. Subcutaneous administration should be performed twice a day, to achieve better control, often with a combination of NPH and regular insulin. Patients on hyperalimentation can receive maintenance insulin by adding it directly to the solution.

40. HYPERKALEMIA

Immediate Actions

1. Severe hyperkalemia (> 6.5 mmol/L) immediate ECG monitoring.
2. Administer 10% calcium gluconate 10–20 mL IV to protect the heart.
3. Begin maneuvers to decrease the potassium levels as noted below.

I. Problem. A patient on the trauma service with a crush injury has a potassium of 7.1 mmol/L on the second hospital day (normal 3.5–5.1 mmol/L).

II. Immediate Questions

A. **What are the vital signs?** Check this first because the cardiac effects of hyperkalemia can result in life-threatening arrhythmias.

B. **What is the patient's urine output?** Renal failure with inability to excrete either endogenous or exogenous potassium load is the most common cause of acute hyperkalemia on a surgical service. Evaluate urine output and recent renal function chemistries. Ensure there is no obstruction to urinary flow.

C. Is the patient receiving potassium in an intravenous solution? A bag of IV solution may contain 20–40 mEq/L of potassium and hyperalimentation solutions may contain more. When beginning the initial evaluation of an abnormal potassium value, stop all exogenous potassium until the problem is resolved.

D. Is the lab result accurate? In the previous example, hyperkalemia is an almost expected outcome. However, abnormally elevated potassium levels are often entirely unexpected or inconsistent. If the lab doesn't notify you, inquire about hemolysis of the specimen, which can falsely elevate the potassium.

E. Is the patient on any medication that could elevate the potassium? If the patient is receiving spironolactone, triamterene, or indomethacin, stop these medications immediately.

III. Differential Diagnosis. The measured laboratory value of extracellular potassium concentration is the level that correlates with the harmful consequences of hyperkalemia. This extracellular level can be increased by redistribution of potassium from intracellular stores (where 98% of the total body potassium is located) or by a real increase in total body potassium.

A. Redistribution
   1. **Acidosis.**
   2. **Insulin deficiency.**
   3. **Digoxin overdose.**
   4. **Succinylcholine.**
   5. **Cellular breakdown.**
      a. **Crush injury (rhabdomyolysis).**
      b. **Hemolysis.**

B. Increased Total Body Potassium
   1. **Renal causes.**
      a. **Acute renal failure.**
      b. **Chronic renal failure:** Potassium will not usually be elevated until endstage disease, typically creatinine clearance < 20 ml/sec.
      c. **Renal tubular dysfunction:** Associated with renal transplant, lupus erythematosus, sickle cell disease, or myeloma.
   2. **Mineralocorticoid deficiency.**
      a. **Addison's disease.**
      b. **Hypoaldosteronism (hyporeninemic).**
   3. **Drug-induced.** Common causes:
      a. **Spironolactone.**
      b. **Triamterene.**
      c. **Indomethacin:** Thought to interfere with renal prostaglandin levels.
      d. **Cyclosporine.**

    e. Potassium supplement excess.

    f. Heparin: Reported to decrease aldosterone synthesis.

C. Pseudohyperkalemia

  1. Hemolysis of the specimen.

  2. Prolonged period of tourniquet occlusion before drawing blood.

  3. **Thrombocytosis/leukocytosis:** White blood cells and platelets release potassium as the clot forms.

IV. Database

A. Physical Exam Key Points

  1. **Cardiac.** Bradycardia, ventricular fibrillation, and asystole with markedly elevated potassium levels.

  2. **Neuromuscular.** Findings of tingling, weakness, flaccid paralysis, and hyperactive deep tendon reflexes. However, cardiac arrest often precedes these symptoms.

B. Laboratory Data

  1. **Electrolytes, BUN, and creatinine.** Hyperkalemia usually diagnosed by this study, and renal failure may be detected.

  2. **Arterial blood gas.** Nonanion gap acidosis associated with hyperkalemia.

  3. **Platelet count, white blood count.** Elevations may yield factitious hyperkalemia. With significant platelet and WBC elevations, order a plasma potassium level.

  4. **Cortisol levels or ACTH stimulation test.**

  5. **Digoxin level** if indicated.

  6. **Myoglobin level in serum/urine.** Useful in crush injury.

C. Radiologic and Other Studies

  1. **ECG.** The second most important test besides the potassium level, and a means to separate pseudohyperkalemia from actual elevations of potassium. Changes seen as potassium increases include peaked T waves, flat P waves, prolonged PR interval, and a widened QRS complex progressing to a sine wave and arrest.

  2. **Ultrasound.** Especially based on renal insufficiency. May show obstructed kidneys or bladder or small kidneys owing to chronic renal disease.

V. Plan. The severity of hyperkalemia as judged by the serum level and the ECG dictate treatment. In general, aggressive treatment of hyperkalemia is indicated for a serum potassium > 6.5–7 mmol/L or if ECG changes are present. The methods of treatment ranked by the rapidity of the response are mechanisms that counteract membrane effects of hyperkalemia, move potassium into cells, and remove potassium from the body.

A. Counteract membrane effects. Counteract membrane effects and protect the heart by using calcium gluconate 10% 10–20 ml IV over 3–5 minutes while on a cardiac monitor. Use with close monitoring in patients on digitalis because arrhythmia may occur.

B. Transfer Potassium to the Intracellular Compartment
   1. **Sodium bicarbonate 1 ampule (44 mEq) IV.** May repeat 1–2 times every 20–30 minutes. Works best in acidotic patients, but also has effects in normal pH patients.
   2. **Insulin/glucose.** One ampule of D50W and 10 units of regular insulin IV given over 5 minutes.
   3. A combination treatment of the above two methods consists of one liter D10W mixed with 3 ampules of sodium bicarbonate. Give over 2–4 hours with regular insulin 10 units s.c. every 4–6 hours.

C. Removal of potassium from the body
   1. **Kayexalate (exchange resin)**
      i. **Oral:** 40 grams in 25–50 ml of 70% sorbitol every 2–4 hours.
      ii. **Rectal:** 50–100 grams in 200 ml water given as a retention enema for 30 minutes every 2–4 hours.
      a. **Dialysis:** Peritoneal or hemodialysis.
      b. **Furosemide:** Monitor urine output and volume status carefully. Administer furosemide IV.
   2. Remove all potassium from intravenous fluids.

D. Any ECG changes should incite prompt transfer to monitored bed.

E. Consider Foley catheter insertion to aid in assessing urine output and eliminate sources of lower urinary tract obstruction.

F. Chronic Therapy. For diseases such as chronic renal failure, use potassium restricted diet (40–60 mEq/d). Addison's disease usually requires glucocorticoid and mineralocorticoid therapy.

41. HYPERNATREMIA

(See also Section II, page 245)

I. Problem. The clinical chemistry lab calls to tell you that an 85-year-old female patient has a serum sodium of 155 mmol/L (normal 136–145 mmol/L).

II. Immediate Questions

A. Is the patient alert and oriented, or is the patient seizing? Symptoms of hypernatremia usually do not appear until the level is >160 mmol/L (irritability, ataxia, anorexia, cramping). Levels >180 mmol/L may result in confusion, stupor, or seizure. The more rapid the change in sodium level, the more likely it will be symptomatic.

B. **What medication is the patient taking?** Diuretics can cause water loss leading to hypernatremia. Many IV antibiotic solutions contain sodium.

C. **What are the intake/output values for the past few days?** A loss of total body water by fluid deprivation (inadequate administration of fluids) can cause hypernatremia.

D. **Are there underlying conditions?** Certain diseases, most notably diabetes insipidus, are associated with hypernatremia. Post CABG patients can have hypernatremia due to water loss secondary to ADH inhibition.

E. **Is the lab value accurate?** As with any unexpected lab result, the error could be in the lab itself. It may be of value to repeat the test.

F. **What is the composition of IV fluids administered?** Check sodium content of fluids. Is the patient receiving adequate free water (usually 35 ml/kg/24h in adult)?

III. **Differential Diagnosis.** The differential diagnosis is best considered in light of the cause of hypernatremia—being a disorder due to a loss of total body water, and rarely associated with an increased total body sodium.

A. **Inadequate Fluid Intake.** Water deprivation (comatose or postoperative patients).

B. **Increased Water Loss.** Most body fluids are hypotonic with respect to sodium, thus excessive losses lead to hypernatremia.
   1. **Nonrenal losses**
      a. **Gastrointestinal losses:** NG suction, diarrhea, fistulas.
      b. **Pulmonary losses:** Insensible losses especially in intubated patients who are not receiving adequate humidification.
      c. **Cutaneous Losses:** Insensible losses increase in the febrile patient 500 ml/24 hours for each degree centigrade increase above 38°C. Air filled or heated beds also increase cutaneous losses.
   2. **Renal losses**
      a. Diuretics.
      b. Hypercalcemic nephropathy.
      c. Hypokalemic nephropathy.
      d. Diabetes insipidus (true vs. nephrogenic).
      e. **Acute tubular necrosis:** Polyuric phase.
      f. **Postobstructive diuresis:** Usually caused by the relief of long-standing bilateral renal obstruction.
      g. **Diabetes mellitus:** Caused by osmotic diuresis (water loss) caused by glycosuria.

        h. ADH inhibition (water loss) via baroreceptor activation.

        i. Drugs: Including lithium, ethanol, phenytoin, colchicine, and mannitol.

  C. Administration of Hypertonic Saline. There are no indications for the routine administration of hypertonic saline in most surgical patients. There are limited uses in some neurosurgical patients.

  D. Increased Mineralocorticoids or Glucocorticoids
    1. Primary aldosteronism.
    2. Cushing's syndrome.
    3. Ectopic ACTH production.
    4. Over-administration of exogenous steroids.

IV. Database

  A. Physical Exam Key Points
    1. Vital signs. Orthostatic blood pressure changes, tachycardia, and decreased weight suggest volume loss.
    2. Skin. Check turgor and mucous membranes—may be dry with volume contraction. Note any "cushingoid" features.
    3. Neurologic exam. Look for signs if patient is irritable, weak, twitches, or experiences seizures.
    4. History. The physical exam and history can give insight into the degree of fluid deficit. With volume loss of 5% or less, the patient may complain only of thirst. With volume loss between 5 and 10%, the patient will be lethargic, with sunken eyes, decreased skin turgor, tears may be absent and will manifest orthostatic hypotension. Above 10% loss, the patient will be hypotensive and hyperventilatory.

  B. Laboratory Data
    1. Serum electrolytes. Often electrolyte disorder involves more than one extracellular ion. Elevated BUN may indicate dehydration.
    2. Serum osmolality. Increased with volume loss.
    3. Urine osmolality. Hypertonic urine suggests extrarenal fluid loss, while isotonic or hypotonic urine suggests renal losses.
    4. Spot urine sodium. If < 20 mEq/L, suggests extrarenal volume losses.
    5. Hematocrit. May be elevated with dehydration because of hemoconcentration.

V. Plan. The overall plan is to replace free water slowly to bring the serum sodium concentration down to normal levels. Volume repletion is especially important in patients showing orthostasis on blood pressure measurement. Correction should be done slowly to prevent the development of cerebral edema, which can precipitate seizures.

A. Determine the volume of free water needed to correct the serum sodium from the actual total body water (TBW).

$$\text{Water deficit} = (0.6 \times \text{weight in kg}) - \text{TBW}$$

$$\text{TBW} = \frac{140}{\text{Serum Na}} \times (0.6 \times \text{weight in kg})$$

Administer the fluids over a 24-hour period as 5% dextrose in water. Alternatively, if a patient is receiving 5% dextrose in 0.45 N saline, the extra free water can be given by increasing the rate of fluid, and changing it to 5% dextrose in 0.2 N saline.

B. Identify and Treat the Underlying Cause of Hypernatremia.

1. Replace unusually large nonrenal losses of free water, such as small bowel or pancreatic fistula drainage (see Section IV, page 337).
2. Treat diabetes mellitus with insulin (see Problem 35, page 121)
3. Treat diabetes insipidus with adequate free water or with vasopressin.

42. HYPERTENSION

I. **Problem.** After vagotomy and antrectomy, a 45-year-old man has a blood pressure of 190/110 in the recovery room.

II. **Immediate Questions**

A. **What is the heart and respiratory rate?** Postoperative pain is often manifested by tachycardia and hypertension; the addition of tachypnea should alert you to the possibility of postoperative hypoxia, especially in the presence of agitation. Bradycardia and hypertension suggests increased intracranial pressure.

B. **Is there a history of hypertension?** Mild blood pressure elevations are often seen in hypertensive patients after large intraoperative fluid infusions; this is rarely worrisome in the absence of other findings.

C. **Is the patient having chest pain?** Severe hypertension often places significant strain on the hearts of patients with a history of coronary artery disease; it can cause angina or infarction and requires rapid control. Aortic dissection is also an emergency and may cause back and chest pain.

D. **What medication is the patient taking?** Sympathomimetic agents at incorrect doses can cause hypertension. Carefully check dilutions and rates of all IV infusions. Steroids and oral contraceptives can elevate the blood pressure. To prevent postoperative hypertension, most cardiac medications and antihypertensives with the exception of diuretics should be given in their usual doses with a small sip of water the morning of the operation.

III. **Differential Diagnosis.** There are six surgically correctable causes of hypertension: coarctation of the aorta, pheochromocytoma, Cushing's syndrome, primary hyperaldosteronism, unilateral renal parenchymal disease, and renovascular hypertension.

   A. **Postoperative**
      1. **Pain-induced.**
      2. **Fluid overload.**
      3. **Hypoxia.**
      4. **Vasospasm.** Loss of body temperature frequently takes place during surgery; this often results in the patient "clamping down" to preserve body heat. May also be seen after aortic cross-clamping.
      5. **Carotid sinus reflex disturbance.** May augment postoperative hypertension following CVA (cerebrovascular accident) and can lead to intracerebral hemorrhage.

   B. **Essential Hypertension.** There is no cause found in 90–95% of patients with chronic hypertension.

   C. **Secondary Hypertension**
      1. **Renal.** Vascular or parenchymal.
      2. **Endocrine.** Pheochromocytoma, Cushing's syndrome.
      3. **Drug-induced.** Oral contraceptives, amphetamines, ketamine, other sympathomimetic causes.
      4. **Pregnancy.** Preeclampsia or eclampsia.
      5. **Coarctation of the aorta.**
      6. **Increased intracranial pressure.** Usually associated with bradycardia. Caused by tumor, subarachnoid bleed, others.
      7. **Polycythemia vera.**
      8. **Baroreceptor stimulation.**

   D. **Factitious.** Using too small a blood pressure cuff on an obese arm may falsely elevate readings.

IV. **Database**

   A. **History.** Careful history reveals previous hypertension and type of treatment, medications, or other predisposing factors.

   B. **Physical Exam Key Points**
      1. **Vital signs.** Measure pressure in both arms. Check the core body temperature, especially in patients in the recovery room.
      2. **HEENT.** Papilledema, retinal hemorrhages, or exudates may be present. Papilledema represents increased intracranial pressure or malignant hypertension.

3. **Lungs.** Listen for rales indicating pulmonary edema and possible heart failure.
4. **Abdomen.** Pulsatile mass with aneurysm or bruit with renovascular hypertension.
5. **Neurologic exam.** Focal changes may represent cerebral ischemia.

C. **Laboratory Data**
1. **Arterial blood gas.** Should be performed if there is any question about hypoxemia.
2. **Urinalysis, BUN, serum creatinine.** Indicate level of renal function because hypertension can accompany renal insufficiency.
3. **Serum catecholamines, urinary VMA, and metanephrines.** Only if one suspects pheochromocytoma.
4. Dexamethasone suppression test can be obtained later to test for Cushing's syndrome (see page 266).

D. **Radiologic and Other Studies**
1. **Electrocardiogram.** Perform routinely in most elderly patients after major cardiac, thoracic, or vascular surgery, and in patients with a history of heart disease after any major operation. In the presence of hypertension, the ECG may show ischemic changes in the absence of symptoms.
2. **Pulmonary artery catheter.** Determination of cardiac output and pulmonary capillary wedge pressure facilitates evaluation of cardiac function in critically ill hypertensive postoperative patients. Its use is not indicated in the vast majority of cases.
3. Although not typically a surgical evaluation, new onset hypertension in patients under 30 and over 60, as well as those failing a variety of drug regimens, should have a thorough evaluation for secondary causes of hypertension. This often includes renal arteriography, selective renal vein renin measurements, renal ultrasonography, determination of urinary catecholamines and VMA, and serum cortisol.

V. **Plan**

A. **Emergent Management.** Severe hypertension (ie, hypertensive encephalopathy, malignant hypertension, and dissecting aortic aneurysm) is usually treated emergently with sodium nitroprusside (Nipride). Other agents can be used to control acute hypertension (diazoxide, labetalol or hydralazine), but do not offer the advantage of titration as Nipride does. With evidence of myocardia ischemia, use IV nitroglycerin.
1. **Sodium nitroprusside 0.5–10 µg/kg/min IV infusion.** Titrate to effect. Monitor for thiocyanate toxicity and methemoglobinemia.

2. **Nitroglycerin 5–100 µg/min.** Titrate to effect.
3. **Nifedipine 10–20 mg PO/SL.** Often a useful oral adjunct to lower blood pressure immediately.

B. **Preoperative.** The goal is to obtain good control of blood pressure before performing elective procedures.
   1. Check ECG for signs of ischemia or failure.
   2. All blood pressure and cardiac medications—except diuretics—can be given on the morning of the operation.
   3. Weight loss and a low-salt diet should be encouraged as the first step.
   4. Typical staged therapy includes starting with a ß-blocker or thiazide diuretic. Thiazides work better in black patients. If a second agent is needed, add the first-line agent that was not used. If there are contraindications to the use of ß-blockers (eg, asthma, heart failure), central antiadrenergic agents (eg, Aldomet, clonidine) or anti-alpha adrenergic agents can be used. Third-line drugs include hydralazine, prazosin, and angiotensin converting enzyme inhibitors (captopril). Hydralazine can cause reflex tachycardia in the non-beta blocked patient. Calcium channel blockers are now frequently used. Drug doses are listed in Section IX, page 388.

C. **Postoperative**
   1. Ensure adequate oxygenation and pain relief and warm the patient with blankets or heating blanket if necessary.
   2. Mild hypertension can be treated with a variety of agents. In the immediate postoperative period, sublingual nifedipine (10–20 mg) is useful, but sometimes causes hypotension. Hydralazine 5–10 mg IV can be used in elderly patients. Sedatives and pain control are often all that are needed to control mild hypertension. Mild persistent hypertension can be further treated by adding a diuretic, such as furosemide, to the treatment regimen temporarily to help excrete mobilized fluids. Hypertension in a pregnant patient is treated with methyldopa, which seems to be safe for the fetus. Always exclude eclampsia before treating hypertension in pregnancy.
   3. Severe hypertension, for example after major vascular surgery, often requires parenteral administration of vasodilators; rarely, parenteral ß-blockers are used if there is a significant history of coronary artery disease and myocardial infarction without heart failure. The vasodilator of choice is sodium nitroprusside.
   4. Newly diagnosed hypertensive patients need appropriate follow-up after discharge.

43. HYPOCALCEMIA

(See also Section II, page 245)

I. **Problem.** A patient admitted to the trauma service with multiple blunt trauma in a motor vehicle accident has a calcium of 7.7 mg/dL (normal 8.5–10.5 mg/dL).

II. Immediate Questions

A. Are there any symptoms relevant to hypocalcemia? Asymptomatic hypocalcemia usually does not require emergency treatment. Signs and symptoms of hypocalcemia may include peripheral and perioral paresthesias, Trousseau's sign (carpopedal spasm), Chvostek's sign, confusion, muscle twitching, tetany, or seizures.

B. Is there a history of neck surgery? Look for scars from a previous neck operation because surgical removal or infarction of the parathyroids is one of the more common causes of hypocalcemia.

C. Does the low calcium level represent the true ionized calcium? Most laboratories report the total serum calcium. However, a decrease in the serum albumin of 1 g/dL will decrease the protein bound calcium by 0.8 mg/dL. Obtain serum albumin values and correct for the total calcium level appropriately or determine the ionized calcium.

corrected Ca = [(normal albumin − patient's albumin) × 0.8] + patient's measured serum Ca

III. Differential Diagnosis.
The causes of low ionized serum calcium can be categorized as parathyroid hormone deficits, vitamin D deficits, magnesium deficiency, and loss or displacement of calcium. The combination of hypocalcemia with a high serum phosphate usually indicates severe hypoparathyroidism.

A. Parathyroid Hormone (PTH) Deficits
1. **Decreased PTH levels**
   a. Surgical excision or injury, including thyroid surgery. Remember that this can occur in the immediate postoperative period—as early as 12 hours postoperatively or as late as 3–5 days.
   b. Infiltrative diseases such as hemochromatosis, amyloid, or metastatic cancer.
   c. Idiopathic.
   d. Irradiation.
2. **Decreased PTH activity**
   a. **Pseudohypoparathyroidism:** Resistance to PTH at the tissue level. PTH level is elevated and can be suppressed by calcium infusion.

B. Vitamin D Deficiency
1. **Malnutrition.**
2. **Malabsorption**
   a. Pancreatitis.

      b. Postgastrectomy.
      c. Short-gut syndrome.
      d. Laxative abuse.
      e. Sprue.
      f. Hepatobiliary disease with bile salt deficiency.

   3. Defective metabolism
      a. Liver disease: Failure to synthesize 25(OH) vitamin D.
      b. Renal disease: Failure to synthesize 1–25 dihydroxy vitamin D.
      c. Anticonvulsive treatment: Phenobarbital and phenytoin produce inactive metabolites of vitamin D.

C. Magnesium Deficiency. Results in decreased PTH release and activity; correcting the magnesium deficit will often correct the calcium level.

D. Calcium Loss/Displacement
   1. Hyperphosphatemia. Increases bone deposition of calcium.
      a. Acute phosphate ingestion.
      b. Acute phosphate release by rhabdomyolysis, tumor lysis.
      c. Renal failure: In chronic renal failure decreased levels of 1, 24 dihydroxy vitamin D also contributes to hypocalcemia.
   2. Acute Pancreatitis.
   3. Osteoblastic metastases. Especially breast and prostate.
   4. Medullary carcinoma of the thyroid. Resulting from increased thyrocalcitonin.
   5. Decreased bone resorption. Agents such as actinomycin, calcitonin, mithramycin.

IV. Database
  A. Physical Exam Key Points
   1. Skin. Dermatitis, eczema with chronic hypocalcemia.
   2. HEENT. Cataracts may be present; laryngospasm is rare but life-threatening. Look for surgical scars on the neck.
   3. Neuromuscular. Confusion, spasm, twitching, facial grimacing, hyperactive deep tendon reflexes, and depression.
   4. Specific tests for tetany of hypocalcemia
      a. Chvostek's sign: Present in 5–10% of patients with normal calcium levels. Tap on facial nerve near the zygoma of patient's jaw and observe for twitch.
      b. Trousseau's sign: Inflate a blood pressure cuff higher than systolic pressure for 3 minutes and observe for carpal spasm.

  B. Laboratory Data
   1. Serum electrolytes. Particularly calcium, phosphate, potassium and magnesium. Calcium must be interpreted in terms of the serum albumin. Hypomagnesemia and hyperkalemia may potentiate the symptoms of hypocalcemia.
   2. Serum albumin. Correction of calcium level as previously noted. Low albumin will not affect the ionized calcium levels.

3. **Renal function tests (BUN and creatinine).** May reveal evidence of chronic renal insufficiency.
4. The combination of hypocalcemia with a high serum phosphate usually indicates severe hypoparathyroidism.
5. Parathyroid hormone levels.
6. **Vitamin D levels.** 25 hydroxy and 1,25 dihydroxy vitamin D levels.
7. **Urinary cyclic AMP levels.** This gives an index of parathyroid function and is increased with elevated PTH levels.
8. **Fecal fat.** To evaluate steatorrhea.

C. **Radiologic and Other Tests**
   1. **ECG.** A prolonged QT interval.
   2. **Bone films.** Bone changes in renal failure or osteoblastic metastases.

V. **Plan.** Assess the patient for tetany, which can potentially progress to laryngeal spasm or seizures and requires acute treatment. Otherwise establish the diagnosis by blood tests of calcium, albumin, magnesium, phosphate, and PTH level and begin appropriate oral therapy.

A. **Acute Treatment.** Give 200–300 mg of elemental calcium rapidly.
   1. **10% calcium gluconate.** One 10 ml ampule contains 90 mg of calcium. Give 20–30 ml total IV.
   2. **10% calcium chloride.** One 10 ml ampule contains 360 mg of calcium. Give 10 ml IV (be careful to avoid extravasation, which can cause a skin slough).

B. **Chronic Treatment.** With primary PTH deficiency the goal is to give 2–4 g of oral calcium daily, then add vitamin D if necessary. In vitamin D disorder, supplement with vitamin D. The use of aluminum phosphate gels (eg, ALTernaGEL) will limit phosphate absorption.
   1. **Calcium carbonate.** 240 mg of calcium per 600 mg tablet.
   2. **Os-Cal-500.** A 1.25 g calcium carbonate tablet provides 500 mg of elemental calcium.
   3. **Dihydrotachysterol vitamin D2.** 0.25–1.0 µg/d.

C. **Magnesium Deficiency**
   1. 1–2 g of 10% magnesium sulfate IV over 20 minutes or 40–80 mEq MgSO$_4$/L IV fluid.
   2. Chronic replacement therapy with magnesium oxide 600 mg 1–2 tablets qd.

44. HYPOGLYCEMIA

(See also Section II, page 245)

I. **Problem.** The nurses tell you that a 40-year-old man with a history of type I diabetes mellitus has a serum glucose of 40 mg/dL (normal fasting 70–105 mg/dL).

II. Immediate Questions

A. Is the patient diabetic and on Insulin? A common cause of hypoglycemia is the inadvertent administration of too much insulin to a diabetic, or the administration of insulin to a patient who is not eating.

B. What medication is the patient taking? Are there any oral hypoglycemic medications being given?

C. What IV fluids are running? Has the patient recently been discontinued from hyperalimentation? This can cause a reactive hypoglycemia, although it is quite rare. If still receiving hyperalimentation, is there insulin in the fluid? Is there dextrose in the IV fluids being administered?

D. What is the patient's diagnosis? There are certain disease states associated with hypoglycemia, such as retroperitoneal sarcoma, insulinoma, and paraneoplastic syndromes (especially squamous cell carcinoma of the lung). Pancreatic transplant recipients can have hypoglycemia secondary to dysfunctional autoregulation postoperatively. Patients who are in the postoperative period after liver resection commonly have hypoglycemia because the liver is the site of stored glycogen.

E. What is the patient's clinical state? Is the patient awake, alert, comatose, or diaphoretic? Diaphoresis and tremulousness are usually a manifestation of catecholamine discharge.

III. Differential Diagnosis

A. Medications

1. **Insulin.** Inadvertent administration of an excessive dose, additional dose, wrong preparation, a dose ordered subcutaneously being given IV, or administration to the wrong patient.

2. **Oral hypoglycemic agents.** Tolbutamide, chlorpropamide, acetohexamide, and others.

3. **Others.** Pentamidine, ethanol, and MAO inhibitors are infrequent causes.

B. Severe Liver Failure/Resection Extensive Hepatic Destruction.

C. Insulinoma. Serum insulin levels can be checked.

D. Sudden Discontinuation of TPN. This is more theoretical than an actual problem. In fact, most patients can easily tolerate sudden discontinuation of TPN.

E. Retroperitoneal Sarcoma. These tumors can cause hypoglycemia

F. **Paraneoplastic Syndrome.** Hypoglycemia can be caused by the secretion of insulin or insulin-like substances by tumors, especially small-cell carcinoma of the lung.

G. **Surreptitious Insulin/Oral Hypoglycemic Administration.**

H. **Reactive Functional Hypoglycemia.**

I. **Alimentary Hypoglycemia.** Found in 5–10% of patients who have undergone partial to complete gastrectomies and resulting from rapid gastric emptying time.

J. **Factitious Hypoglycemia.** A rare but possibly confounding diagnosis, it is caused by the utilization of glucose in the red top tube by leukocytes, and found in patients with WBC > 40,000. These patients will have asymptomatic hypoglycemia. Thus, any patients with very high WBC counts should have serum glucose determinations from blood collected in tubes that contain sodium fluoride, which inhibits white cell metabolism.

K. **Hormone Deficiencies.** Glucocorticoids, growth hormone, thyroid hormone, glucagon, panhypopituitarism.

L. **Miscellaneous.** Sepsis, alcoholism or severe malnutrition.

IV. **Database**

A. **Physical Exam Key Points**
    1. **Vital signs.** Tachycardia may be caused by adrenergic response to decreasing glucose levels.
    2. **Skin.** Diaphoresis is also an adrenergic response.
    3. **Neurologic exam.** Orientation, level of consciousness may be altered.

B. **Laboratory Data**
    1. **Serum glucose.** The most important diagnostic test is the serum glucose level. Values < 50 mg/dL are diagnostic in the presence of symptoms. Rapid glucose measurements using reagent strips, glucometers, and fingerstick blood samples may be helpful but should be confirmed with a serum level.
    2. **Urine glucose levels.** Usually of little help in this setting.
    3. **Serum insulin levels.** If insulinoma is suspected, or to detect surreptitious insulin administration.
    4. **C peptide levels.** Detects endogenous insulin production. Elevated C-peptide, with elevated serum insulin levels suggest insulinoma. If the serum insulin is increased and the C peptide level is decreased, insulin overdosage or surreptitious insulin administration is likely.

C. **Radiologic and Other Studies.** May be indicated to diagnose tumors as suspected from the clinical picture. Arteriography is often more useful than CT in localizing pancreatic insulinoma.

V. Plan. In acute cases, increase the serum glucose and eliminate symptoms, then identify the cause.

   A. Administer Glucose. Do not await the results of the serum glucose (drawn before treatment) if you strongly suspect the diagnosis. The mainstay of initial therapy is glucose, given orally if the patient is awake, alert, and able to take fluids or intravenously otherwise.

      1. Oral. Give orange juice with or without additional sugar.

      2. Parenteral. 1 ampule of D50 (dextrose 50%) IV push. If there is no change, repeat the ampule of D50. A failure to respond at this point should lead the clinician to question the diagnosis, especially if the results of a serum glucose determination are not available yet to prove hypoglycemia is the cause of the problem.

      3. When IV access is not possible, glucagon 0.5–1 mg IM or s.c. may be given immediately. Vomiting may occur.

      4. Start maintenance IV of D5W at 50–100 ml/hr to help prevent recurrence of hypoglycemia and follow-up with serial glucose measurements after the initial episode.

   B. Adjust Medications. Reevaluate the current dosing schedule of insulin or other oral hypoglycemic agents.

   C. Workup of Hypoglycemia. After treating the acute episode, diagnostic tests are required to evaluate the patient for the cause of the hypoglycemia. Serum insulin levels, C peptide levels, liver function tests, glucose tolerance tests, and appropriate radiographic tests are to be considered.

   D. Liver Resection. Patients after liver resection should be maintained on IV fluids containing 10% dextrose with frequent serum glucose determinations.

45. HYPOKALEMIA

(See also Section II, page 245)

I. Problem. A 72-year-old man on long-term diuretics for heart failure develops abdominal distention and an ileus. His serum potassium is 2.5 mmol/L (normal 3.5–5.1 mmol/L).

II. Immediate Questions

   A. What medication is the patient taking? Loop diuretics with furosemide—the most typical example—are kaliuretic and cause significant renal potassium wasting. Thiazide diuretics can cause hypokalemia, but the level is rarely dangerous, except when digoxin is used concomitantly. Hypokalemia will potentiate digitalis toxicity. Amphotericin B causes potassium wasting by direct renal toxic effects.

B. Is there a history of vomiting, NG suction, or diarrhea? Gastrointestinal losses are common causes of hypokalemia in the surgical patient.

C. What are the vital signs? Look for irregular pulse, which in the postoperative patient could represent new premature atrial or ventricular contractions (PACs and PVCs) due to increased myocardial irritability.

D. Is the patient symptomatic? Symptoms of hypokalemia include weakness, nausea, vomiting, and abdominal tenderness.

III. Differential Diagnosis

A. Potassium Losses

1. Gastrointestinal

   a. Prolonged NG suction without replacement can cause hypokalemia through direct losses, induced renal losses, and through potassium shifts into cells due to the development of metabolic alkalosis.

   b. Intractable vomiting (same mechanism as NG suction).

   c. Bowel obstruction can result in hypokalemia through the pooling of secretions and inefficient potassium absorption.

   d. Diarrhea, fistula, villous adenoma.

2. Renal

   a. Diuretics: Especially loop diuretics, such as furosemide.

   b. Renal tubular acidosis results in hypokalemia when K^+ is secreted and H^+ is absorbed.

   c. Antibiotics: Carbenicillin, others. Amphotericin B may also cause magnesium wasting.

   d. Postobstructive diuresis or the diuretic phase of acute tubular necrosis (ATN).

B. Potassium Redistribution

1. Alkalosis. Cation balance requires that as H^+ moves out of cells to correct alkalosis, K^+ moves in.

2. Insulin. Insulin administration results in glucose and potassium transport into cells.

C. Inadequate Intake.
Most often iatrogenic (administration of potassium free IV fluids over a prolonged time period). In the absence of other losses, normal daily potassium requirements with normal renal function are 40–60 mEq/24h.

IV. Database.
Because potassium is the principal intracellular cation, hypokalemia usually represents a significant loss of body potassium.

Thus, serum levels of 3.0 mEq/L (mmol/L) often represent total deficits of 100–200 mEq in the adult.

A. Physical Exam Key Points
  1. **Cardiac.** Irregular pulse may represent new arrhythmias (PAC, PVC) or digoxin toxicity.
  2. **Abdomen.** Look for evidence of distention and listen for bowel sounds. Obstruction can cause hypokalemia; rarely, ileus results from hypokalemia and thus exacerbates the condition. Vomiting may cause hypokalemia or indicate digitalis toxicity.
  3. **Neurologic exam.** Severe hypokalemia can cause blunting of reflexes, paresthesias, and paralysis.

B. Laboratory Data
  1. **Serum electrolytes.** Hypocalcemia and hypomagnesemia may coexist.
  2. **Arterial blood gas.** Severe electrolyte abnormalities often have accompanying acid-base defects. Renal tubular acidosis and metabolic alkalosis often result in hypokalemia.
  3. **Urine electrolytes.** Useful only in the patient not taking diuretics, renal wasting can be evaluated by simple "spot" determinations of urine K^+, Na^+, and osmolality (see page 292).
  4. Digoxin level if appropriate.

C. Radiologic and Other Studies. ECG and rhythm strip should be done on the patient with evidence of digitalis toxicity, new PACs, and new PVCs as manifested by a new irregular pulse. T wave flattening, U waves, and S-T segment changes also occur with hypokalemia.

V. Plan. More severe cases of hypokalemia, usually levels < 3.0 mmol/L, or those cases associated with ECG abnormalities should be treated aggressively because of the potential for life-threatening arrhythmias. Aggressive potassium replacement should only be performed after good renal function has been documented.

A. Parenteral Replacement
  1. **Indications.** Should be considered in the following patients: digoxin toxicity or significant arrhythmia, severe hypokalemia (< 3.0 mmol/L), and those who cannot take oral replacement (NPO, ileus, nausea and vomiting). Parenteral administration is ideally given via a central venous catheter. Most hypokalemia can be safely corrected in a slow, controlled fashion with oral supplementation.
  2. **Replacement.** Maximum concentrations of KCl used in peripheral veins should generally not exceed 40 mEq/L because of damaging effects of high concentrations of KCl on the veins, although in an emergent situation 60 mEq/L can be attempted. Between 10 and 20 mEq KCl diluted in 50–100 mL D5W or NS

can be infused over 1 hour through a central line safely, and doses repeated as needed when severe depletion or life-threatening hypokalemia is present. Special care must be taken to ensure slow infusion of these high doses. For lesser degrees of hypokalemia that require parenteral replacement, 10–40 mEq/h can be infused peripherally.

3. **Monitoring.** Check serum levels frequently to avoid hyperkalemia, every 2–4 hours depending on clinical response. ECG/ICU monitoring is required for arrhythmias or for rapid infusions of KCl.

B. **Oral Replacement** (see also Section IX, page 388). Generally indicated for asymptomatic, mild levels of potassium repletion (K usually > 3.0 mEq/L). Oral replacements include liquids and powders. Slow release pills typically contain < 10 mEq/tablet and thus are not usually appropriate for repletion therapy. Replacement doses should be 40–120 mEq/d in divided doses depending on patient's weight and level of hypokalemia. Maintenance therapy, if needed, should be given in doses of 20–40 mEq daily using the preparation best tolerated by the patient. In patients with normal renal function, it is difficult to induce hyperkalemia by the oral administration of potassium. Another important exception is to avoid the use of potassium supplements in patients on potassium sparing diuretics (eg, triamterene, spironolactone, amiloride) to prevent hyperkalemia.

C. **Replace Ongoing Losses.** Large amounts of nasogastric aspirate should be replaced ml for ml with D5 1/2NS with 20 mEq/L KCl every 4–6 hours.

D. **Refractory Cases.** Rarely, hypokalemia may not be correctable because of concomitant hypomagnesemia or hypocalcemia. Replace calcium as described in Problem 39, page 134.

46. HYPONATREMIA

(See also Section II, page 245)

I. **Problem.** An elderly woman admitted for a mastectomy has a sodium of 119 mmol/L on routine admission labs (normal 136–145 mmol/L).

II. **Immediate Questions**

A. **Does the patient have any CNS symptoms relevant to the hyponatremia?** Symptomatic hyponatremia manifests primarily CNS symptoms as brain cells become edematous in a hypo-osmotic state. Inquire about lethargy, agitation, disorientation, or obtundation.

B. Are there any recent prior sodium levels to document the chronicity of the hyponatremia? The rate of development of hyponatremia correlates directly with the severity of symptoms it produces. Acute changes in sodium are more likely to produce severe symptoms.

C. Does the patient take diuretics? A common single cause of hyponatremia is chronic diuretic use.

D. Is the hyponatremia real, or is it a laboratory artifact? Osmotic agents and space-occupying compounds at high concentrations can alter the reported laboratory value of sodium. Note the concentration of glucose and triglycerides and adjust the measured sodium up to true levels as below.

E. Is the patient receiving IV fluids? Overhydration with excess free water is the most common cause of hyponatremia in the surgical patient.

F. Has the patient had recent surgery? Surgery and anesthesia often result in temporary inappropriate ADH secretion and transient hyponatremia.

III. Differential Diagnosis. The initial differentiation is between true hyponatremia and laboratory artifact. Hyponatremia may be classified according to the volume status of the patient: hypovolemic, euvolemic, or hypervolemic. Hypovolemic hyponatremia may be further classified by serum and urine chemistries.

A. Laboratory Artifact (Pseudohyponatremia)
1. **Osmotic agents.** Hyperglycemia is most common. Adjust the serum sodium up 1.6 mEq/L for every excess 100 mg/dL of glucose over the normal value of 100 mg/dL.
2. **Space-occupying compounds.** Lipids (hyperlipidemia) are the most common. The lab can ultracentrifuge the specimen to find the corrected plasma level.

B. Hypovolemic Hyponatremia
1. **Spot urinary Na < 10 mEq/L**
   a. **GI fluid losses:** Vomiting or diarrhea. In surreptitious vomiting or bulimia the urinary chloride is usually < 10 mEq/L.
   b. **Third space fluid loss:** Such as pancreatitis or peritonitis.
   c. Burns.
2. **Urinary Na > 10 mEq/L**
   a. **Diuretic usage:** Caused by thiazides (eg, hydrochlorothiazide) and loop (furosemide) diuretics and often associated with hypokalemia and alkalosis; with surreptitious diuretic use, urinary chloride is > 20 mEq/L.
   b. **Renal disorders:** Medullary cystic disease, polycystic disease, and chronic interstitial nephritis can result in hyponatremia.

      c. Addison's disease: Hyperkalemia and low urinary potassium are also found.

      d. Osmotic diuresis: Most commonly owing to glucose, mannitol, or ketones (as in diabetic ketoacidosis [DKA]).

C. Euvolemic Hyponatremia

  1. SIADH. The diagnosis of SIADH (Syndrome of Inappropriate Antidiuretic Hormone) is based on the finding of low serum osmolality, elevated urine sodium, and slightly concentrated urine (osmolality near sodium).

    a. Postoperative: Anesthesia and surgical procedures cause increased ADH. The transurethral resection of the prostate (TURP) syndrome is caused by excessive fluid absorption during transurethral surgery.

    b. Tumors: Small-cell lung cancer most common.

    c. Pulmonary infections: Such as TB and other bacterial pneumonia.

    d. CNS disorders: Trauma, tumors, and infections.

    e. Stress: Including perioperative stress.

    f. Drugs: Oral hypoglycemics, chemotherapeutics (cyclophosphamide, vincristine), psychiatric drugs (haloperidol, tricyclic antidepressants), and clofibrate.

  2. Hypothyroidism.

  3. Hypopituitarism.

D. Hypervolemic Hyponatremia

  1. Congestive heart failure.

  2. Cirrhosis.

  3. Renal disease.

    a. Chronic renal failure.

    b. Nephrotic syndrome.

  4. Psychogenic polydipsia.

IV. Database

A. Physical Exam Key Points. As apparent by the differential diagnosis, close attention should be paid to the assessment of the volume status.

  1. Vital signs. Evaluate for orthostatic blood pressure changes. Measure supine and standing blood pressures. A drop in blood pressure > 10 mm Hg or a pulse increase of > 10 BPM is highly suggestive of volume depletion. Tachypnea may suggest volume overload and pulmonary edema.

  2. Skin. Tissue turgor will be diminished and mucous membranes dry with dehydration. Edema suggests volume overload. Evidence of cirrhosis is jaundice and caput medusae.

  3. HEENT. Evaluate the internal jugular vein with the bed up at 45 degrees (veins flat with volume depletion and markedly engorged with volume overload).

4. **Lungs.** Rales may be heard with volume overload.
5. **Heart.** An S3 gallop murmur suggests volume overload.
6. **Abdomen.** Hepatosplenomegaly, other evidence of cirrhosis or ascites may be present. A hepatojugular reflex may be present in CHF.
7. **Neurologic exam.** Hyperactive deep tendon reflexes, altered mental status, confusion, coma, or seizures usually indicate a sodium level of < 125 mmol/L.

B. **Laboratory Data**
   1. **Electrolytes.** All electrolyte abnormalities may involve several key electrolytes on the SMA-7.
   2. **Spot urine electrolytes and creatinine.** Obtain before any diuretic treatment.
   3. **Urine and serum osmolality.** Serum osmolality will be normal in cases of laboratory artifact but decreased in true hyponatremia.
   4. **Liver function tests.** To detect liver disease.
   5. **Arterial blood gases.** Acidosis/alkalosis may be present.
   6. Thyroid function.
   7. Cortisol levels, ACTH stimulation test.
   8. Cultures (blood and sputum).

C. **Radiologic and Other Studies**
   1. **Chest x-ray.** Evidence of CHF or a lung tumor.
   2. **Head CT scan** if indicated.
   3. **Water load test.** Bring the serum sodium to a safe level by fluid restriction then challenge with 20 ml/kg of water PO, collect urine hourly for 5 hours. If < 75% of intake volume is excreted or if urine osmolarity fails to decrease to less than 200, then SIADH is present.

V. **Plan.** The underlying cause of the hyponatremia as well as the presence and severity of symptoms guide therapy. Aggressive therapy for severe symptoms (eg, coma) will be discussed as well as specific therapies for certain diagnoses.

A. **Acute Therapy**
   1. **Normal saline and furosemide 1 mg/kg IV.** Use the combination of normal saline and diuretics to achieve a net negative volume balance. Document carefully volume in and volume out. Supplement fluids with potassium as needed.
   2. **Hypertonic saline (3%) is rarely, if ever, needed.** Some institutions have banned its use entirely because of possible serious complications.

B. **Specific Therapies**
   1. **Hypovolemic hyponatremia**
      a. For almost all causes, treat by repleting volume and sodium. (Normal saline IV infusion).

   b. For diuretic abuse repletion of lost body potassium is also needed.

  2. Euvolemic hyponatremia. The patient is not edematous.

    a. SIADH: Water restriction between 800 and 1000 ml daily. Demeclocycline for increased urine Na or urine osmolarity.

    b. Hypothyroidism: Treat with thyroid replacement.

    c. Hypopituitary: Treat with hormone replacement.

  3. Hypervolemic hyponatremia. Patient is edematous. Restrict IV and oral fluids. Check urine sodium—urine sodium low (< 10 mEq/L)

    a. CHF: Treat with digoxin, diuretics, water restriction.

    b. Nephrotic syndrome: Steroids, water restriction, increased protein intake commonly used.

    c. Cirrhosis: Water restriction, diuretics, and portosystemic shunt if indicated. Urine sodium >20 mEq/L.

    d. Renal failure: Treated with water restriction and dialysis if indicated.

47. HYPOTENSION (SHOCK)

Immediate Actions

1. Assess airway and breathing. Intubate if necessary.
2. Assure large bore IV access and begin 500 mL LR bolus.
3. Control external hemorrhage (if present) with direct pressure.
4. Trendelenburg position.
5. See Figure I–12, page 160.

I. Problem. A 40-year-old female who underwent total abdominal hysterectomy earlier that day has a blood pressure of 80/50 mm Hg.

II. Immediate Questions

  A. What is the patient's pulse? In surgical patients particularly, where there is often an induced hypovolemic state, the pulse can give clues as to the cause of hypotension. A high pulse rate indicates cardiovascular response to hypovolemia, whereas a normal pulse is less suggestive of a hypovolemic state.

  B. What have been the blood pressure readings preoperatively? Be sure this is not the patient's resting BP. Again, looking at the pulse helps discern this important point. Always double check any arterial line blood pressure readings with a careful cuff determination.

  C. When was the patient's surgery? If this is the first night postop, then hypovolemia or active bleeding is especially likely.

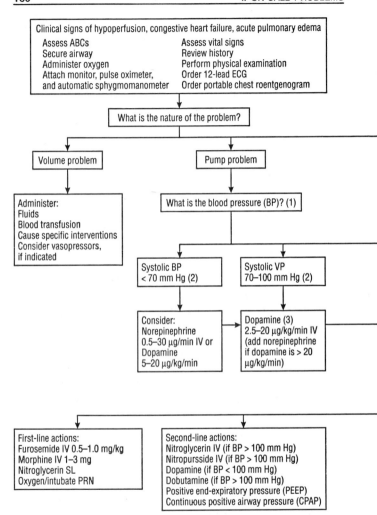

Figure I–12. Algorithm for hypotension, shock, and acute pulmonary edema. *(Reproduced, with permission, from Adult Advanced Cardiac Life Support. JAMA 1992;268, No. 16.)*

Footnotes
(1) Base management after this point on invasive hemodynamic monitoring if possible.
(2) Fluid bolus of 250–500 mL normal saline should be tried. If no response, consider sympathomimetics.
(3) Move to dopamine and stop norepinephrine when BP improves.
(4) Add dopamine when BP improves. Avoid dobutamine when systolic BP < 100 mm Hg.

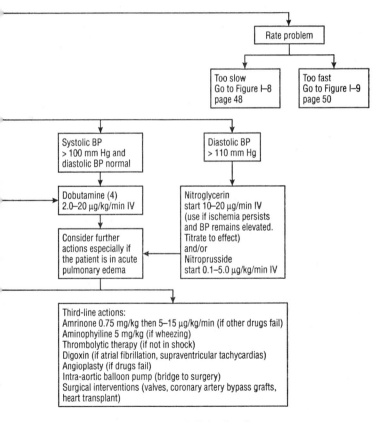

Figure I–12. (*continued*)

D. What is the cardiac rhythm? Abnormal rhythms can cause hypotension, especially atrial fibrillation or flutter. Hypotension with bradycardia suggests heart block.

E. What is the patient's mental status? See if the hypotension is affecting critical organ perfusion.

F. What medication is the patient taking? A patient on ß-blockers can have a lower pulse, which will worsen hypotension by blunting reflex tachycardia. Narcotics and some sedatives can induce hypotension. Anaphylactic reactions may be caused by medications or intravenous contrast agents (see Problem 5, page 19). Epidural anesthesia may occasionally cause hypotension.

G. What is the fluid balance? Urine output gives a clue to the volume status of the patient. A decreasing urine output with hypotension suggests poor renal perfusion. Be sure that the patient has been adequately hydrated and that excessive losses (such as NG drainage) are being replaced.

H. Is there any obvious bleeding source? Inquire about blood on the dressings, bloody NG drainage, increased chest tube, or mediastinal tube output.

I. Addisonian Crisis (Adrenal Insufficiency). Especially after adrenal surgery or radical nephrectomy. Any patient who has taken steroids over the last year may have blunted adrenal response to the stress of surgery.

III. Differential Diagnosis. As a rule of thumb, a blood pressure of < 90 mm Hg in an adult is considered hypotension. Hypotension may cause shock, a state characterized by inadequate tissue perfusion. Shock can be classified as hypovolemic, neurogenic, vasogenic, and cardiogenic. Each type is presented below:

A. Hypovolemic. A condition often seen in surgical patients.

1. **Hemorrhagic**

   a. **Traumatic:** Patients in shock often have significant blood loss that either may not be readily apparent (chest, abdomen, retroperitoneal; into fracture sites such as the pelvis, long bones; or into soft tissues) or obvious external bleeding.

   b. **Postoperative:** Internal hemorrhage postoperatively or direct exsanguination through surgically placed drains, etc.

   c. **Others:** Disseminated intravascular coagulation, GI tract bleeding, ruptured aneurysms. Ruptured ovarian cyst or ectopic pregnancy should be suspected in female patients.

2. **Fluid losses.** Severe vomiting, diarrhea, sweating, extensive burns, and "third space losses" (eg, pancreatitis, bowel obstruction). It can also be a result of inadequate hydration during

surgery with continued vasodilatation and evaporative losses from an open abdomen.

B. Neurogenic. Seen in patients with spinal cord trauma characterized by hypotension and a normal pulse. These patients will usually have normal urine output after fluid administration. They may require large amounts of fluid owing to loss of sympathetic tone.

C. Vasogenic. Septic shock, anaphylactic reactions, or adrenocortical insufficiency may cause decreased vascular tone (low systemic vascular resistance, see page 329). In surgical patients, septic shock is most frequently this type; usually a hyperdynamic state with high cardiac output and low peripheral vascular resistance.

D. Cardiogenic. "Pump failure" (usually due to MI or cardiomyopathy), arrhythmia (atrial fibrillation, complete heart block), tension pneumothorax, or pulmonary embolus can lead to cardiogenic shock. Lesions such as pericardial tamponade, aortic valve disease (late), and septal rupture can also present with hypotension.

IV. Database

A. Physical Exam Key Points

1. **Vital signs.** Confirm arterial line pressure readings with a cuff pressure to rule out technical errors. Tachycardia is the usual response to hypotension, with bradycardia suggesting heart block. Irregularity of the pulse suggests an arrhythmia. Tachypnea may indicate hypoxia or acidosis resulting from poor perfusion or early sepsis. Fever might suggest sepsis; however, elderly or immunosuppressed patients may be afebrile in the face of sepsis. Occasionally, hypothermia may be a sign of sepsis.

2. **Skin.** Good skin turgor and moist mucous membranes are clinical signs of hydration; cool, clammy skin may indicate shock.

3. **Neck.** Check for jugular venous distention. Bulging neck veins are compatible with congestive failure, pericardial tamponade, or tension pneumothorax.

4. **Chest.** Rales suggest congestive heart failure; wheezing and stridor with anaphylaxis; decreased breath sounds may indicate hemothorax or pneumothorax. Rib fractures may be associated with hemo- or pneumothorax and sternal tenderness with pericardial tamponade (such as in steering wheel trauma).

5. **Cardiac.** Check for new murmurs, arrhythmias, or rubs. Heart sounds may be muffled with cardiac tamponade.

6. **Abdomen.** Distention, pulsatile mass, flank ecchymoses, or active bleeding at drain sites or wound dressings may suggest the cause.

7. **Rectal exam.** Gross (hematochezia) or occult blood.
8. **Pelvic exam.** Pelvic fractures can result in a large amount of blood loss. Pelvic exam in females may reveal gynecologic cause.
9. **Extremities.** Absent or "thready" pulses are consistent with shock; long bone fractures (especially femur) may result in significant bleeding into soft tissues. Examine IV sites for evidence of infection. Edema is often seen with CHF.
10. **Neurologic exam.** Mental status alterations suggest poor central perfusion. Loss of motor and sensation functions with spinal cord trauma.

B. Laboratory Data
1. **Hemogram.** Serial hematocrit determinations are essential, because the hematocrit may not drop for some time after an acute bleed.
2. **Serum electrolytes.** Addisonian crisis causes hyperkalemia with hyponatremia.
3. **Coagulation panel (PT, PTT, platelet count).** If excessive bleeding due to DIC is suspected, fibrinogen and fibrin split products.
4. **Arterial blood gases.** Early sepsis may result in respiratory alkalosis; acidosis may indicate inadequate tissue perfusion; hypoxia may require ventilatory support.
5. **Cardiac injury panel.** CPK (q8h times 3) and LDH (q12h times 3) isoenzymes may reveal evidence of myocardial injury (see Section II, page 245).
6. **Pregnancy test.** Especially if a ruptured ectopic pregnancy is suspected.
7. **Blood.** Should be set up immediately. Type and cross.

C. Radiologic and Other Studies
1. **Chest x-ray.** Look for evidence of CHF, cardiac enlargement, pneumothorax, or hemothorax.
2. **ECG.** Myocardial ischemia may show flipped T waves or S-T segment depression; arrhythmias may be noted.
3. **Pulmonary artery catheter.** A PA catheter is helpful in managing the patient in whom fluid overload would be particularly dangerous. By using a PA catheter, filling pressures are measured directly, avoiding iatrogenic pulmonary edema. Can also help differentiate cardiogenic from hypovolemic or vasogenic causes. For diagnostic and insertion details, see Section III, page 295.
4. **Angiogram.** May help identify bleeding sites (especially for GI tract bleeding). A pulmonary angiogram may be needed to diagnose pulmonary embolism with an equivocal V/Q scan.
5. **Nuclear ventilation/perfusion (V/Q) scan.** To diagnose pulmonary embolus.
6. **Echocardiogram.** To examine valves (mitral stenosis, aortic insufficiency, etc), pericardial fluid, and intracardiac thrombi.

      7. Blood, sputum, urine cultures. In cases of suspected sepsis.

      8. Peritoneal tap, thoracentesis, or culdocentesis if indicated (see Section III, page 295).

V. Plan. Reestablish adequate tissue perfusion as soon as possible if the patient is in shock. In general, a blood pressure of > 90 mm Hg and urine output of at least 0.5 mL/kg/min is acceptable.

  A. Emergency Management. See Figure I–12 page 160 for useful algorithm.

    1. Control external hemorrhage with direct pressure.

    2. Establish good venous access, and closely monitor the patient in shock.

    3. Trendelenburg position (supine with feet higher than head) may improve cerebral perfusion and blood pressure immediately. Pneumatic antishock garment (PASG or MAST suit) is useful in the trauma patient with acute blood loss.

    4. Except for cardiogenic shock, replace volume immediately with IV crystalloid (normal saline, lactated Ringer's, etc).

    5. Foley catheter for urinary output monitoring

    6. Supplemental oxygen or ventilatory support if needed. Correct severe acidosis with IV sodium bicarbonate.

    7. CVP line or PA catheter to better manage volume replacement and accurately diagnose the cause of the shock.

  B. Hypovolemic Shock. Restore intravascular volume.

    1. Place two large bore (18 gauge or larger) IVs.

    2. Administer fluids. Use blood if the hematocrit is low or crystalloids (normal saline or lactated Ringer's) if blood is not available or if hematocrit is "acceptable" (ie, > 35%).

    3. Titrate fluids by following blood pressure and urine output.

    4. A PA catheter may help guide fluid administration. A CVP line is useful for following trends in the pressure reading. Avoid using central venous lines as resuscitation lines. A short, large bore peripheral line will allow a much faster rate of fluid administration.

    5. Do not use pressor agents (eg, dopamine) unless there is persistent hypotension despite adequate cardiac filling pressures ("a full tank," wedge pressure > 12 mm Hg). Hypotension with low filling pressures (wedge pressure < 6 mm Hg) are initially treated with intravenous fluids. A CVP or PA catheter is necessary for monitoring when using pressor agents.

    6. With good filling pressures and adequate cardiac output, the next step is peripheral vasoconstrictors such as epinephrine or Levophed in a patient who is still hypotensive.

  C. Neurogenic Shock

    1. Use moderate IV fluids to avoid volume overload.

   2. Low dose vasopressors (dopamine) may help support blood
   pressure.
   3. A major neurologic injury may not be obvious at the time of presentation in an unconscious trauma patient.
 D. Vasogenic Shock
   1. Septic shock. Treatment is directed at the underlying sepsis.
      a. Measure cardiac output and systemic vascular resistance
      (typically high cardiac output with low systemic resistance)
      with a PA catheter (see Section III, page 295).
      b. Administer IV fluids to support pressure and urine output.
      c. Culture aggressively to identify source.
      d. Treat the underlying cause of sepsis. Initiate appropriate an-
      tibiotics, consider laparotomy or percutaneous drainage of
      an abscess if indicated.
      e. Use pressors as needed. First line is often dopamine.
      Dopamine is discussed in Section IX, page 388. The lowest
      effective dose of dopamine to maintain blood pressure and
      urine output should be used. Physiologic effects of
      dopamine are as follows:

         3–5 µg/kg/min - Renal and splanchnic vasodilatation via
            dopamine receptors
         5–10 µg/kg/min - Positive inotrope via ß-1-receptors
         > 10 µg/kg/min - Peripheral vasoconstriction via α-
            receptors.

   2. Anaphylactic shock, see Problem 5, page 19.
 E. Cardiogenic Shock
   1. Cardiac output is maximized by the judicious use of inotropic
   (dopamine or dobutamine) agents. Dobutamine is the drug of
   choice for pump failure. The severe pulmonary edema is
   treated with diuretics (eg, furosemide) and vasodilators (eg, nitrates).
   2. Myocardial ischemia is treated with oxygen, pain relief (morphine), and nitrates acutely.
   3. Arrhythmia is identified and treated appropriately to return to
   normal sinus rhythm.
   4. Pulmonary embolus (see Problem 24, page 91).

48. HYPOXIA

 I. Problem. An intubated patient has become hypoxic after the morning
   chest x-ray and is not responding to 100% FIO_2.

 II. Immediate Questions
   A. Are the monitoring devices accurately connected? Visually inspect the patient for cyanosis and respiratory distress. Cardiac
   monitor and continuous pulse oximeter should be applied.

B. **Is the airway secure?** With repositioning the patient for chest x-ray, the endotracheal tube may have been advanced into the right mainstem bronchus, or the cuff may be ruptured or above the vocal cords necessitating repositioning the endotracheal tube or reintubating the patient.

C. **Are the breath sounds equal?** Absence of breath sounds indicates lung collapse, pneumothorax, or mucous plug.

D. **Is the chest moving symmetrically?** Pain from rib fracture, lung injury, or incision can cause splinting and decreased air movement.

E. **Does the patient have a history of pulmonary disease or congestive heart failure?** Knowledge of prior pulmonary disease or medications may be helpful.

F. **Is the patient alert?** Severe hypoxia will alter mental functions. Opioid overdose may cause hypoventilation.

III. **Differential Diagnosis.** Alveolar-arterial (A-a or A-aDO$_2$) gradient is useful to determine the cause as well as the severity of the oxygenation defect (see following section, "Database"). It is of most use in the ventilated patient.

A. **Low Inspired Oxygen Tension.** Seen in high altitude situations such as mountain climbing or improper ventilator settings. Normal A-a gradient.

B. **Hypoventilation.** Central nervous system depression from drug overdose or CVA, spinal cord injury, chest wall failure from circumferential burns, splinting, neuromuscular disease (Guillain-Barré, myasthenia gravis, tetanus), as a compensatory mechanism for metabolic alkalosis, airway obstruction. Normal A-a gradient.

C. **Diffusion Impairment.** Carbon monoxide poisoning, pulmonary fibrosis. Increased A-a gradient.

D. **Ventilation.** Perfusion imbalance. There is perfusion of nonventilated alveoli pulmonary embolism, fat emboli, pneumonia, COPD, ARDS, pulmonary contusion, asthma, atelectasis, TB, pneumothorax. Increased A-a gradient.

E. **Right to Left Shunt.** Pulmonary edema, nitroglycerin, cardiac anomalies (PDA = patent ductus arteriosus; PFO = patient foramen ovale; ASD = arterial septal defect; VSD = ventricular septal defect.) Increased A-a gradient.

IV. **Database**

A. **Physical Exam Key Points**

1. **Vital signs.** Is the hypoxia associated with tachy- or bradycar-

dia? What is the respiratory rate? Is the patient hypo- or hypertensive? Tachypnea, tachycardia, and hypertension are common early indicators of respiratory distress.

2. **Chest.** Careful auscultation for equal breath sounds to identify pneumothorax, intubation of right mainstem bronchus, consolidation, or mucus plugging. Poor air movement and wheezing with asthma. Palpate for rib fractures.

3. **Heart.** Murmur suggesting valvular disease, signs of CHF.

4. **Skin and nailbeds.** Look for cyanosis, signs of emboli.

5. **CNS.** Confusion and agitation are signs of inadequate CNS perfusion.

6. **Respiratory equipment.** Inspect for loose connections, incorrect settings.

B. Laboratory Data

1. Arterial blood gas and mixed venous blood gas.

2. **Hematocrit.** Check for anemia.

3. **Cardiac enzymes** if MI suspected.

4. **Alveolar-arterial gradient** (A-a or A-aDO$_2$) is a useful calculated value that determines the difference in the alveolar oxygen and the arterial oxygen content in the pulmonary capillary bed. Normal is 20–65 mm Hg on 100% O$_2$

   a. Place patient on 100% O$_2$ (FIo$_2$ = 1.0) for 20 minutes.

   b. Obtain peripheral ABG.

   c. A-a gradient in mm Hg = Atmospheric pressure (760 mm Hg) minus partial pressure of H$_2$O (47 at 37°C) minus arterial Pco$_2$ minus arterial Po$_2$.

   d. The larger the gradient the more severe the defect. Gradients greater than 400 mm Hg are severe.

C. Radiologic and Other Studies

1. **Chest x-ray.** To evaluate pneumothorax, pleural effusion, pulmonary edema, and to check position of endotracheal tube.

2. **ECG.** Acute myocardial infarction will decrease cardiac output, right heart strain may indicate pulmonary embolism.

3. Nuclear ventilation-perfusion scan, followed by pulmonary angiography if pulmonary embolism is suspected.

4. **Chest CT.** If indicated. Obviously this should be obtained only after a complete evaluation and correction of the acute problem and stabilization of the patient.

V. Plan. Overall, the underlying cause should be ascertained while improving patient oxygenation. The patient should be transferred to a monitored setting.

A. Increase FIo$_2$. Numerous respiratory aids are available to provide any desired oxygen level, for example, nasal cannula, ventimask, or face tent. If there is any question about the patient's ability to protect their airway or maintain sufficient ventilation on their own, the patient should be intubated and mechanical ventilation begun. When an acceptable level of oxygenation has been achieved, wean the F_{IO_2} back as tolerated. Remember that oxygen at high concentrations can lead to atelectasis (by eliminating nitrogen from alveoli) and oxygen toxicity.

B. Pneumothorax or other mechanical problems should be diagnosed and treated as rapidly as possible. Chest tube and endotracheal tube insertion or manipulation should be followed by a chest x-ray to ensure proper position.

C. Airway Care. Suctioning, postural drainage.

D. Atelectasis. Chest physiotherapy, incentive spirometry, increase tidal volume, PEEP.

E. Bronchodilators. Relieve bronchospasm and increase clearance of secretions. Inhalational metaproterenol, IV theophylline and oral or subcutaneous terbutaline are the most commonly used agents. Asthma refractory to these may require steroids.

F. Other Medications. Antibiotics, inotropic agents, anticoagulation as indicated.

49. INABILITY TO VOID (URINARY RETENTION)

I. Problem. A 66-year-old man with severe suprapubic pain presents to the emergency room after not being able to void for almost 24 hours.

II. Immediate Questions

A. What are the patient's vital signs? Fever and tachycardia may be signs of acute bacterial prostatitis.

B. What medication is the patient taking? Pharmacologic causes of acute urinary retention are common and discussed further below.

C. Is there any history of voiding problems, such as hesitancy, urgency, frequency, or nocturia? These symptoms are suggestive of bladder outlet obstruction in males (prostatic hypertrophy, stricture). If gross hematuria is present, it may suggest possible clot retention.

D. Has the patient had recent surgery? Patients who have had recent prostate or bladder surgery may rebleed in the postoperative period and develop clot retention; patients who have had abdominoperineal resection can develop a neurogenic bladder. In general, after any surgical procedure (but especially with her니orrhaphy or anorectal surgery) the patient may develop retention due to pain and increased sympathetic outflow (closes bladder neck) in the immediate postop period.

E. Is there a history of neurologic problems? Disk herniation, spinal cord injury, and stroke can affect bladder function.

III. Differential Diagnosis

A. Pharmacologic. Medications that cause retention include major tranquilizers (phenothiazines), antihypertensives (ganglionic blockers, methyldopa), anticholinergic agents (cold preparations), and narcotics.

B. Neurologic. Pelvic or lumbar spine trauma can result in urinary retention (detrusor contraction is dysfunctional while bladder sensation is intact). Causes, in addition to trauma, are after pelvic surgery (APR), and in neuromuscular diseases, and these often resolve with time. Other common situations where temporary acute urinary retention is seen are after spinal anesthesia and following operative procedures performed in the inguinal or genital region.

C. Anatomic. In the elderly man with acute retention, prostatic enlargement, either benign or malignant, should be immediately considered. Other anatomic causes include acute prostatitis (obtain history of perineal pain and fever) and urethral stricture (history of episodes of sexually transmitted diseases or instrumentation), especially in young patients. A psychiatric patient may present with foreign body obstruction. With a history consistent with urolithiasis (flank pain radiating to the groin, nausea and vomiting) consider an obstructing calculus at the bladder neck. Gross hematuria can result in clot retention. Usually owing to pelvic fracture, urethral disruption (eg, blood at the meatus, "floating prostate") may cause retention in the trauma patient.

IV. Database. History should include medications, infections, previous operative and urologic procedures, psychiatric history, and recent trauma or injury.

A. Physical Exam Key Points
1. **Rectal exam.** Specifically determine the presence of focal or generalized prostatic enlargement. Tenderness may indicate prostatitis. Note quality of anal sphincter tone as an indicator of pelvic nerve function. A high riding "floating" prostate may indicate urethral disruption.
2. **Genital exam.** Look for purulent (infectious) or bloody (traumatic) meatal discharge.

3. **Abdomen.** Gentle palpation and percussion of the lower abdomen will reveal bladder distention.
4. **Neurologic.** Determine presence of normal deep tendon reflexes, cremasteric reflex, and of normal local sensation, presence of the "anal wink" (squeezing the glans penis will result in involuntary contraction of the anal sphincter, indicating an intact pelvic reflex arc).

B. **Laboratory Data**
   1. **Hemogram.** WBC elevation may indicate infection (prostatitis).
   2. **Serum electrolytes, BUN, creatinine.** Long-standing and acute retention can lead to renal dysfunction.
   3. **Urinalysis and urine culture.** Note the presence of blood or crystals. A positive urine culture is almost always seen in acute bacterial prostatitis.
   4. Culture urethral discharge.

C. **Radiologic and Other Studies**
   1. **Excretory urography.** Especially if blood is found on urinalysis or if urolithiasis is suspected. If the creatinine is elevated, ultrasound is a better test to evaluate for upper tract obstruction.
   2. **Retrograde urethrogram.** Indicated to evaluate for urethral stricture or urethral disruption.
   3. **Cystoscopy.** Indicated in most patients with anatomic and neurologic causes for retention. Usually performed after Foley catheter decompression.

V. **Plan**

A. **Catheterization (see page 298).** First, attempt decompression by passing a 16–18 Fr Foley catheter gently. If this fails, a coude tip (elbow tip) catheter sometimes passes more readily in males. Injection of 30 mL of water soluble jelly into the urethra may also help pass the catheter. Rarely will filiform and followers or a suprapubic cystostomy be required. Complete decompression should be performed gradually. Catheterization must not be performed in the trauma patient unless urethral disruption has been ruled out with a retrograde urethrogram.

B. **Antibiotics.** Urinary tract infections or sepsis and acute prostatitis will require treatment with appropriate antibiotics. Cultures should be obtained before initiating treatment.

C. **Fluid and Electrolyte Management.** Care should be taken to monitor serum electrolytes, especially if postobstructive diuresis follows decompression of the urinary tract obstruction. This will not be a significant concern with acute retention caused by spinal anesthesia, operation, or prostatitis, but it is seen especially in the setting of chronic obstruction resulting from prostatic hypertrophy.

Patients with elevated BUN and creatinine are more prone to this problem. The diuresis is due to impaired concentrating ability of the chronically obstructed kidneys and the osmotic diuresis caused by the chronic retention of waste products. Untreated postobstructive diuresis can result in vascular collapse due to hypovolemia. After the bladder is decompressed, monitor urine output and vitals closely. Initially, use maintenance IV fluids without potassium. Physiologic diuresis is common, but significant urine output associated with hypotension suggests a postobstructive problem. Check electrolytes and replace mL/mL with IV fluid similar to the urine electrolyte profile. Then gradually change to ½ mL/mL and taper IV from there.

D. Postoperative. Once ambulatory, many patients will be able to void without difficulty. This is especially true in patients who have undergone painful groin or anorectal procedures. Limiting pain medications may help. Alpha-blockers (terazosin, doxazosin) may help relax the bladder neck and help return voiding pattern.

E. Cystoscopy. Cystoscopy and urodynamic studies are usually performed in this setting, but are rarely needed in acute cases.

50. INSOMNIA

I. Problem. A patient hospitalized for 14 days of intravenous antibiotics for fasciitis complains of lying awake for hours at night.

II. Immediate Questions

A. Is the patient bothered by pain? Most surgical patients experience some degree of pain, either postoperatively or related to the admission diagnosis. Painful stimuli coupled with the disruptive situation of being in the hospital (noise, interruptions, roommates, strange bed) can understandably produce insomnia. Make sure a patient is receiving adequate pain medication in addition to sleeping medication.

B. What are the patient's sleep habits during the day? Certainly if a patient sleeps for extended periods during the day, he or she won't be able to drop off to sleep at night. Discuss this matter with the patient and with the social service and recreational therapy departments (if available).

C. Does the patient routinely take sleeping medications? Virtually all sleeping medications show a tolerance effect and a disruption of the sleep patterns that can lead to less restful sleep with chronic usage. Take a detailed drug history to evaluate the contribution of withdrawal or tolerance to the insomnia.

D. Does the patient have difficulty lying down? Ask specifically about shortness of breath (orthopnea) and calf pain (ischemic rest pain) as causes for disrupted sleep.

E. What is the patient's sleep pattern? Early morning awakening is associated commonly with depression. Anxiety usually causes difficulty in getting to sleep.

III. Differential Diagnosis

A. Medical Causes
1. **Pain.** Inadequate control is often correctable.
2. **Congestive heart failure.** Orthopnea is the hallmark.
3. **Peripheral vascular disease.** Ischemic rest pain indicates advanced disease.
4. Hyperthyroidism.
5. **Sleep apnea syndrome.** Most often seen with morbid obesity. Patients often awaken with a sense of panic and complain of chronic lethargy.

B. Drug/Toxin
1. Tolerance to sleeping medications or tranquilizers.
2. **Alcohol abuse.** With secondary chronic disruption of appropriate sleep patterns.

C. Psychiatric
1. **Depressive illness.** Either bipolar or unipolar.
2. Anxiety.

D. Situational
1. **Noise.** Close to nursing station or a noisy roommate.
2. **Anger.** Unexpressed anger towards staff or family.
3. **Anxiety.** Either appropriate or inappropriate anxiety about medical condition, possible operation or discharge.

IV. Database. The most important portion of the database in insomnia is the history, including an evaluation of the mental status of the patient. Other studies add little except in rare cases.

A. Physical Exam Key Points
1. **Neurologic exam.** Mental status. Evaluation for anxiety or depression.
2. **Cardiopulmonary.** Evidence of rales, displaced PMI, gallop rhythm to suggest CHF.
3. **Extremities.** Decreased or absent pulses, pallor on elevation, dependent rubor.

B. Laboratory Data. Many times the cause of insomnia will be determined without the use of laboratory tests.
1. **Screening chemistries.** Include hepatic and renal function.

     2. Thyroid hormone levels. If clinically indicated.

C. Radiologic and Other Studies
1. Chest x-ray if indicated for cough or CHF.
2. Ankle/brachial blood pressure or other vascular studies if indicated.
3. Sleep lab for chronic sleeping difficulty and to rule out sleep apnea.

V. Plan

A. Etiology. Attempt to determine the cause of the insomnia, whether medical, psychologic, or situational causes. Most cases will be secondary to a situational cause or just being in the hospital. For this reason it is wise to include a prn sleeping medication order with all admission and postop orders unless specifically contraindicated. Any specific medical problem should be treated and pain should be adequately controlled.

B. Specific Treatments
1. **Oral sleeping medication.** Frequently used agents are:
   a. Diphenhydramine (Benadryl) 25–50 mg PO
   b. Temazepam (Restoril) 15–30 mg.
   c. Flurazepam (Dalmane) 15–30 mg. Used to be standard order. Found to have prolonged and cumulative effects and triazolam is becoming new standard.
   d. Chloral hydrate 500–1000 mg.
   e. Triazolam (Halcion) 0.125 or 0.25 mg PO. Use 0.125 for elderly.
   f. Zolpidem (Ambien) 5 or 10 mg PO. A new nonbenzodiazepine agent that does not distort the natural sleep cycle.
2. **Nonoral sleeping medications**
   a. Chloral hydrate 500–1000 mg per rectum.
   b. Nembutal 100 mg per rectum.
3. **Nonmedical treatments.** Often as effective and may include discussing apprehensions with the patient or having the patient's room changed.
4. **Sleep apnea** is usually managed by nighttime nasal CPAP support.

51. IRREGULAR PULSE

Immediate Actions
1. Assess Airway, Breathing, Circulation. Intubate if necessary. Check vital signs. Administer O_2.
2. Assess impact on hemodynamic stability. Hypotension associated with arrhythmia requires rapid action.
3. Assure IV access.

I. **Problem.** On routine check of vital signs, a nurse discovers that a 75-year-old man, status post BK amputation, has an irregular pulse.

II. **Immediate Questions**

A. **What is the pulse rate?** The pulse rate can give clues to the nature of the arrhythmia. For instance, the ventricular rate in atrial fibrillation is rarely greater than 150, whereas supraventricular tachycardias are usually greater than 150.

B. **What are the other vital signs?** You must know if the irregular pulse is associated with hemodynamic instability (hypotension).

C. **What medication is the patient taking?** Be especially careful to note cardiac medications or diuretics, which can induce hypokalemia.

D. **Is there a history of cardiac disease?** Prior heart disease may be a clue to the cause. Check for history or previous documentation of irregular rhythm. Postoperative arrhythmias are rare in individuals younger than ages 40–45. Mitral stenosis is often seen with atrial fibrillation.

E. **Is the rhythm regular, irregular, irregularly irregular?** The rhythm can give a clue about the nature of the problem. While an ECG is necessary to formally evaluate rhythm, a quick check of the pulse is helpful.

III. **Differential Diagnosis.** Remember that an irregular pulse is a result of a disease process, not a diagnosis.

A. **Impulse Formation Disorders**
1. **Premature atrial and ventricular contractions.**
2. **Sinus arrhythmia.** A benign variation of pulse.
3. **Escape beats.** Seen especially in bradycardias.
4. **Extrasystoles.** Has a constant interval between a sinus beat and the extrasystole. Abolished by exercise.
5. **Atrial fibrillation.** Commonly associated with many types of underlying heart disease (ischemic, valvular). Absent P waves on the cardiogram, as well as an irregularly irregular ventricular rate, and flutter waves may also be seen.
6. **Pacemaker malfunction.**
7. **Sick sinus syndrome.**
8. **Paroxysmal atrial tachycardia with variable block.** The atrial rate is 140–250 with a variable ventricular response.

B. **Conduction Disorders**
1. **Sinoatrial block.** Can be associated with ischemia or caused by digoxin.
2. **Partial AV block.** Mobitz type I (Wenckebach) or type II second degree block.

       3. Pulsus alternans. Regular rhythm with alternation in amplitude of equally spaced beats.

  C. Myocardial Ischemia. The first evidence of asymptomatic ischemic myocardium (or infarction) is often an arrhythmia.

  D. Pulmonary Disease. Pulmonary embolus can present as atrial fibrillation or other arrhythmia.

  E. Pericardial Disease. Constrictive pericarditis and tamponade can cause irregular pulse.

IV. Database

  A. Physical Exam Key Points

    1. Vital signs. Pulse regularity and rate; tachypnea may suggest pulmonary embolism.

    2. Heart. A rub is associated with pericarditis or a transmural infarction, murmurs suggest valvular disease.

    3. Neck. Look for jugular atrial waves, venous distention.

    4. Blood pressure. Check for pulsus paradoxus—associated with constrictive pericarditis, pericardial tamponade, or severe asthma. The pulse appears grossly irregular at first, but is easily related to respiratory variations. A positive test shows a greater than 10 mm Hg fall in blood pressure with inspiration, measured by cuff.

  B. Laboratory Data

    1. Electrolytes. Electrolyte abnormalities, especially potassium, can cause a variety of arrhythmias.

    2. Arterial blood gases. Hypoxia can cause arrhythmias and may be associated with pulmonary embolism.

    3. Cardiac Panel (CPK, LDH, isoenzymes, AST). To look for evidence of myocardial ischemia.

    4. Digoxin level. In the patient already on digoxin.

    5. Other drug levels (quinidine, procainamide) as indicated.

    6. Thyroid hormone levels. Hyperthyroidism can lead to arrhythmias (T_4, TSH).

  C. Radiologic and Other Studies

    1. 12-lead electrocardiogram. This is essential to evaluate any arrhythmia. Atrial fibrillation will be an obvious diagnosis on ECG. Look for signs of acute ischemia. Compare to old ECGs.

    2. Chest x-ray. Look for signs of congestive failure, cardiomegaly, primary pulmonary disease, pneumothorax, etc.

    3. ECG. Identify intracardiac mural thrombus in a patient with chronic atrial fibrillation, valvular disease, or pericardial effusion.

    4. Nuclear ventilation/perfusion (V/Q) scan. If pulmonary embolus is suspected.

V. Plan

  A. Overall Plan. Eliminate the arrhythmia by treating the underlying cause. It is imperative to rapidly treat any patient who is hemodynamically compromised (hypotensive) or symptomatic (shortness of breath or chest pain) from the arrhythmia. An otherwise stable patient can be treated more conservatively.

  1. Start O_2 on any patient with an arrhythmia.

  2. IV access should be established if not already present.

  B. Specific Plans. Drug dosages are discussed in detail in Section IX, page 388.

  1. Sinus arrhythmia. No treatment needed.

  2. Atrial fibrillation

  a. Treat underlying electrolyte imbalance or hypoxia.

  b. Administer digoxin.

  i. Give 1.0 mg over 24 hours in divided doses as 0.5 mg, then 0.25 mg, then 0.25 mg.

  ii. Follow with a maintenance dose.

  iii. If rate control is imperative, the 1.0 mg may be given more rapidly.

  iv. Adjust dose for patient size as well as patients in renal failure.

  c. Administer verapamil 0.25 mg IV push; can repeat in 10 minutes if rate control still not achieved.

  d. Pronestyl can be used for chemical cardioversion after treatment with digoxin. Quinidine can be useful. These medications may be helpful in maintaining a sinus rhythm also.

  e. A patient with hemodynamic compromise should be electrically cardioverted.

  3. Pulmonary embolus

  a. Diagnosed by nuclear ventilation/perfusion scan.

  b. If a question of pulmonary embolus exists with a negative or "low probability" scan, then obtain a pulmonary angiogram—the "gold standard" of diagnosis of pulmonary embolus.

  c. Treat with heparin (bolus followed by constant drip to maintain PTT > 1.5.2 times control) or streptokinase.

  4. Myocardial infarction. The usual supportive therapy is indicated: monitor, oxygen, pain relief (morphine), nitrates, and prophylactic lidocaine.

52. INTRAVENOUS ACCESS PROBLEMS

  I. Problem. A 40-year-old intravenous drug abuser enters the hospital with abdominal pain and protracted vomiting. No veins on the arms are usable for rehydration due to scarring.

II. Immediate Questions

A. What is the nature of the patient's illness? Patients requiring immediate IV access (eg, hypotension with shock) should undergo percutaneous central line placement or cutdown in the absence of large peripheral veins. Do not waste time looking for small peripheral veins.

B. Is there a history of IV drug abuse or history of prolonged hospitalization and loss of venous access? What routes of access were used on other occasions? Chronically hospitalized patients often lose usable peripheral veins because of multiple IV and venipunctures.

III. Differential Diagnosis. Peripheral intravenous access may be poor in the following situations:

A. Intravenous Drug Abuse.

B. Obesity.

C. Prior Chemotherapy.

D. Prolonged Hospitalization. Numerous IV Lines in the Past.

E. Lymphedema. After mastectomy or axillary lymphadenectomy for other reasons.

F. Anasarca.

G. Hypotension and Hypovolemia.

IV. Database

A. Physical Exam Key Points

1. **Upper extremities.** Look for needle marks indicating previous IV access. Look for antecubital vein.
2. **Vital signs.** Hypotension or other signs of shock often cause peripheral veins to collapse.

B. Laboratory Data. Usually are not helpful in solving the problem.

V. Plan. IV access should be approached in the following order in both elective and emergent situations. In emergencies, evaluation should be undertaken quickly to provide rapid access (see also Section III, pages 300, 312, 332).

A. Peripheral (Arm). Start distally and work proximally. These are standard IV lines, and are the lines of choice in trauma situations because 14–16 gauge catheters allow for massive fluid repletion, more so than central lines. Antecubital lines can be used, although the immobilization of the elbow can result in discomfort. For elective IV line placement, the following can be attempted: Use a blood pressure cuff inflated to just above systolic for 5–10 minutes and then release. This often causes a reflex that dilates the extremity veins. Alternatively, place warm towels or a heating pad on the arm for a few minutes to dilate the veins. Lower extremity lines should be avoided because they do not work well or last for more than a few hours with patients who are ambulatory and have a higher incidence of thrombophlebitis.

B. External Jugular. Simple 1–2″ angiocatheters can be placed in the external jugular vein without difficulty and with little or no patient risk. Placing the patient in the Trendelenburg (head down) position and gently occluding the vein just above the clavicle will usually dilate it.

C. Central Lines. Percutaneous puncture should be attempted in the following order:
   1. Internal jugular (IJ).
   2. Subclavian.
   3. Femoral (technically not central).
   Experience with a particular route of access, however, is also an important determinant.

   IJ and subclavian lines are useful for measuring central venous pressure. Many people believe that femoral lines should be used rarely because of the risk of infection, and in arrest situations owing to poor lower extremity circulation during CPR; they are adequate for short-term use for fluid resuscitation.

D. Cutdowns. Three veins are readily accessible by cutdown techniques, which are described on page 332.

E. Other. In children with no intravenous access, a technique has been described whereby tibial puncture with a large needle (interosseous line) allows infusion of fluid and medication. This clearly represents a technique of last resort in pediatric patients near death. The incidence of osteomyelitis in survivors is relatively high.

F. Clotted Catheter. Occasionally, clotted catheters can be cleared by gentle irrigation with agents such as urokinase (see page 499).

53. NAUSEA/VOMITING

I. Problem. A patient complains of nausea and then vomits repeatedly 1 week following a colectomy for diverticulitis.

II. Immediate Questions

A. Are there any associated symptoms, particularly gastrointestinal? Nausea and vomiting may accompany a wide spectrum of illnesses covering most body systems. Inquire about related concurrent symptoms to focus the differential diagnosis. Specifically ask about abdominal pain, abdominal distention, diarrhea, or constipation/obstipation associated with the nausea and vomiting.

B. What is the appearance and odor of vomitus? Sometimes the vomited material can give clues to the nature of the underlying dysfunction. First, look and test for blood (see Problem 34, page 118). Feculent vomitus indicates stasis or distal obstruction. Bilious vomit merely implies a patent pyloric channel. A change in the vomit from bilious to bloody may indicate a Mallory-Weiss tear.

C. How is the vomiting related to eating or specific medications? In the postoperative setting note if the vomiting correlates with beginning or advancing an enteral diet. Vomiting 1–2 hours after eating (especially if the vomit is partially digested food) points to gastric stasis or gastric outlet obstruction. Vomiting concurrent or immediately after eating is often psychogenic. Certain medications can cause vomiting, such as narcotics or nonsteroidal anti-inflammatory drugs (NSAIDs).

D. Is the vomiting projectile? Projectile vomiting is often associated with CNS dysfunction. However, it may also occur with certain types of food poisoning.

E. Does the patient have a nasogastric drainage tube in place? Confirm proper functioning and positioning.

III. **Differential Diagnosis.** The following differential list is structured around the primary system involved in the underlying cause of nausea and vomiting.

   A. Gastrointestinal
   1. **General**
      a. Peritonitis.
      b. Postoperative ileus.
      c. Mechanical obstruction at any level.
      d. Gastroenteritis.
   2. **Stomach**
      a. Gastric outlet obstruction.
      b. Peptic ulcer disease.
      c. Gastric atony.
   3. **Hepatobiliary/pancreas**
      a. Biliary colic or acute cholecystitis.
      b. Pancreatitis.
      c. Hepatitis.
   4. **Colon**
      a. Diverticulitis.
      b. Malignant obstruction from colorectal cancer.
      c. Appendicitis.

B. Metabolic
1. Uremia.
2. Hepatic failure.
3. Metabolic acidosis.
4. **Electrolyte abnormalities**
   a. Hypercalcemia.
   b. Hyperkalemia.

C. Endocrine
1. **Diabetes.** Gastroparesis.
2. Adrenal insufficiency.
3. Hypothyroidism.

D. Drug/Toxin
1. Alcohol abuse.
2. Botulism.
3. Food poisoning (eg, staphylococcal).
4. Food or drug allergy.
5. Narcotics, especially codeine.
6. Nonsteroidal anti-inflammatory drugs (eg, ibuprofen).
7. Chemotherapeutic agents.

E. Cardiopulmonary
1. **Acute myocardial infarction.** Particularly inferior MI.
2. Congestive heart failure.

F. Genitourinary
1. Renal colic.
2. Pelvic inflammatory disease.
3. Pregnancy.

G. Nervous System
1. Space-occupying CNS lesion; increased intracranial pressure.
2. Migraine headache.
3. Labyrinthitis.

H. Acute Febrile Illnesses. Particularly in the pediatric age group.

IV. Database

A. Physical Exam Key Points
1. **Vital signs.** Orthostatic signs, fever, tachycardia.
2. **HEENT.** Pharyngitis, otitis, or other evidence of acute infections, papilledema.
3. **Skin.** Turgor, mucus membranes to estimate volume status. Jaundice.
4. **Abdomen.** Evaluate for bowel sounds, abdominal distention, peritoneal signs, areas of tenderness. Pain out of proportion to physical findings may indicate ischemic bowel.
5. **Rectal exam.** Evidence of impaction, positive fecal occult blood, mass, or fluctuance (suggestive of abscess).

   6. Neurologic exam. Mental status changes may signify CNS lesion or severe electrolyte disorder.
   7. Pelvic exam. Consider if PID suspected.

B. Laboratory Data
   1. Hemogram. For signs of infection or blood loss.
   2. Urinalysis and urine culture. May reveal infection or blood seen with stones.
   3. Chemistries. General screening includes electrolytes, BUN/creatinine, liver function tests.
   4. Amylase.
   5. Arterial blood gases if indicated.
   6. Urinary HCG to diagnose pregnancy.

C. Radiologic and Other Studies
   1. KUB and upright abdominal films. Obtain abdominal films in most patients with vomiting and in all patients with abdominal distention.
   2. Chest x-ray. To aid in the diagnosis of pneumonia, CHF, and evidence of aspiration. Pleural effusion can be seen with pancreatitis. Look for free air on upright film.
   3. ECG. If possibility of ischemic heart disease.
   4. Abdominal ultrasound/HIDA scan. If possibility of biliary colic.
   5. UGI series/upper endoscopy. If likely significant obstruction. Use water soluble contrast (Gastrografin) instead of barium.
   6. Barium enema/colonoscopy. If evidence of colonic pathology or obstruction.
   7. CT of the head. If an intracranial lesion is suspected.

V. Plan

A. Overall Plan. Assess the patient for level of hypovolemia and begin appropriate fluid resuscitation. Make the patient NPO. Screen for drug allergies/reactions. Narcotics are common offenders in the postoperative surgical patient.

B. Abdominal Causes. Always make the patient NPO and treat with IV fluids. Place nasogastric tube if there is persistent vomiting, mechanical obstruction, or abdominal distention. Proceed with diagnostic work-up.

C. Nonabdominal causes, such as metabolic disorders, labyrinthitis, minor infections (eg, acute viral gastroenteritis). Assess volume status, administer intravenous fluids if indicated, treat the underlying disorder, and treat vomiting with antiemetics. Frequently used antiemetics include:
   1. Prochlorperazine (Compazine) 10 mg IM/PO every 6 hours.
   2. Trimethobenzamide (Tigan) 250 mg PO every 6–8 hours, 200 mg IM/PR every 6–8 hours.

3. Promethazine (Phenergan) 12.5–25 mg PO every 8 hours, or 25 mg IM every 8 hours.
4. Meclizine (Antivert) 25–50 mg PO every 8–12 hours. Useful for nausea in labyrinthitis or vertigo.
5. Metoclopramide (Reglan) 10 mg IV/PO every 6 hours. Particularly useful in diabetics or other situations with poor gastric emptying not due to obstruction.
6. Granisetron hydrochloride (Kytril) 10 μg/kg IV over 5 minutes before chemotherapy. Related agents may help chemotherapy induced nausea and vomiting.

54. NASOGASTRIC TUBE MANAGEMENT— BLOODY DRAINAGE

I. **Problem.** A 43-year-old male has bloody output from his nasogastric tube 2 days after small bowel resection for a Meckel's diverticulum.

II. **Immediate Questions**

A. **How long has the NG tube been in place?** A tube that has been placed recently may have bloody drainage from the trauma of insertion or gastric surgery. An old tube may show blood from local mucosal irritation.

B. **How much bloody drainage has there been?** A tube that passes large amounts of bright red blood is obviously a more critical situation than one that passes a few red streaks.

C. **Has the patient had recent or remote upper gastrointestinal surgery?** If the surgery is recent, there may be bleeding at a newly formed anastomotic site, or there may be a marginal ulcer at an old anastomotic site.

D. **Is the patient receiving antacids? What is the pH of the fluid?** The presence of acidic gastric secretions increases the likelihood of the development of gastritis. Specifically, the pH should be > 4.0 for mucosal protection.

III. **Differential Diagnosis**

A. **Insertion Trauma.** Usually nasopharyngeal in nature.

B. **Mucosal Irritation.** Often from a tube that has been in place for some time. There is usually an associated acidic pH.

C. **Suture Line Disruption or Hemorrhage.** Especially in a patient recently operated on.

D. **Swallowed Pharyngeal Blood.** From an upper source of bleeding perhaps unrelated to the nasogastric tube.

  E. Ulceration (Curling, Cushing, preexisting). Look for associated conditions: burns, head injury, etc.

  F. Gastric erosion/gastritis/esophagitis/variceal bleed.

  G. Coagulopathy.

IV. Database

  ### A. Physical Exam Key Points
  1. **Vital signs.** Look for tachycardia and hypotension as evidence of sepsis or excessive blood loss.
  2. **Abdomen.** Look for peritoneal signs, epigastric tenderness or gastric distention.
  3. **HEENT.** Evidence of pharyngeal bleeding.

  ### B. Laboratory Data
  1. **Hemogram.** To check for excessive blood loss.
  2. **PT/PTT and platelet count.** To rule out coagulopathy.

  ### C. Radiologic and Other Studies
  1. **Upright chest x-ray.** To look for free intra-abdominal air. Look at the mediastinum and both lung fields for air that may be a result of esophageal perforation after forceful vomiting (Boerhaave's syndrome).
  2. **pH.** Check the pH of the gastric fluid. Is it < 4.0?

V. Plan

  ### A. Overall Plan. To determine whether the cause of bleeding is serious enough to require specific aggressive therapy.

  ### B. Specific Plans
  1. For life-threatening upper GI bleeding, establish venous access and begin fluids. A CVP line may be helpful, especially in the elderly. Hypotensive patients will require vigorous blood and fluid replacement.
  2. **Begin antacid therapy.** Use Maalox 30 mL every 2 hours via NG tube. Intravenous H_2-receptor blockers (cimetidine, etc) may also be used. Sucralfate can also be helpful.
  3. **Irrigate the NG tube with saline.** Room temperature is adequate for the saline, but the temperature is not important. Irrigation enables diagnosis of further bleeding as well as the therapeutic maneuver of removing clots from the stomach, which lead to distention and persistent bleeding.
  4. The presence of peritoneal signs or new free intra-abdominal air require emergency laparotomy.
  5. Perform upper GI endoscopy if bleeding persists (see Problem 34, page 118).

55. NASOGASTRIC TUBE MANAGEMENT—CHANGE IN AMOUNT OF OUTPUT

I. Problem. A 56-year-old woman with pancreatitis has a sudden increase in the amount of nasogastric tube aspirate on the fifth hospital day. Another patient has minimal NG aspirate after small bowel resection 3 days ago.

II. Immediate Questions

A. Is there associated abdominal distress? If the patient developed a generalized ileus or a distal obstruction, the amount of aspirate will increase.

B. Is the output bilious? Bilious NG output indicates a more distal problem with bile reflux into the stomach or a nasogastric tube placed distal to the pylorus.

C. Is the tube functioning? Tubes often become obstructed with mucous or antacids. Listen for whistle on sump tube indicating patency. Is the suction functioning?

D. Is the patient passing flatus or stool? Often, decreased NG output correlates with return of bowel function.

E. Is an NPO patient surreptitiously taking in fluid? Can be seen in patients with psychiatric histories. Often "ice chips" given to patients with NG tubes can be excessive and cause high NG tube outputs.

III. Differential Diagnosis

A. Increased Output

1. **Tip of tube distal to pylorus.** Tube aspirates all biliary and pancreatic secretions as well as gastric output.
2. Distal bowel obstruction or gastric outlet obstruction.
3. Return to higher secretory state after discontinuation of H_2-receptor blockers, eg, cimetidine.
4. **Surreptitious ingestion.**

B. Decreased Output

1. Return of normal bowel motility and function.
2. Obstructed/kinked tube.
3. Use of H_2-receptor blocker, which decreases gastric secretion or agents that improve motility and gastric emptying, eg, metoclopramide.
4. Tip of tube above GE junction or coiled in the oropharynx.

IV. Database

  A. Physical Exam Key Points
   1. **Abdomen.** Listen for bowel sounds and their quality. No sounds may indicate ileus or far advanced obstruction. High-pitched, hollow sounds indicate obstruction. Distention may mean obstruction or ileus.
   2. **Mouth.** Look for tube coiled or kinked in mouth or throat.
   3. **Rectal exam.** Determine presence or absence of stool.
   4. **Tube.** Check patency and function by flushing with air or saline.

  B. Laboratory Data
   1. **Serum electrolytes.** Carefully monitor hydration status and potassium and bicarbonate levels during nasogastric suction.
   2. **Nasogastric aspirate.** A pH > 6 indicates use of antacids, or the tip of catheter is distal to pylorus.

  C. Radiologic and Other Studies
   1. **Upright chest x-ray.** Look for a large stomach bubble, indicating poor gastric emptying. Check position of the tube tip.
   2. **Upright and flat abdominal x-rays.** Show distended bowel indicating ileus or obstruction.
   3. **Contrast swallow.** When partial bowel obstruction or upper GI obstruction is contemplated, Gastrografin or dilute barium can be swallowed. Serial x-rays will show normal or delayed emptying and passage of contrast. Contrast should **not** be used in the presence of ileus or complete obstruction.

V. Plan. The first priority is to determine that the nasogastric tube is functioning properly and in a proper position. **Note:** Manipulation of all nasogastric tubes must be performed with the full understanding of why the tube has been placed and the nature of the surgical procedure.

  A. Position. Based on x-ray and acidic aspirate.

  B. Function. Sump tubes should whistle continuously on low suction. Most tubes need to be flushed with saline (30 mL) every 3–4 hours to maintain patency. Flush tube with 40 mL of air while auscultating over the gastric area to determine function and positioning.

  C. Increased Output
   1. **Poor gastric emptying (no obstruction).** Try metoclopramide 10 mg IV every 6 hours.
   2. **Distal obstruction.** Continue NG suction; consider further work-up and operation to relieve obstruction.
   3. **Ileus.** Patience and a period of observation are necessary, especially if immediately postop. Correct electrolyte abnormalities, especially hypokalemia, with parenteral solution. Continue NG suction. Prolonged ileus may indicate intra-abdominal sepsis.

D. Decreased Output
1. Most often indicates return of bowel function. Correlate with physical examination and passage of flatus or stool. Remove the tube if appropriate.
2. Irrigate tube to clear it, or advance tube into stomach if it is not positioned correctly.

56. OLIGURIA/ANURIA

I. **Problem.** A patient has sequential hourly urine outputs of 22, 15, 9, and 4 ml via an indwelling Foley catheter 1 day following an aortic aneurysm repair.

II. **Immediate Questions**

A. **What is the patient's volume status?** The most common cause of oliguria in the postoperative setting is hypovolemia. The most important and most frequent differential diagnosis is acute tubular necrosis (usually secondary to ischemia), which is also related to hypovolemia. Assess the volume status by left-sided pressures from a pulmonary artery catheter, central venous pressures, weight change, and physical exam. Do not let elevated weight dissuade you if other assessments point to a decreased intravascular volume. Be sure that hypovolemia is not a result of hemorrhage.

B. **Did the patient suffer any periods of documented hypotension?** As previously mentioned, ischemic acute tubular necrosis is a cause of oliguria on a surgical service. Review the operative record of the anesthesiologist noting any episodes of hypotension intraoperatively.

C. **What is the baseline renal function?** Look at the admission BUN and creatinine and any subsequent chemistries. Any insult to the kidneys will be amplified by baseline chronic renal dysfunction.

D. **Is the patient taking any renal toxic drugs?** Aminoglycosides are the major offenders. Send off appropriate drug levels and hold the next dose until the levels return. Also consider IV contrast dye from radiologic procedures as a potential nephrotoxin.

E. **Is the patient taking any medication that is excreted by the kidneys?** Digoxin and antibiotics are the most important medications in this category. Either modify or hold the dose until renal function improves or drug levels become available.

F. **Is the Foley catheter patent?** Most nurses will think of this before you do, but flush the catheter at least once to make sure the oliguria is a reflection of renal function (see Problem 32, page 113).

III. Differential Diagnosis. The differential diagnosis for acute oliguria is identical to that of acute renal failure and may be viewed as prerenal, renal, or postrenal causes.

A. Prerenal (Renal Hypoperfusion)
  1. Shock/hypovolemia
    a. Hemorrhage: Traumatic or as a postop complication.
    b. Inadequate fluid administration.
    c. Sepsis.
  2. Apparent intravascular hypovolemia, a relative decrease in the effective circulating volume.
    a. "Third space" losses: Very common in the initial postoperative period following major operations or with major burns.
    b. Congestive heart failure.
    c. Cirrhosis may have associated hepatorenal syndrome.
    d. Nephrotic syndrome.
  3. Vascular
    a. Renal artery occlusion (acute or chronic).
    b. Aortic dissection.
    c. Emboli (eg, cholesterol).

B. Renal
  1. Acute tubular necrosis
    a. Ischemic: Secondary to shock, sepsis.
    b. Toxins: Medications (aminoglycosides), contrast media, heavy metals.
  2. Acute interstitial nephritis
    a. Drugs: ß-lactamase resistant penicillins, NSAIDs.
    b. Hypercalcemia: Can cause nephrocalcinosis.
  3. Acute glomerular disease
    a. Malignant hypertension.
    b. Immune complexes.
    c. Systemic diseases (Wegener's, TTP, SLE, Goodpasture's).

C. Postrenal
  1. Urethral obstruction (prostatic hypertrophy, catheter obstruction).
  2. Bilateral ureteral obstruction (carcinoma or retroperitoneal fibrosis).

IV. Database

A. Physical Exam Key Points
  1. Vital signs. Weight change, orthostatic signs to document fluid loss.
  2. Skin. Tissue turgor, mucus membranes, or edema.
  3. Cardiopulmonary. Rales, elevated venous pressure, cardiac gallop, or JVD.
  4. Abdomen. Determine if there is ascites, or if the bladder is distended.

     5. Extremities. Assess perfusion by color and temperature.

B. Laboratory Data

    1. Electrolytes, BUN, and creatinine. If BUN/creatinine > 20:1 then likely prerenal; if BUN/Cr < 15:1 then likely renal. Hyperkalemia can be life-threatening and may accompany acute renal insufficiency.

    2. Urinalysis. Protein, red blood cell casts support glomerular disease. Eosinophils are associated with hypersensitivity reactions. WBC casts may indicate glomerulonephritis.

    3. Spot or random urine electrolytes and creatinine. Obtain before giving diuretics. Urinary sodium < 20 mEq/L indicates prerenal cause; urinary sodium > 20 mEq/L is suggestive of renal cause. Calculate renal function index as urinary sodium × plasma creatinine divided by the urine creatinine. If the RFI is > 1, it is likely a renal cause; if RFI is < 1, it is likely prerenal (see also Section II, page 245).

    4. Hemogram. For evidence of infection or anemia.

    5. Drug levels. Evaluate for any renal toxic drugs (eg, aminoglycosides), or any medications cleared through the kidneys (eg, digoxin).

C. Radiologic and Other Studies

    1. Chest x-ray. May reveal congestive failure.

    2. Central venous pressure line or PA catheter. Will give useful information about volume status.

    3. KUB. May reveal obstructing renal calculi.

    4. IVP. A combination of ultrasound, renal scan, and retrograde studies will give equivalent information plus more without renal toxic contrast media.

    5. Ultrasound. Examines the bladder and upper urinary tract for signs of obstruction; also estimates renal size.

    6. Renal scan. Technetium labeled DTPA or MAG-3 nuclear medicine study to assess blood flow to the kidneys, especially if embolus is a concern.

    7. Angiogram. To visualize vascular anatomy, but rarely needed acutely.

    8. Renal biopsy. Occasionally needed to determine specific diagnosis of renal cause of oliguria. This is not needed immediately to treat oliguria.

V. Plan

A. Overall Plan. As a general rule, the minimal acceptable urine output in an adult is 0.5 ml/kg/hr. As previously stated, oliguria in most surgical patients results from hypovolemia. In almost every case it is appropriate to give the patient a potassium free volume challenge (eg, 500 ml of normal saline). In patients with fragile cardiorespiratory status, smaller boluses and central venous catheters should be used to monitor volume status. Also review the patient's medications and stop or alter all nephrotoxic or renally excreted drugs and remove potassium from the IV fluids.

B. Prerenal
1. Treat with volume boluses to increase urinary output and adjust baseline IV rate up.
2. Monitor volume replacement with central lines, if needed.
3. **Follow hourly urine output.** Give specific criteria to be notified for (eg, call house officer for urine output < 25 ml/hour).

C. Renal
1. Monitor volume status with central lines.
2. Remove potassium from IV solutions unless it is abnormally low.
3. Attempt to increase urine output once volume status is corrected.
   a. **Furosemide:** Use escalating doses to obtain response of increased urine output. One method is to start with 80 mg IV, then 160 mg IV, and 320 mg IV.
   b. **Mannitol:** 12.5–25 g (50–100 ml of a 25% solution) to induce an osmotic diuresis.
   c. **Dopamine:** 3–5 µg/kg/min to increase renal blood flow.
4. **Review medications.** Adjust doses or stop nephrotoxic drugs.
5. **Monitor electrolytes.**

D. Postrenal. Usually requires urologic consultation. Ureteral stents or percutaneous nephrostomy may be needed. A blocked Foley catheter can be treated as outlined in Problem 32, page 113.

57. PARESTHESIAS

I. Problem. A 62-year-old male patient is complaining of paresthesias (tingling or "pins and needles") 1 day after right radical neck dissection.

II. Immediate Questions

A. Where are the paresthesias? A patient with paresthesias in an extremity and with known or likely peripheral vascular occlusive disease presents a different clinical dilemma than one with circumoral paresthesias.

B. Does the patient have peripheral vascular disease? Paresthesias are one of the "five Ps" of peripheral vascular occlusive disease—the others being pain, pallor, pulselessness, and paralysis. Find out if the patient has any of these other signs of vascular occlusive disease.

C. Has the patient had these symptoms before? It is important to determine if the condition was present preoperatively or a consequence of the recent surgical procedure.

D. Did the paresthesia appear suddenly or gradually? Find out if they can be linked to a particular event, such as an operation.

III. Differential Diagnosis. Paresthesias may be reported as tingling, "pins and needles," or numbness.

A. Vascular Insufficiency. It is important to determine if vascular occlusive disease is the cause, because paresthesias may be one of the early symptoms of vascular compromise, and early action may be necessary to save the affected extremity.

B. Hypocalcemia. Paresthesias primarily involve the lips, tongue, fingers, and feet. An especially significant symptom after thyroid or parathyroid surgery (see Problem 43, page 146 for further suggestions regarding patient evaluation and therapy).

C. Operating Room Causes. People (eg, tired residents and students) leaning on the patient for prolonged periods in the operating room may lead to postoperative paresthesias in a peripheral nerve distribution. Improper positioning and padding of extremities during a case is also a preventable cause. Check placement of pneumatic compression boots.

D. Neuroma. Would occur weeks postoperatively as a result of nerve injury during surgery.

E. Hyperventilation. Results in bilateral hand and finger tip numbness, thereby reproducing the symptoms.

F. Transient Ischemic Attack (TIA). Often bilateral extremity numbness that may accompany speech and sight difficulties. Carotid bruit may be present and residual neurologic deficits are rare.

G. Peripheral Neuropathy. Often classic "glove and stocking" distribution seen in patients with diabetes, alcoholism, or chronic renal insufficiency.

H. Nerve Compression. Such as carpal tunnel syndrome or a dressing that is applied too tightly.

I. CNS tumors, neurosyphilis.

IV. Database

A. Physical Exam Key Points

1. **Vital signs.** Tachypnea associated with hyperventilation.
2. **Peripheral pulses.** Especially in an affected extremity.
3. **Look for causes of pressure in the area.** Dressings, casts, etc.

   4. Check for physical signs of hypocalcemia. Chvostek's and
      Trousseau's sign (see Problem 43, page 146).
   5. Carotid bruit may be present to suggest TIAs.
   6. Neurologic exam. Signs of peripheral neuropathy include
      symmetric loss of pinprick sensation. Reflexes are decreased
      with nerve compression.

B. Laboratory Data
   1. Serum electrolytes and calcium. To rule out hypocalcemia,
      renal failure, diabetes.
   2. Arterial blood gases. Hyperventilation can occasionally cause
      paresthesias as seen in a respiratory alkalosis.

C. Radiologic and Other Studies
   1. ECG. Look for atrial fibrillation, which predisposes to thrombus
      and embolization.
   2. Nerve conduction velocities. Assist with the diagnosis of
      nerve compression.
   3. Doppler blood flow determination may reveal blood flow in an
      extremity with a nonpalpable pulse.

V. Plan

   A. Vascular Insufficiency with Paresthesias is a serious symptom
      and requires rapid therapy to save the extremity. Reoperating on
      a clotted graft or angiographic study of an acutely obstructed ves-
      sel is indicated (see Problem 62, page 201).
   B. Hypocalcemia. In the patient with paresthesias following thy-
      roidectomy, repletion of serum calcium is indicated with oral or IV
      calcium (see Problem 43, page 146).
   C. Transient ischemic attacks. TIAs are often treated surgically to
      remove carotid plaques.
   D. Peripheral Neuropathies For example, alcoholism, and diabetes
      are most often chronic and irreversible.
   E. Dressings and Casts should be revised as appropriate.

58. PHLEBITIS

I. Problem. A 32-year-old woman had an exploratory laparotomy for
   ovarian cancer. An IV in her arm has not been changed for 5 days and
   the site is now red and painful.

II. Immediate Questions

   A. What are the patient's vital signs? Fever can develop from both
      superficial thrombophlebitis and deep venous thrombosis.

    B. Can pus be expressed from the site? Pus indicates a local infection, and sepsis with pus may indicate suppurative thrombophlebitis. Look for red streaks proximal to IV site.

    C. What medications are being administered through the line? Agents such as potassium, and calcium can cause phlebitis.

III. Differential Diagnosis. Acute venous inflammation or occlusion can occur in superficial or deep veins. Deep venous thrombosis usually does not have a significant inflammatory component and rarely is infected. This discussion will be limited to inflammation and infection of superficial veins.

    A. Superficial Thrombophlebitis. Acute inflammation without infection is the most common presentation.

        1. Site of intravenous catheter, especially upper extremity.

        2. Extravasation of irritant medications, such as chemotherapeutic agents.

        3. Unknown cause, especially lower extremities.

    B. Suppurative Thrombophlebitis. Persistent fever, sepsis, and positive blood cultures indicate significant infection of the affected vein. Pus is expressed, and there may be daily increases in the length of vein involved despite local treatment. Superficial thrombophlebitis occurs rarely at upper extremity IV sites, and slightly more commonly at emergent cutdown sites, especially in the lower extremities.

    C. Other

        1. Deep venous thrombosis (see Problem 65, page 209).

        2. Septic thrombophlebitis of subclavian vein.

IV. Database

    A. Physical Exam Key Points

        1. Vital signs. With close attention to sepsis.

        2. Extremities. Old intravenous sites should be examined in the febrile patient. Palpate the calves for tenderness. Gently squeeze erythematous IV sites in an attempt to express pus.

    B. Laboratory Data

        1. Hemogram. Leukocytosis is present in suppurative superficial thrombophlebitis.

        2. Culture and gram stain of pus from old IV site.

    C. Radiologic and Other Studies. Venography is indicated very rarely if central vein infection or deep venous thrombosis are suspected in the septic patient (usually *Staphylococcal* species) with no known source.

V. Plan. Prevention of thrombophlebitis by frequent rotation of IV sites should keep this problem at a minimum.

A. Superficial Thrombophlebitis
1. Local heat, dry or moist.
2. Limb elevation.
3. Nonsteroidal anti-inflammatory drugs (NSAIDs).
4. Consider administering heparin if patient is an acceptable anti-coagulation candidate.

B. Suppurative Thrombophlebitis
1. Local care.
2. Analgesics and anti-inflammatory agents.
3. **Intravenous antibiotics.** Usually broad-spectrum with good anti-staphylococcal coverage (nafcillin, etc).
4. Persistent or progressing infection mandates exploratory venotomy and venectomy of the entire involved segment of vein. This may need to be done in the operating room. Segments of vein should be sent to the pathology and microbiology departments, and the wound should be left open and packed.
5. Consider administering heparin if patient is an acceptable anti-coagulation candidate.

C. Other. Suppurative thrombophlebitis of a subclavian vein requires resection in the operating room and intravenous antibiotics.

59. POSTOPERATIVE PAIN MANAGEMENT

I. Problem. The night of an open lung biopsy the patient threatens to pull out his chest tube and leave the hospital because of severe incisional pain.

II. Immediate Questions

A. Is there any evidence of a wound infection, hematoma, or other problem? Early wound infections (*Clostridium, Streptococcus*) may be a factor in early postop pain that is more than expected. Also, a wound hematoma may amplify expected postop pain.

B. What is the current pain medication regimen—what drug, what dose, and how often has it been given? If a patient complains of excruciating postop pain, then the current pain medication is obviously inadequate. Titrate the dose up to relieve pain, make certain the frequency is appropriate, and ensure the nurses are administering the medication appropriately. Expect thoracotomy, midline abdominal, flank, and orthopedic incisions to cause the most pain, especially in young, muscular patients.

C. Is there any history of narcotic use or abuse? Patients frequently have taken narcotics either preoperatively for chronic pain or illicitly. Tolerance to narcotics is a real phenomenon and these patients need their doses elevated sometimes to alarmingly high levels to achieve pain control in the immediate postop period.

III. Differential Diagnosis. Discussions of postoperative pain almost always mean incisional pain.

A. Inadequate Analgesic Regimen

1. **Too small a dose.** When writing postop orders, take into account the size and age of the patient and the type of operation. If a wide range of medication dose is given in the orders, nurses will frequently use the lower end of the scale, so as not to overmedicate.

2. **Too long between doses.** Dosing schedules should be set by the half-life of the drug, which is usually 3–4 hours in narcotics given intramuscularly or subcutaneously. Also make certain a patient knows to request a medication that is administered as needed.

3. **Patient controlled analgesia.** Dosing may be too low or lockout too long.

B. Wound Complications

1. **Infections.** Be alert for aggressive life-threatening infections (*Clostridium, Streptococcus,* necrotizing fasciitis) that may only initially present with pain.

2. Hematoma.

3. Dehiscence.

4. Nerve entrapment or excessive pressure from a dressing postop.

5. Compartment syndrome developing in an extremity.

C. Drug-seeking Behavior. Usually, a patient's complaint of pain should be treated in the immediate postoperative period. However, if reported pain persists or increases as times passes, a contributing factor, including drug-seeking behavior, should be considered. Look for signs of drowsiness and disorientation due to overmedication.

IV. Database

A. Physical Exam Key Points

1. **Vital signs.** Fever and tachycardia suggest an infection. Early postoperative tachycardia with hypertension suggests pain.

      2. Wound. Look for signs of infection (erythema, purulence, crepitation, margination, drainage) or developing hematoma. Make sure the dressing is not the cause of the pain.

      3. Neurologic exam. Observe for posturing, grimacing, splinting, and other body movements consistent with pain. Disorientation or obtundation is consistent with narcotic overdose or sepsis.

  B. Laboratory Data

      1. Hemogram if infection is suspected.

      2. Wound culture if it is the suspected source.

  C. Radiologic and Other Studies. Chest x-ray if indicated.

V. Plan

  A. Overall Plan. Realize that pain management is part of the complete care of the surgical patient. Let the patient know you are concerned and are taking actions to improve pain control. Follow-up on any changes made in pain medication regimen.

  B. Pain Medications. Medications are discussed in detail in Section IX, page 388.

      1. Morphine sulfate. Gold standard for postop pain. Dose is 8–12 mg s.c. every 3–4 hours in most cases. In thoracic and orthopedic patients 12–15 mg are commonly needed. In ICU, patients may be given 1–4 mg IV every 1–3 hours.

      2. Demerol. 75–125 mg IM every 3 hours.

      3. Dilaudid. 2–4 mg IM every 3–4 hours.

      4. Percocet, Percodan, or Tylenol with codeine are fairly standard oral analgesics used postop. Given as one or two tablets PO every 4–6 hours as needed.

      5. Hydroxyzine (Atarax, Vistaril). Use as adjunct to parenteral narcotics 25–50 mg every 8 hours. It is useful to potentiate the pain relieving action and minimize nausea associated with narcotics.

  C. Alternative Methods of Pain Control

      1. Epidural narcotics. An epidural catheter is left in place by the anesthesia team and is usually managed by the anesthesiologists. Always confirm who is to help with the catheter (particularly at night). Find out what medications can be given in addition to the epidural.

      2. Self-controlled IV pumps. Infuses either boluses, continuous IV morphine, or both and is controlled to some extent by the patient. This is called "PCA-Patient Controlled Analgesia." Orders are given for number of milligrams per dose, lockout time (ie, minimum time interval between doses), and maximum dose per 4 hours. A typical order is 3 mg, 15 min lockout maximum 30 mg per 4 hrs.

3. **Nerve blocks.** For certain incisions (thorax, flank) that can be extremely painful especially in the first few hours postop, infiltration with a long-acting anesthetic in the operating room at the end of the case can be helpful. For example, bupivacaine (Marcaine) can be used to infiltrate the intercostal nerves at the end of a thoracotomy.

60. PRURITUS

I. Problem. Three days after a low anterior resection a 49-year-old male is complaining of severe pruritus (itching) of both legs.

II. Immediate Questions

A. What is the duration of the symptom? An acute condition can more often be related to an exact cause, such as a change in laundry soap, new medication, etc.

B. Has the patient recently started taking any new medications, eating different foods, wearing different clothing, using new detergents or soaps? These are common causes of itching, especially postoperative analgesics.

C. Is there an associated rash or lesions? These may also give clues to the cause.

III. Differential Diagnosis

A. Skin Disorders. Pruritus associated with visible skin lesions
1. Papulosquamous skin diseases.
2. Vesicobullous diseases.
3. Allergic reactions, eg, contact dermatitis (most commonly caused by soaps, detergents, etc).
4. Infestations, eg, scabies.
5. Infection, eg, viral exanthemas.

B. Systemic. Itching can be associated with a variety of systemic conditions without an associated rash
1. **Dry skin.** Especially in the elderly, may be related to cold weather.
2. **Liver disease.** Often with jaundice and cholestasis.
3. **Uremia.** May be unrelated to BUN.
4. Hypothyroidism.
5. Hyperparathyroidism.
6. Diabetes mellitus.
7. Gout.
8. Hodgkin's disease, leukemias.
9. Intestinal parasites, such as pinworms or hookworms.
10. Drug reactions.

11. Pregnancy.
12. Polycythemia vera.

C. **Psychosomatic Pruritus.**

D. **Neurologic and Circulatory Disturbances.**

IV. Database

A. **Physical Exam Key Points.** Check the patient's skin (not just the affected area); examine the distribution of rash and any skin lesions—carefully record distribution and appearance. What looks like a rash may be a skin breakdown secondary to severe scratching of the pruritic area. Examine skin carefully near IV sites.

B. **Laboratory Data**
1. **Liver function tests.** To help rule out liver disease.
2. **BUN and creatinine.** May reveal renal insufficiency and uremia.

C. **Radiologic and Other Studies.** Chest x-ray may show a new lung malignancy, which can present with pruritus.

V. Plan

A. **Overall Plan.** Pruritus does not require immediate treatment, unless caused by a significant systemic disease or early anaphylaxis. It is important to rule out major illness as a cause. The primary goal is to enhance the patient's comfort until the definitive diagnosis is available to dictate therapy.

B. **Specific Measures**
1. **Dry skin.** Skin hydration by daily bathing in warm water, followed immediately by applying skin moisturizer cream (Aquaphor, Eucerin) will give some relief, especially if xerosis is the cause. Adding salt to the water may be of added benefit. Creams should not be applied in cases of chronic pruritus in the absence of a rash.
2. **Uremic pruritus.** In uremic pruritus, UV light and lidocaine IV may help.
3. **Cholestasis.** Cholestyramine may also help in pruritus secondary to hepatic disease.
4. **Medical treatment.** There are three oral medications useful in the treatment of symptomatic pruritus
   a. **Diphenhydramine (Benadryl)** 25–50 mg PO or IV every 8 hours.
   b. **Cyproheptadine (Periactin)** 4 mg PO tid.
   c. **Hydroxyzine (Atarax)** 25 mg PO tid or qid.
   Topical steroids range from mild (hydrocortisone), to midpotency (triamcinolone [Kenalog]), high potency (halcinonide

[Halog]), and the highest potency (betamethasone dipropi-
onate [Dipro-lene]).
5. Discontinuation of medication causing pruritus, if possible.

61. PULMONARY ARTERY CATHETER PROBLEMS

(Technique of pulmonary artery catheterization is discussed in Section III,
Bedside Procedures, page 295)

I. **Problem.** A pulmonary artery (PA) catheter inserted into a septic patient will not "wedge."

II. **Immediate Questions**

   A. **Has the catheter ever been in good "wedge" position?** Be sure
   that the catheter has worked in the past. Check the tip position on
   x-ray. It may reveal the catheter is not in proper position (see below).

   B. **Is the balloon working properly, or is there any problem with
   the monitor or transducer system?** Balloons can occasionally
   rupture. A pulmonary artery pressure tracing suggests that the
   transducer system is otherwise intact.

III. **Differential Diagnosis**

   A. **Placement Problem.** The most frequent sites of catheterization
   are the internal jugular and subclavian veins. Fluoroscopy will help
   in certain cases, such as in patients who have undergone pneumonectomy where careful placement is mandatory. Placement
   problems include:
      1. Passage into internal jugular or out contralateral subclavian
      vein.
      2. Looping in right ventricle.
      3. Knotting of catheter.

   B. **Functional Problems.** Functional problems develop relatively frequently after successful placement of a PA catheter.
      1. **No wave form.** A thrombus may occlude the catheter.
      2. **Cannot "wedge" catheter.** This is perhaps the most common
      problem. A small amount of repositioning is usually adequate to
      restore function and is particularly easy if the flexible plastic
      sheath was used at the time of original placement.
      3. **Balloon rupture.** Never use more than 1.5 mL of air to inflate
      the balloon. Make sure the wave form changes from a pul-
      monary artery tracing to a wedge as the balloon is inflated.

C. Complications
   1. Pneumothorax/hemothorax, usually related to initial line placement.
   2. Infection.
   3. Pulmonary artery perforation, either immediate or delayed (very rare).
   4. **Arrhythmias.** Usually ventricular as the catheter passes through the ventricle. Patients with left bundle branch block may develop complete heart block if the PA catheter causes right bundle branch block.
   5. Pulmonary infarction, most often caused by a catheter tip that remains in a small pulmonary artery with the balloon inflated.

IV. Database
A. Physical Exam Key Points
   1. **Look at the catheter and check all connections.** Make sure the patient's heart is level with the measuring apparatus.
   2. **Check how much of catheter is in the patient.** Even in large patients, a wedge waveform will be present by the time 60 cm is used. If much more is used (for a subclavian approach), suspect that the catheter is not proceeding as desired. **Do not proceed beyond 60 cm.**
B. Laboratory Data. Usually not needed.
C. Radiologic and Other Studies
   1. **Check catheter position on chest x-ray.** The tip usually is in the right main pulmonary artery. There should be a gentle curve as the catheter passes from right atrium, through tricuspid valve into ventricle and out into the pulmonary artery. The catheter should lie in a smooth curve and not be further than 5 cm from the midline. There is a greater incidence of pulmonary artery perforation when the catheter tip is in the left main pulmonary artery.

V. Plan.
Placement of a pulmonary artery catheter should be done with careful monitoring. The catheter should be flushed and tested before placement. The balloon should be inflated with 1 mL of air and then deflated. The catheter should be connected to the transducer before placement to test the electronic aspects of the entire system. Once connected the tip of the catheter should be briskly tapped, revealing high frequency, high amplitude waveform on the pulmonary artery.

A. Placement
   1. Inflate the balloon in the superior vena cava to allow blood flow to carry the catheter out the right ventricular outflow tract. This is usually at about 20 cm via subclavian approach.

    2. Be sure that the balloon is **deflated** whenever the catheter is being withdrawn and **inflated** when advancing the catheter.

    3. As the catheter passes into the right ventricle, ventricular arrhythmias may develop and should be treated if persistent or associated with hemodynamic compromise. Some clinicians think it is safest to withdraw the catheter into the right atrium and bolus the patient with lidocaine before replacing the catheter. These rhythm abnormalities are usually short-lived and rarely persist after placement of the catheter into the PA.

B. Functional Problems. These problems typically occur after a variable period of catheter use. If still needed, a nonfunctioning catheter should be replaced after certain maneuvers have been performed, even if the catheter has just been placed. Most functional problems develop because of thrombosis at the catheter tip or at other ports.

    1. Flush nonfunctional ports frequently.

    2. Test balloon. If the balloon is intact you should be able to remove the same volume of air carefully placed into the balloon. During use, however, passive deflation is safest.

    3. Reposition the catheter further distally with balloon inflated if unable to "wedge" the balloon.

C. Complications

    1. Pneumothorax requires tube thoracostomy.

    2. Infected catheter should be immediately removed. Antibiotics may be required with positive blood cultures.

    3. Arrhythmias are treated with lidocaine, use 1 mg/kg bolus. Withdraw the catheter into the right atrium until the drug is given.

62. PULSELESS EXTREMITY

I. Problem. Two days after a coronary artery bypass, a nurse examines an elderly patient and reports that he has no pulses in his right leg.

II. Immediate Questions

A. Is this an acute change for the patient? Look at the admission history and physical for prior documentation of pulses. Unfortunately, a complete vascular exam (at a minimum femoral and pedal pulses) is often a neglected portion of the admit note. Ask the patient if he noted any acute changes in the extremity.

B. Are there any associated symptoms of pain or numbness in the involved extremity? Pain, pallor, pulselessness, paresthesias, and paralysis are the "Five Ps" of diagnosis of an acute arterial occlusion. Most patients have pain and pallor. Paresthesias are an early sign, and paralysis is a late sign of ischemic injury to the leg. Ask if these symptoms are new, and if so, how rapidly they developed (see also Problem 57, page 190).

C. Is there any history of claudication or any previous vascular surgery? Significant peripheral vascular atherosclerosis may be the underlying cause of an acute arterial occlusion. Also, the degree of chronic obstruction determines the amount of collateral circulation to the extremity that has developed. This may have an effect on how well an acute occlusion is tolerated.

D. What are the pulses in the other leg? Chronic peripheral vascular occlusive disease is usually bilateral, and comparison of pulses between the extremities may indicate baseline status of the extremity in question. Some acute events may also be bilateral (eg, saddle embolus).

E. Any history of palpitations or atrial fibrillation? Atrial fibrillation is one of the leading causes of embolic arterial occlusion. Even if a patient is found to be in a sinus rhythm, ask about history of arrhythmias or digoxin use. A recent conversion to sinus rhythm may be the cause of an acute embolic event.

III. Differential Diagnosis. The majority of acute arterial occlusions occur in the lower extremity, and the majority are due to embolic phenomenon. However, thrombosis, vasculitis, and even venous disease may cause an acute occlusion.

 A. Embolic Causes
  1. Cardiac sources
   a. Coronary artery disease. Prior myocardial infarction with mural thrombi.
   b. Atrial fibrillation.
   c. Rheumatic heart disease. Usually mitral stenosis with atrial fibrillation.
   d. Prosthetic cardiac valves.
   e. Endocarditis.
   f. Atrial myxoma.
  2. Peripheral sources
   a. Aortic. Aneurysm with mural thrombi.
   b. Atheroemboli. Often associated with invasive procedures (cardiac catheterization) or from peripheral sources (aortic, iliac, popliteal); this phenomenon is known as blue toe syndrome or "trash foot."
   c. Paradoxical emboli through a patent foramen ovale or other type of right to left shunt.
 B. Thrombotic Causes. Almost always some degree of atherosclerotic occlusive disease with contributing factors of hypovolemia/low flow and hypercoagulable states.

        1. Arterial occlusive disease.
        2. Hypovolemia/low flow
           a. Trauma and resultant shock.
           b. Dehydration.
           c. Fever.
           d. Sepsis.
        3. Hypercoagulable
           a. Malignancy.
           b. Polycythemia.
           c. Estrogen use.
           d. Heparin-induced thrombosis.

C. Arterial Dissection.

D. Trauma. Either blunt or penetrating.

E. Vasculitis
    1. Takayasu's disease. Often causes upper extremity occlusions.
    2. Thromboangiitis obliterans. In young smokers (Buerger's disease).

F. Acute Femoral/Iliac Vein Occlusion. Phlegmasia cerulea dolens.

IV. Database

A. Physical Exam Key Points
    1. Vital signs. Look for orthostatic hypotension for hypovolemia or irregular pulse of atrial fibrillation.
    2. Cardiac. Murmur of valvular diseases or endocarditis, rhythm disturbances.
    3. Abdomen. Abdominal bruits, palpable aneurysm.
    4. Extremity exam. Pulses and temperature at all levels compared to the contralateral side. Examine for skin pallor or mottling, and look for a cutoff for the level of ischemia. Look for changes of chronic ischemia, such as hair loss or skin atrophy. Look also for areas of well demarcated ecchymoses in feet suggesting "trash foot." Do not forget to feel for popliteal and femoral artery aneurysms. Use a Doppler probe if pulses are not readily palpable.
    5. Neurologic exam. Focal signs, paresthesias indicate significant ischemia. Paralysis indicates likely limb loss.

B. Laboratory Data
    1. Chemistries. Hyperkalemia may be associated with tissue damage from ischemia.
    2. Hemogram.
    3. PT/PTT. Especially if a patient is on anticoagulant therapy to verify if therapeutic (see pages 280 and 282).
    4. Arterial blood gas. Acidosis may be seen with poor perfusion.

5. **Urinalysis.** The presence of hemoglobin in absence of RBCs suggests myoglobinuria.
6. Myoglobin level for rhabdomyolysis suggests tissue loss.

C. **Radiologic and Other Studies**
   1. **Chest x-ray.** To evaluate for cardiac or thoracic aorta pathology.
   2. **ECG and rhythm strip.** For arrhythmia recognition.
   3. **Noninvasive vascular study.** Always check nonpalpable pulses with the Doppler. If a more sophisticated noninvasive lab is available, it can also be used.
   4. **Echocardiogram.** Looking for valvular disease, ventricular aneurysm, mural thrombi, or akinesis.
   5. **Cardiac thallium scan.** This scan evaluates for prior infarct, but not usually needed in acute cases.
   6. **Angiogram.** This documents level of obstruction, collaterals, occasionally shows aneurysms and other unrecognized visceral emboli. May show a source of peripheral emboli.
   7. **Abdominal ultrasound.** To evaluate for abdominal aneurysmal disease. Ultrasonography is also useful for peripheral aneurysms.

V. **Plan**

A. **Overall Plan.** An acute arterial occlusion is a surgical emergency requiring prompt diagnosis and early treatment to save the extremity. Evaluate for evidence of paresthesias and paralysis as signs of advancing ischemia and impending limb loss. Treat with anticoagulation, volume as needed, and prepare for the operating room. Evaluate the need for an angiogram. An angiogram is usually obtained, but in some cases the diagnosis and the level of obstruction is obvious and the patient may go directly to the operating room.

B. **Correct Volume Deficit.** If hypovolemia is a contributing factor, treat with IV fluid boluses. Monitor urine output and central filling pressures to guide therapy.

C. **Anticoagulation.** If there is any delay prior to surgery or an angiogram, load with 10,000 units of heparin IV, then give a continuous infusion of 10 U/kg/hr to prevent thrombus progression. Follow the PT/PTT (see Section II, page 245). Some centers may use thrombolytic therapy (streptokinase, tissue plasminogen activator) as a first line treatment. Some debilitated patients who are judged to have significant operative risk may be managed conservatively with anticoagulation only.

D. **Antibiotics.** Especially if the patient has prosthetic graft material in place.

   E. Protection of the Ischemic Extremity. Position the limb in a mild dependent position. Protect it from trauma.

   F. Operation. Alert the appropriate senior staff, anesthesia, and patient's family as most acute occlusions will be managed by either embolectomy or some type of reconstruction.

   G. Postoperatively, observe for acidosis, hyperkalemia, myoglobinuria, compartment syndrome, which may develop after extremity reperfusion. Also, monitor pulses and neurologic exam every 2 hours.

63. SEIZURES

Immediate Actions

   1. Assure **A**irway, **B**reathing, and **C**irculation. Do not force anything into the mouth of a seizing patient.

   2. Prevent self-inflicted injuries.

   3. Obtain IV access.

   4. Single seizures usually end before therapy can be started urgently. A patient in status epilepticus needs therapy. Start with Diazepam (Valium) 10 mg slow IV push (see following section, "Plan").

I. Problem. A 25-year-old male is found seizing in bed 1 day after appendectomy.

II. Immediate Questions

   A. Has the patient ever had seizures before? A patient with a history of seizures is often on an antiseizure medication (or is supposed to be). In these patients, a common cause of seizures is the failure to take the prescribed medication.

   B. Is the patient taking any anticonvulsant medications? Has the patient been put back on all medications he was taking before admission? If the patient is NPO, be sure that an appropriate parenteral form is given. Check for other medications, as some of these can affect the blood levels of antiseizure medication, particularly diphenylhydantoin (Dilantin).

   C. Does the patient have a history of alcohol abuse or diabetes? This may be confused with alcoholic withdrawal or severe hypoglycemia.

   D. Was the seizure generalized or focal? Focal seizures suggest a central nervous system cause.

   E. What are the results of the most recent lab tests? May reveal an obvious electrolyte abnormality.

   F. Were there any witnesses? Observers may indicate a prodrome, or if the patient suffered any specific injury or fall.

III. Differential Diagnosis. The hallmark of the seizure is rigid stiffening of the muscles, loss of bladder control, and cyanosis with a postictal phase consisting of confusion, myalgia, lethargy, and headache.

   A. Idiopathic Epilepsy. The most common cause of seizures, but must be a diagnosis of exclusion in the acute situation.

   B. Tumors. Either primary brain tumors or metastatic lesions can be responsible. Frequent lesions include carcinoma of the breast, lung, or kidney, melanoma or lymphoma.

   C. Infection. In adults, intracranial infection can cause seizures, whereas in children any infectious process with systemic reaction (fever) can cause seizures.

   D. Trauma. A careful history must be obtained. Was the patient found on the floor? Are there signs of skull fracture?

   E. Alcohol/Drug Withdrawal. This is common in patients hospitalized, causing sudden withdrawal (see Problem 25, page 93).

   F. Chronic Renal Failure. With uremia.

   G. Anoxia. Evaluate arterial blood gases.

   H. Electrolyte Abnormalities. Including hypoglycemia, hypomagnesemia, hypocalcemia, and hyponatremia with rapid correction.

   I. Collagen Vascular Disease.

   J. Hallucinations.

   K. Hypothyroidism.

   L. Degenerative Disease (Tay Sachs).

   M. Vascular Lesions. Infarcts, emboli, hypertensive encephalopathy, carotid sinus disease, subarachnoid hemorrhage.

   N. Syncope. Often what is thought to be a seizure is just a syncopal attack. Get a careful description from both nurses and patient about the event.

   O. Hysteria. Such as psychiatric pseudoseizures.

   P. Inadequate level of prescribed anticonvulsants. Especially phenytoin (Dilantin) where the level can be altered by the addition of almost any drug (aspirin, others).

IV. Database

   A. Physical Exam Key Points

   1. **Vital signs.** Fever suggests an infection; febrile seizures may be seen in children. Check blood pressure and palpate pulse to be sure the patient is stable.

   2. Do not interfere if the patient is spontaneously breathing. Specifically, do not try to force something into the patient's

mouth like a tongue depressor. This can lead to injury to the patient or yourself and is unnecessary.
3. Check for aspiration.
4. **Neurologic exam.** Look for focal signs that may help diagnose the cause. Perform a complete exam including all cranial nerves, sensation, strength, DTRs, and mental status. There may be transient deficits after the seizure (the postictal state).
5. Is there evidence of fecal or urinary incontinence?

B. **Laboratory Data**
1. Serum electrolytes, calcium, magnesium, creatinine, glucose to rapidly screen for metabolic causes.
2. **Arterial blood gases.** To rule out hypoxia as a cause.
3. Drug levels of anticonvulsants being taken. Do this immediately as a patient seizing with adequate drug levels will need to have new therapy instituted.
4. CSF fluid analysis, if indicated (see Section III, page 295.)

C. **Radiologic and Other Studies**
1. **Head CT scan.** If this episode represents new onset seizures and there is no obvious cause, then CT scan of the head is indicated. However, the scan does not need to be done emergently, unless other evidence suggests a space occupying lesion that may require emergent treatment.
2. Lumbar puncture may help if there is evidence of meningeal irritation. Be sure to check for increased intracranial pressure before the spinal tap.

V. Plan

A. **General Plan.** Support life functions (the ABCs of CPR), and prevent self-inflicted injury during the seizure. This is followed by a careful workup to determine the cause and institute appropriate therapy.

B. **Specific Measures** (see Section IX, page 388, for a discussion of drugs listed below).
1. Vital functions, especially airway, must be monitored and supported.
2. Establish IV access as soon as possible.
3. A single seizure will usually finish before the onset of action of any IV medication, and therefore does not need to be specifically treated. However, to treat a second seizure, or status epilepticus (repeated seizures with no regaining of consciousness between seizures), diazepam (Valium) IV may be given, usually as 5 mg IV push (slowly), repeating at 10–15 minute intervals as needed to control seizure activity.
4. Phenytoin (Dilantin) may be used if Valium fails, or to prevent recurrence of seizures if Valium has given temporary control. It

    must be given slow IV push, no faster than 50 mg/min, directly
    into the vein. Check levels daily after first starting the drug.
    Loading dose is 15–18 mg/kg IV.

5. Phenobarbital may also be used. It is given slow IV usually with
a 120–240 mg (10–20 mg/kg in children) loading dose.
Maintenance doses are given IV, IM, or PO to maintain therapeutic levels.

6. Be alert for the complications of aspiration and hyperthermia.

7. Anticonvulsants are not indicated for alcohol withdrawal
seizures, but Librium may be useful to control other symptoms
of delirium tremens.

8. Refractory seizures that do not respond to the above management may require general anesthesia.

C. Treat Underlying Condition. After the acute seizure episode is
controlled, treat the underlying condition. Treat electrolyte abnormalities as outlined in the specific on call problem. Treat CNS lesion as appropriate.

64. SUPRAPUBIC CATHETER PROBLEMS

I. Problem. A patient has a suprapubic catheter that has stopped
draining.

II. Immediate Questions

A. Does the patient have a full bladder? Determined by palpating
suprapubic fullness with associated tenderness.

B. Is the total urine output adequate? Gradual decrease in urine
may suggest oliguria as opposed to an obstructed tube.

**C. Is urine draining around the suprapubic tube, and is there
blood or clots?** Suggests that the tube is blocked or pulled out of
the bladder.

D. Why does this patient have a suprapubic catheter? Suprapubic cystostomy drains are placed surgically or percutaneously
for bladder decompression. Temporary tubes placed emergently
(ie, Cystocath, Stamey type, which have a small diameter [ie,
12–14 Fr]) can dislodge if not carefully secured. Tubes placed in
the operating room intended for long-term use are usually of the
Malencot variety and of larger caliber (22–24 French). They are
placed for a wide range of indications such as bladder injury, urethral injury and obstruction, transplant neoureterocystostomy obstruction or stricture.

E. How long has the catheter been in place? A long-standing
suprapubic tube usually will have a mature tract into the bladder,
whereas a recently placed tube may not.

III. Differential Diagnosis

A. Systemic Causes. For detailed discussion of low urine output (oliguria), see Problem 56, page 187.

B. Catheter Obstruction. Can be caused by blood clots or occasionally by debris (stone encrustation). Long-standing tubes can become coated with calcium deposits.

C. Catheter Tip Dislodgement. More of a problem with a recent suprapubic tube because the tract may be immature.

IV. Database

A. Directed History and Physical Exam. Attention to fluid status, vital signs, temperature, abdominal exam, catheter exit site, and catheter suture.

B. Laboratory Data. Lab studies usually not necessary in acute cases.

V. Plan. The approach to a poorly functioning tube depends primarily on the age of the tube.

A. Recently Placed Tube. Attempt to flush the tube. Tube change probably should be done in the operating room because the tract is immature.

B. Chronically Indwelling Tube. A new tube of similar size can be placed because the tract is mature. If a tube is no longer needed, and the patient can void via the urethra, the tract will typically close within 48 hours. Chronic tubes are generally replaced every 4–8 weeks to prevent encrustation. Annual KUB x-ray is needed in these patients to evaluate for stone formation. Unless symptomatic, the colonization that accompanies a chronic suprapubic tube is generally not treated. The notable exception is that any colonization with stone-forming organisms (eg, proteus) must be treated.

65. SWOLLEN EXTREMITY

I. Problem. Three days after a knee replacement, a 49-year-old obese woman develops a swollen left calf and right ankle.

II. Immediate Questions

A. What are the vital signs? Tachycardia and fever may represent infection. Tachycardia and tachypnea may be manifestations of pulmonary embolus.

B. Is the patient short of breath? Complaints of not getting enough air in a patient with a swollen extremity should be evaluated for pulmonary embolus or congestive heart failure.

C. Is the extremity or just the joint swollen? This would limit the diagnostic possibilities.

III. Differential Diagnosis

A. Venous Obstruction. Deep venous thrombosis (DVT), most of which remain clinically silent, occurs in a high percentage of immobile postoperative patients. Thrombus can form anywhere from the level of the calf to the pelvis. The major risk of DVT is pulmonary embolus (PE) and pulmonary infarction, which are significantly life-threatening. Superficial thrombophlebitis can also occur in the upper or lower extremity (see Problem 58, page 192).

B. Lymphatics

    1. Obstruction. Typically a result of a tumor involving the inguinal nodes, obstructed lymphatics produce diffuse, nontender swelling of the entire leg.

    2. Destruction. Operative destruction of draining lymph nodes can produce extremity swelling acutely or years later, as typified by arm swelling after axillary node dissection. Radiation can also ablate lymphatic channels.

C. Infection. Cellulitis of the lower extremity, especially the "diabetic foot," can produce swelling to any level depending on the extent of the infection. A foreign body with associated infection can also produce leg swelling.

D. Congenital. This is usually lymphedema, either lymphedema tarda or praecox.

E. Other. Causes of edema, such as renal failure, liver disease, and congestive heart failure, typically produce bilateral swelling, though early disease may manifest as a unilateral problem. Joint swelling may be a result of infectious or inflammatory arthritis.

IV. Database

A. Physical Exam Key Points

    1. Vital signs. Tachypnea is a sign of pulmonary embolus.

    2. Extremities. Check both extremities for swelling. Look for evidence of infection (eg, cellulitis, lymphangitis, or tender superficial veins). Feel for calf tenderness and palpable cords, which are suggestive of DVT. Measure calf and thigh circumferences from a well marked constant point on both legs as a baseline.

    3. Chest. Listen for rales (congestive heart failure).

    4. Abdomen. Look for ascites (liver disease).

5. **Axillary and inguinal nodes.** Has a lymphadenectomy been performed? Are nodes palpable (tumor)? Has there been recent breast surgery, or is there a breast mass?

B. **Laboratory Data**
   1. **Hemogram.** Especially if infection is suspected.
   2. **Serum electrolytes and glucose.** Inflammatory processes can affect the therapy of diabetics and patients with chronic renal failure.
   3. **Coagulation panel (PT, PTT, platelet count).** As a baseline before anticoagulant therapy; occult thrombocytosis may be evident, as well as evidence of DIC.

C. **Radiologic and Other Studies**
   1. **Venogram.** The invasive standard for evaluating DVT.
   2. Noninvasive venous studies such as impedance plethysmography (IPG) are sometimes useful. Venous Doppler studies are also helpful, but expert interpretation is mandatory.
   3. **Bone radiographs.** These may be useful if "diabetic foot" and cellulitis are suspected. Evaluates for presence of soft tissue air and osteomyelitis, as well as foreign bodies.
   4. CT scan of the abdomen and pelvis looking for a mass causing obstruction of the iliac veins or vena cava is recommended.

V. Plan

A. **Venous Obstruction**
   1. Bedrest with elevation of involved extremity.
   2. Baseline platelet count and activated partial thromboplastin time (PTT) should be sent. Heparin rarely causes thrombosis and thrombocytopenia. However, the physician must follow the patient's serial platelet counts to identify who may become thrombocytopenic.
   3. **Heparin.** 5000–10,000 U IV bolus followed by 1000–1500 U/hr continuous infusion to maintain PTT at 2–2.5 times control value.
   4. **Coumadin.** The administration of Coumadin can begin approximately 3–5 days after starting therapeutic heparin and should be continued for 6–12 months or longer for recurrent episodes. Prothrombin time should be maintained at 1.5–2.5 times control values (INR 2–4.5).
   5. **Prevention.** Minidose heparin is useful in preventing DVTs when started preoperatively in high risk patients, eg, those undergoing pelvic or orthopedic procedures, obese patients, or patients with a history of DVT. The dosage is 5000 U given subcutaneously every 8–12 hours. Pneumatic stockings are available, which intermittently inflate around the calves presumably reproducing muscle contractions that are effective in preventing DVT. Early ambulation also helps prevent DVT.

   6. **Superficial thrombophlebitis.** Typically treated with local heat
      and nonsteroidal anti-inflammatory agents (see problem 58,
      page 192).

B. **Lymphatic Disease.** Local measures, such as heat and elevation,
   are of little benefit. Custom-made elastic stockings (eg, Jobst) are
   of some use. Intermittent pneumatic compression, such as at bedtime, may also give some relief.

C. **Infection.** Antibiotics should be started, covering for *Staphylococcal* and *Streptococcal* species in the upper extremity, as well as
   for gram negative and anaerobic species in the lower extremity.
   Blood cultures should be obtained in the toxic patient. It may be
   difficult to differentiate cellulitis from DVT.

66. SYNCOPE

I. **Problem.** A patient undergoing a preoperative evaluation for a mitral
   valve replacement has a syncopal episode in the radiology department.

II. **Immediate Questions**

A. **What was the patient doing when the episode occurred?**
   Vasovagal syncope or fainting from orthostatic hypotension can
   occur only in a sitting or standing position. Syncope while lying flat
   is almost always cardiac in origin. Vasovagal attacks have associated factors of heat, anxiety, pain, or closed space. Syncope with
   exertion is often cardiac. Also ask the patient about coughing, turning or twisting the head, or getting up quickly.

B. **Was the syncope observed, and was there any seizure activity?** In determining the cause of loss of consciousness a seizure
   is always in the initial differential diagnosis. Ask observers about
   seizure activity, examine for bites to the tongue, and evaluate rate
   of return to baseline consciousness. Syncopal patients recover
   quickly, whereas seizure patients have a postictal period.
   Incontinence is indicative of a seizure.

C. **How did the patient feel immediately before the loss of consciousness?** Patients with vasovagal syncope normally have a
   presyncopal complex consisting of sweating, lightheadedness,
   and abdominal queasiness. Cardiac syncope and orthostatic hypotension are usually sudden in onset. Seizure episodes may
   have a preceding aura.

D. **Did anyone take the patient's pulse during the episode?**
   Vasovagal attacks are associated with bradycardia; orthostatic hy-

potension with tachycardia; and cardiac syncope with variable heart rates ranging from severe bradycardia in heart block to tachycardia as the cause for the syncope.

E. Is the patient a diabetic? Insulin dependent? Hypoglycemic events are an infrequent but readily treatable cause of syncope.

F. What medications is the patient taking? MAO inhibitors and antihypertensives can cause orthostatic hypotension if the dose is large enough.

III. Differential Diagnosis

A. Cardiovascular

1. **Reflex syncope**
   a. Vasovagal (simple faint).
   b. Orthostatic often associated with volume depletion or medications (ie, α-blockers such as terazosin).
   c. Carotid sinus syncope.
2. **Cardiac**
   a. Mechanical
      i. Aortic stenosis.
      ii. Myocardial infarction.
      iii. Mitral stenosis.
      iv. Cardiomyopathy.
      v. Pulmonary embolism.
   b. **Electrical (dysrhythmias)**
      i. AV block
      ii. SVT/Ventricular arrhythmias
      iii. Sick sinus syndrome
      iv. Pacemaker-related

B. Noncardiovascular

1. **Neurologic.** Subclavian steal, seizure (see Problem 63, page 205).
2. **Metabolic.** Hypoxia, hypoglycemia, hyperventilation.
3. **Psychiatric.** Hysteria, panic.

IV. Database

A. Physical Exam Key Points

1. **General exam.** Is the patient confused, lethargic, or anxious? Is there any obvious injury? Evidence of incontinence suggests a seizure.
2. **Vital signs.** Orthostatic changes, heart rate and rhythm. Discrepancy in blood pressure between both arms > 20 mm Hg is suggestive of subclavian steal syndrome.

3. **Neck.** Carotid bruits, carotid upstroke.
4. **Chest.** Murmurs of aortic stenosis, IHSS, rhythm. Crackles and wheezes may indicate aspiration associated with the episode or CHF.
5. **Rectal exam.** Heme positive stools or other evidence of an acute bleed.
6. **Neurologic exam.** Dysarthria, focal signs, mental status.

B. **Laboratory Data**
   1. **Hemogram.** With close attention to the hematocrit.
   2. **Chemistry panel.** For electrolytes and glucose.
   3. **Blood gas.** Hypoxia or hyperventilation (decreased CO_2, decreased pH) may be present.

C. **Radiologic and Other Studies**
   1. **Chest x-ray.** Note especially the cardiac silhouette for evidence of heart failure or effusion.
   2. **ECG with a rhythm strip.** Short PR intervals, delta waves, or any other obvious signs of rhythm disturbance.
   3. **Cardiac echo.** May reveal myoxoma, valvular lesions or mural thrombi.
   4. Reproduce syncope with maneuvers such as coughing, turning the head, hyperventilation, or carotid massage.
   5. **Holter monitor.** Useful for evaluation of dysrhythmias.

V. **Plan**

A. **Overall Plan.** Causes for syncope range from an inconsequential vasovagal attack to the emergency of heart block. Therefore, treatment is dictated by the correct diagnosis. Always assess the patient for injury from a fall during syncope.

B. **Specific Treatments**
   1. **Vasovagal.** Instruct the patient to put his head down at the onset of presyncopal symptoms.
   2. **Orthostatic hypotension**
      a. Assess for volume loss (paying close attention for possible GI bleed) and treat accordingly.
      b. Instruct the patient to change positions slowly.
   3. **Cardiac**
      a. **Treat the arrhythmia:** If tachyarrhythmia is causing hypotension, treat as outlined in Problem 67, page 215. Cardiac arrest rhythms are treated as in Problem 11, page 37.
      b. **Monitor the patient:** Often, a 24-hour Holter needs to be obtained for diagnosis.

67. TACHYCARDIA

I. **Problem.** On a routine check of vital signs, a 68-year-old woman is found to have a pulse of 155 two days after sigmoid colectomy.

II. **Immediate Questions**

A. **What is the patient's normal pulse?** It is important to have a frame of reference for evaluating tachycardia.

B. **What are the other vital signs?** A tachycardia along with hypotension in a postoperative patient is an important clue to possible hypovolemia. Similarly, a fever can cause tachycardia. Tachycardia above 150 BPM with significant symptoms (eg, decreased consciousness, significant hypotension, chest pain or shortness of breath, immediate pharmacologic or cardioversion) may be indicated.

C. **Does the patient have underlying heart disease?** Is the rhythm regular or irregular (atrial fibrillation).

D. **What medication is the patient taking?** If the patient is on an antiarrhythmic, has the patient been receiving the appropriate doses? Diuretics and potassium supplements may cause electrolyte abnormalities and arrhythmias.

III. **Differential Diagnosis**

A. **Sinus Tachycardia**
   1. **Thyrotoxicosis.** Weight loss, irritability, and tremor are associated symptoms.
   2. **Pheochromocytoma.** Associated with headache, abdominal pain, hypertension, and sweating.
   3. **Anxiety/Pain.** Normal physiologic response related to catecholamine release.
   4. **Drug-related.** Sympathomimetics, such as epinephrine, can cause tachycardia.
   5. **Hypotension.** With associated hypovolemia.
   6. **High-output states.** A rise in right atrial pressure from any cause such as thyrotoxicosis, A/V fistula, anemia, pregnancy, or severe Paget's disease.
   7. **Cardiac failure.** A drop in pulse pressure along with increased right atrial pressure leads to tachycardia.
   8. Fever related.
   9. Sepsis.
   10. Pneumothorax/pericardial effusion.

B. Ectopic Tachycardia

1. **Paroxysmal atrial tachycardia.** Often accompanied by palpitations and lightheadedness, with a rate of 140–250 BPM.

2. **Atrial flutter.** Rates are faster than in atrial or junctional tachycardia (rate 250–350 BPM).

3. **Ventricular tachycardia.** Usually associated with ischemic heart disease, including acute MI; also can be a forerunner of ventricular fibrillation.

IV. Database

A. Physical Exam Key Points

1. **Vital signs.** Check pulse rate and regularity as well as for fever. Hypotension is a major threat to life.

2. **Cardiac.** Look for evidence of failure, neck vein distention, S_3, etc.

3. **Lungs.** For evidence of cardiac failure, rales, or pneumothorax.

4. **Extremities.** Check for edema or cyanosis.

B. Laboratory Data

1. **Serum electrolytes.** Especially potassium.

2. **Arterial blood gases.** To rule out hypoxia.

3. **Hemogram.** To evaluate for sepsis or anemia.

4. **Thyroid function tests.** If indicated.

C. Radiologic and Other Studies

1. **ECG.** The most important piece of information will be the electrocardiogram because this allows correct diagnosis of the particular tachycardia in that patient.

2. **Chest x-ray.** Looking for signs of cardiac failure or primary pulmonary problems.

V. Plan

A. General Plan. Establish the correct diagnosis. Remember that even late at night, a medical colleague usually will be glad to help read a confusing cardiogram.

B. Specific Plans

1. **Ventricular tachycardia.** Perhaps most important because it can lead to cardiac arrest and death rapidly (see Problem 11, page 37 and Figure I–9).

2. **Atrial flutter and fibrillation**

   a. If the patient is hemodynamically compromised, immediate treatment with synchronized electrical cardioversion is indicated (20–50 joules) along with IV diazepam sedation.

   b. Initially, attempt carotid massage to slow rate and visualize flutter waves.

   c. If the patient is stable, then pharmacologic therapy is indicated.

      i. The first goal is to slow the ventricular response. This is accomplished with digoxin or verapamil intravenously.

      ii. The second goal is to restore normal sinus rhythm. Quinidine may be used to do this once the ventricular response is lower. Procainamide is an alternative to quinidine (see Problem 51, page 174).

      iii. Digoxin and verapamil should not be used in patients with the Wolff-Parkinson-White syndrome.

      iv. Patients with chronic atrial fibrillation may not be convertible to sinus rhythm. While verapamil acts faster than digoxin, its rapid clearance from the blood may require more frequent dosing.

3. Paroxysmal atrial tachycardia. This condition can be treated in a variety of ways.

   a. Vagal maneuvers such as an ice bag on the face, induced vomiting, or carotid massage should be tried first. Be careful performing carotid massage in patients with carotid disease.

   b. Verapamil given IV is also effective, usually starting with 2.5 mg IV push and giving added doses of 2.5 mg every 5 minutes or so to a total dose of 10 mg.

   c. Combined verapamil with carotid massage is often effective. Intravenous propranolol is also effective.

   d. Synchronized DC cardioversion is also an effective therapy.

4. Sinus tachycardia. In the surgical patient, fever and hypovolemia are common causes of this condition. The key to therapy of sinus tachycardia is treatment of the underlying condition. Hypovolemia will be associated with oliguria in the surgical patient.

68. TRANSFUSION REACTION

I. Problem. During a transfusion of packed red blood cells, a patient's temperature rises to 38.5°C.

II. Immediate Questions

   A. Vital signs. Hypotension should be ruled out. Tachypnea is a sign of a significant reaction. Fever is the most common manifestation of a transfusion reaction.

   B. Does the patient have back or chest pain? Acute coagulopathy can develop from a major transfusion reaction. Chest pain may develop during hemodynamic stress. Other symptoms may include chills, diaphoresis, hypersensitivity reactions (hives, wheezing, pruritus) or exacerbation of congestive heart failure.

C. Has the transfusion been stopped? If not, do so, and maintain an open IV line with normal saline.

III. Differential Diagnosis. Differentiating a fever due to a transfusion reaction from other causes of postoperative fever is difficult. Assuming no other source, the following transfusion reactions are possible, in order of decreasing likelihood and increasing severity:

   A. White Cell Antigens. Unlike washed red cells, packed cells contain relatively large numbers of leukocytes. Febrile responses to these cells are usually accompanied by urticaria.

   B. Minor Protein Reactions. Allergic reactions to transfused serum proteins can cause fever. Sometimes, anaphylaxis or acute pulmonary edema can occur.

   C. ABO Incompatibility. This represents a potentially life-threatening problem, but it occurs rarely. Signs are seen after transfusion of relatively small quantities of blood.

   D. Contaminated Blood. Bacterial contamination is rare but should be suspected when high fever and hypotension develop early during a transfusion because it is often fatal.

IV. Database

   A. Physical Exam Key Points
   1. **Lungs.** Listen for rales and wheezing.
   2. **Cardiac.** Examine for tachycardia and new flow murmur.
   3. **Abdomen.** Evaluate for pain, especially in the flanks.
   4. **Skin.** Look for rash or hives.

   B. Laboratory Data
   1. **Blood bank specimen.** Two freshly drawn clot tubes (red top tubes) should be returned to the blood bank with the remaining untransfused blood. A repeat crossmatch will be performed. In addition, most blood banks require a heparinized specimen to perform an indirect Coombs' test, looking for previous sensitization.
   2. **Urinalysis.** Hematuria after a transfusion reaction represents hemoglobinuria after hemolysis from a major ABO incompatibility.
   3. **Hemogram.** Schistocytes may be present in a transfusion reaction; a worsening anemia may develop in the face of massive red cell destruction.
   4. **Serum for free hemoglobin and haptoglobin.** Free hemoglobin will be present with a reaction and haptoglobin will be decreased.

    5. Other lab tests. Coagulation studies and thrombocytopenia may indicate DIC. Monitor renal function by obtaining BUN and creatinine along with serum electrolytes. Arterial blood gases rarely are indicated (cardiovascular collapse).

C. Radiologic and Other Studies. Not routinely needed, but ordered it clinically indicated.

V. Plan

A. Immediately Stop Transfusion. Consultation with the blood bank pathologist usually is indicated to evaluate the reaction as well as to discuss any further transfusions.

B. Maintain IV Access. Monitor urine output and vital signs closely.

C. Send Blood Bank Appropriate Specimens. See preceding section, "Laboratory Data." Make sure the bag is returned to the blood bank immediately.

D. Mild Reactions. Usually fever without any evidence of more severe symptoms or hemolysis.
    1. Antihistamines (diphenhydramine 25–50 mg IM or IV) and acetaminophen may reverse mild allergic and febrile reactions.
    2. Transfusion can usually be restarted.

E. Severe Reactions. Usually signifies acute hemolysis has taken place. One of the major goals is to prevent renal failure.
    1. Circulatory support. Maintain adequate blood pressure with volume or pressors. Diuresis with furosemide or mannitol with usually D_5W should be started to prevent renal injury in the setting of marked hemolysis. Also consider alkalinization of the urine with bicarbonate to further protect the kidneys.
    2. Antibiotics. These will be needed if examination of the remaining untransfused unit reveals evidence of bacterial contamination. The organisms are usually gram-negative bacilli.

F. Known Reactions. In patients with known febrile reactions to blood products, the patient can be pretreated with antihistamines (Diphenhydramine) or antipyretics or steroids to avoid the reaction. Blood bank products are discussed in Section VI, Blood Component Therapy.

69. TRAUMA ASSESSMENT & RESUSCITATION

Immediate Actions
Start with the ABCs of trauma:

    1. Airway. Check for clear airway. Evaluate C-spine and assume injury until cleared with x-ray. Intubate if necessary. Perform cricothyrotomy if needed.

2. **B**reathing. Administer O_2, ventilate, and vent (14 gauge needle) any suspected pneumothorax.
3. **C**irculation. Obtain two large bore (14–16 gauge) IVs in the upper extremities and begin crystalloid infusion (LR) as fast as possible. Draw routine blood work.
4. Evaluate response to initial resuscitation. Begin secondary survey once stabilized.
5. **D**isability. Rapid neurologic assessment.
6. Examine. Remove all clothing and quickly inspect the patient.
7. Begin ECG monitoring.

I. Problem. An 18-year-old female involved in a motor vehicle accident has a blood pressure of 90/50 mm Hg and is combative.

II. Immediate Questions

A. **Is the patient able to talk?** Airway obstruction and major chest injuries are rapidly fatal and therefore are addressed first. If the patient is unable to talk, but is making ventilatory efforts, sweep the oropharynx with gloved fingers to remove debris. Suction the oropharynx. Grasp the symphysis (chin) and displace it anteriorly. Ventilate with a well fitting mask and 100% oxygen for 2–3 minutes. If unsuccessful (saturation < 90%, no clinical improvement), then intubate with a No. 7 or No. 8 cuffed endotracheal tube. Rarely patients who present with severe maxillofacial injury cannot be intubated orally and require immediate tracheostomy. A cricothyroidotomy made between the laryngeal cartilage and cricoid is preferred over a formal tracheostomy because it is faster and safer. Maintain axial traction with an assistant during all airway maneuvers to minimize cord injury.

B. **Has the patient's ventilatory status improved?** Frequently, reevaluation is essential in trauma management to identify missed injuries. A patient in severe respiratory distress that has not improved with intubation should have chest tubes placed immediately, before chest x-ray is performed. Flail chest, tension pneumothorax, bronchial discretion are lethal injuries that are treatable.

C. **How long ago was the injury?** Assessing the degree of shock to plan fluid resuscitation is the next priority. If the injury occurred 2 hours ago and the degree of shock is mild, then massive or ongoing hemorrhage is less likely.

D. **What is the blood pressure?** Blood pressure does not fall until more than 20% of intravascular blood volume is lost. Compensatory mechanisms of vasoconstriction and increased heart rate and contractility occur early, allowing blood pressure to be maintained in early shock.

E. What is the heart rate? Tachycardia above 120 BPM should be considered a sign of hypovolemic shock in the trauma setting.

F. Is the skin cool and moist? Vasoconstriction of muscle and skin is an early compensatory mechanism. Epinephrine release causes sweating. Cool, moist skin is a reliable clinical sign of impending shock.

G. What is the urine output? Any patient with serious trauma should have their urine output monitored. Visceral vasoconstriction with resulting decreased renal blood flow is reflected in diminished urine output.

H. Are the external jugular veins distended? A trauma patient who appears to be in hypovolemic shock by other parameters, but who has distended neck veins most likely has cardiac tamponade.

III. Database

A. Physical Exam Key Points. History and physical examination performed with the patient fully immobilized and completely exposed. It is particularly important to perform a thorough head-to-toe initial examination in order to avoid missed injuries such as unsuspected entrance and exit sites in penetrating injuries.

1. **Lungs.** Evaluate breath sounds considering the possibility of pneumothorax.
2. **Heart.** Listen for tachycardia, muffled heart sounds.
3. **Abdomen.** Evaluate for distention (possible site of significant bleeding) and peritonitis.

B. Laboratory Data. Send complete blood count, coagulation studies, chemistries, toxicology screen, urinalysis, type and cross-match sample from blood drain while placing first intravenous line. Send arterial blood gas.

C. Radiologic Studies. Lateral C-spine with collar on, flat pelvis film, upright chest x-ray and other x-rays as indicated.

IV. Plan

A. Fluid Resuscitation. With moderate to severe hypovolemic shock, treatment is initiated before a complete assessment. Large bore, peripheral intravenous lines are started—two is the minimum required. The upper extremities are used preferably.

1. Cutdowns are placed easily in the saphenous vein at the ankles or the brachial and cephalic veins at the antecubital crease. The use of large bore lines (No. 8 or cut IV tubing to allow the administration of 2 L crystalloid in < 15 minutes. Short catheters allow more rapid infusions (thus subclavian CVP lines are not used at all).

2. Avoid placing percutaneous subclavian or internal jugular lines. The added risk of iatrogenic pneumothorax is not warranted.
3. Transfusion of red blood cells is used to improve oxygen carrying capacity in patients with hemorrhage. Type specific blood is preferred, but if unavailable, universal type O should be given. Packed red blood cells are more viscid than whole blood. To increase delivery rate of packed cells they can be injected into the vein with the crystalloid.

B. Secondary Assessment. If the initial resuscitation and assessment result in a hemodynamically stable and neurologically intact patient then a more thorough secondary assessment and reevaluation occur. If shock persists despite resuscitation, then ongoing hemorrhage is present and immediate operative intervention may be indicated.

C. Observation. Once the patient is stabilized, placement of an NG tube and Foley catheter are undertaken. Be careful about initiating urinary drainage if there is any possibility of a urethral injury (eg, pelvic fracture). Observe for blood at the meatus or a free floating prostate on rectal exam. In these cases, urinary catheter placement is only performed after radiographic evaluation of the urethra (urethrogram and cystogram). Peritoneal lavage may be indicated at this time. Temperature monitoring should be started.

D. Patients who remain in shock despite aggressive resuscitation must be rapidly assessed as to the cause. Hypovolemic shock usually results from blood loss within the chest or abdomen, or from a massive pelvic injury. Cardiogenic shock may be due to tension pneumothorax or hemopericardium, both of which are easily treated once suspected. The detailed secondary survey is begun once the patient is stabilized during the initial resuscitation phase. This includes a comprehensive examination and reevaluation of the patient.

70. VAGINAL BLEEDING

I. Problem. A young woman admitted for observation for possible appendicitis develops vaginal bleeding.

II. Immediate Questions

A. Is there any evidence of shock? Vaginal bleeding can be profuse. In some cases the visible blood loss may represent only a fraction of the actual blood loss. Assess the patient for hypovolemia or shock.

Is there any pain associated with the bleeding? The most serious condition in the differential diagnosis of acute vaginal bleeding 's ectopic pregnancy, and pain is always a predominant part of the patient's complaints. Other causes of vaginal bleeding are also associated with pain and other gastrointestinal symptoms.

C. When was the patient's last period, and has she been sexually active since that time? Inquire about specific details of menstrual history, regarding the most recent period, and any abnormal bleeding in the past. Obtain a complete sexual history including contraceptive use and any associated symptoms of early pregnancy (morning sickness, fluid retention, etc).

D. Attempt to quantitate the blood loss. The rate of bleeding has both diagnostic and therapeutic implications. If a volume estimate of blood loss cannot be given, ask about number of pads or tampons used and degree of saturation.

III. Differential Diagnosis

A. Normal Menstrual Period. Clearly the most commonly encountered cause.

B. Dysfunctional Bleeding (Related to Menstrual Cycle)
1. Perimenopausal.
2. Inadequate luteal phase.
3. Oral contraceptives.
4. Endometriosis.

C. Pregnancy Related
1. Ectopic pregnancy.
2. Threatened or spontaneous abortion.
3. Retained products of gestation.

D. Neoplasia
1. Uterine fibroids.
2. Cervical polyps.
3. Carcinoma
   a. Endometrium.
   b. Cervix.
   c. Ovarian.

E. Infection
1. Pelvic inflammatory disease.
2. Vaginitis.

F. Trauma

G. Bleeding Diathesis. Bleeding is usually present at other sites as well.

IV. Database

A. Physical Exam Key Points
1. **Vital signs.** Check orthostatic signs for excessive blood loss; fever is a sign of infection.

2. **Skin.** Pallor suggests significant blood loss. Bruising and petechiae suggest bleeding diathesis.
3. **Abdomen.** Observe for peritoneal signs, tenderness, distention.
4. **Pelvic exam.** Examine for mass in vagina, cervix, uterus, or adnexa. Areas of tenderness including cervical motion pain. Evaluate source and rate of bleeding, and if the cervical os open or closed, with or without tissue fragments.

B. **Laboratory Data**
1. **Hemogram.** To look for leukocytosis, falling hematocrits or thrombocytopenia.
2. **PT/PTT.** If coagulopathy is suspected. Check fibrinogen and fibrin split products if DIC is suspected.
3. **Blood.** Type and crossmatch blood if indicated.
4. **Serum/urine HCG.** A pregnancy test will be positive with an ectopic pregnancy.
5. Pap smear of cervix.
6. Cervical culture.

C. **Radiologic and Other Studies**
1. **Culdocentesis.** If ectopic pregnancy is possible.
2. **Pelvic ultrasound.** Evaluates intrauterine and intratubal lesions and valuable for possible ectopic pregnancy or any pelvic mass.
3. **CT scan of pelvis.** Good method to detect any mass lesion. Usually not as obtainable in emergencies as an ultrasound. Be sure there is no salvageable intrauterine pregnancy before obtaining a CT scan.

V. **Plan.** Most vaginal bleeding does not require specific treatment because it represents normal menstrual bleeding.

A. **Overall Plan**
1. Resuscitate the patient from the acute blood loss as needed.
2. Establish large bore IVs, administer crystalloid, type and crossmatch for blood, monitor urine output, and follow serial hematocrits. Also make the patient NPO as urgent operative procedures may be indicated.

B. **Specific Treatment.** Virtually all the causes of significant vaginal bleeding require evaluation by the gynecology service. Ongoing bleeds require emergency consultation, while spotting or a bleeding episode that has resolved can be evaluated as above and seen on an elective basis—depending on the diagnosis.

C. **Ectopic Pregnancy.** If lower abdominal pain is a part of the symptom complex and the patient is of child-bearing age, ectopic pregnancy must be ruled out even if the pregnancy tests are normal. The diagnostic procedure of choice is a pelvic ultrasound; if ultrasound is not available, then use culdocentesis.

71. VENTILATOR MANAGEMENT: AGITATION

(Ventilators are discussed in detail in Section VII, page 366)

I. Problem. A patient—status postcraniotomy for a cerebellar lesion on a ventilator in the ICU—has become agitated and is "bucking" the ventilator.

II. Immediate Questions

A. What are the most recent blood gases? Hypoxia may be evident as well as hypocarbia from tachypnea.

B. When was the most recent chest x-ray? Be sure there is a recent chest x-ray. A new pneumothorax, perhaps secondary to positive pressure ventilation, can cause hypoxia resulting in agitation. Placement of the ETT into the right mainstem bronchus can also cause agitation.

C. What is the patient's respiratory rate? Tachypnea is a common cause of "bucking" the ventilator.

D. What are the ventilator settings (mode, rate, PEEP, F_{IO_2}, TV)? IMV delivers a fixed number of breaths per minute. Assist control will cause the ventilator to deliver a full tidal volume with each patient initiated breath.

III. Differential Diagnosis

A. Respiratory Decompensation. This must be ruled out first.
1. Pneumothorax or tension pneumothorax.
2. Improper positioning of the endotracheal tube. Either proximally or distally (usually down the right mainstem bronchus).
3. **Mucous plugging.** Tenacious secretions can obstruct the tube.
4. **Ventilator malfunction.** Verify with the nursing staff respiratory therapist that the ventilator is working properly and delivering the preset parameters.
5. **Aspiration.** Usually around a partially inflated cuff.
6. **Sepsis.** Systemic sepsis can cause agitation.
7. **Other causes.** CHF, pulmonary embolus, hiccups.

B. Inadequate Tidal Volume. Is the preset tidal volume sufficient for the patient (10–15 mL/kg)?

C. Insufficient Pain Medication or Sedation.

D. Status Epilepticus. May be confused with agitation.

E. Tetanus.

IV. Database

A. Physical Exam Key Points

1. **Vital signs.** Especially blood pressure, respiratory rate.
2. **Neck.** Distended neck veins or tracheal deviation may suggest pneumothorax.
3. **Lungs.** Examine for bilateral breath sounds, wheezing, or evidence of congestive heart failure.
4. **Chest.** Look for subcutaneous emphysema and symmetric excursion.
5. Verify that the cuff is inflated properly and listen for any air leaks.

B. Laboratory Data

1. **Arterial blood gases.** Look for hypoxia, CO_2 retention.
2. **Serum electrolytes** to complete acid-base workup.

C. Radiologic and Other Studies.
A chest x-ray is necessary to check endotracheal tube placement, rule out pneumothorax, effusions, etc. Therapy should not be delayed because of a pending x-ray.

V. Plan

A. Obtain a new set of arterial blood gases and a STAT portable chest x-ray.
This should be the first step in any patient on positive pressure ventilation.

B. Manually ventilate the patient with a bag and 100% O_2.

1. If the patient is easily ventilated, check for a mechanical ventilator problem.
2. If there is increased resistance to ventilation, consider pneumothorax. Be sure to check for bilateral breath sounds, etc. If there is evidence of a pneumothorax do not wait for the x-ray; place a chest tube immediately if the patient is unstable.
3. If there is no evidence of pneumothorax, check ET tube for obstruction. Consider replacing the tube if the obstruction cannot be relieved. If there is no obstruction then consider sepsis, CHF, pulmonary embolus, or aspiration as a cause of decompensation.

C. Treat Pain Appropriately.
Sedation may also be helpful with diazepam (Valium) IV. Use 2–5 mg IV every 2 hours as a start. Other agents include lorazepam (Ativan), midazolam (Versed) and others.

D. Patients "fighting" the ventilator can sometimes be calmed by increasing the tidal volume.

E. Remember that IMV mode delivers a fixed tidal volume at preset intervals, regardless of the patient's own respiratory rate.
The use of IMV has been beneficial in managing patients with an increased respiratory drive Assist control will give a full breath at

a preset tidal volume when the patient triggers the ventilator with an inspiration. Thus, a patient making small inspiratory efforts will trigger the ventilator for a full breath, which can lead to fighting the ventilator. Controlled ventilation should not routinely be used on conscious patients because it will not allow the patient to initiate any breaths on his own; the use of this modality in the conscious patient may lead to agitation.

F. If the patient is alert, reassure the patient by carefully explaining the mechanical ventilator. Often this helps relieve the fears of an otherwise frightened patient and assists in ventilator management.

G. Paralysis must be used with extreme caution, if at all. Only in patients with extremely critical respiratory compromise or tetanus does this have a definite role. Paralytic agents such as succinylcholine or pancuronium bromide must be used with adequate sedation.

72. VENTILATOR MANAGEMENT: HIGH F$_{IO_2}$

(Ventilators are discussed in Section VII, page 366)

I. Problem. A mechanically ventilated trauma patient is maintaining a P$_{O_2}$ of only 75 mm Hg on 90% inspired oxygen.

II. Immediate Questions

A. What are the arterial blood gas values? An elevated P$_{CO_2}$ indicates hypoventilation. When ventilation, as reflected by minute ventilation, is not adequate to maintain P$_{CO_2}$ in a normal range and there is concomitant lung disease, hypoxemia may result.

B. What does the chest x-ray show? Significant atelectasis, pneumonia, pneumothorax, pleural effusion, pulmonary edema, and ARDS can cause hypoxemia and result in high oxygen concentration requirements.

C. What is the endotracheal tube status? Mucous plugging could be occluding the tube. A cuff leak may not be allowing adequate inflation. If the tube is in too far it may be down the right mainstem bronchus.

D. What are the ventilator settings? Poor oxygenation may sometimes be corrected by increasing PEEP.

III. Differential Diagnosis. Causes of hypoxia can be classified into two main categories: problems causing poor matching between ventilation and perfusion (V/Q mismatch, shunt, and diffusion abnormalities) and pure hypoventilation (see also Section II, page 250).

A. Ventilation and Perfusion Mismatches. Most common cause of hypoxemia and high oxygen requirements. A 100% mismatch is termed a physiologic shunt.

1. Reactive airways (COPD, asthma).
2. Pneumonia.
3. Atelectasis.
4. Pulmonary embolus.
5. Pneumothorax.
6. Physiologic shunting seen in ARDS and pulmonary edema.
7. Anatomic shunting seen in congenital heart disease.
8. Sepsis in the face of mild to moderate mismatch of ventilation and perfusion through lowering of mixed venous oxygen.
9. Mainstem bronchus endotracheal tube. An endotracheal tube may migrate down the right mainstem bronchus.

B. Hypoventilation. Rare cause of hypoxemia.

1. Very low minute ventilation (low tidal volume, low rate, or both).
2. Increased dead space (unavoidable part of mechanical ventilation).
3. Muscle weakness in nonventilated patient.
4. Cuff leak.

IV. Database

A. Physical Exam Key Points

1. **Vital signs.** Fever, tachycardia, and hypotension may indicate sepsis.
2. **Cardiac.** Presence of S_3 and tachycardia may indicate heart failure as cause of pulmonary edema.
3. **Lungs.** Careful exam can indicate pulmonary edema (rales), decreased sounds (atelectasis, effusion, pneumothorax), egophony (pneumonia), wheezing (asthma). Confirm with chest x-ray.
4. **Neck.** Look for jugular venous distention.

B. Laboratory Data

1. **Arterial blood gas.** Follow serially.
2. **Hemogram.** Verify that hemoglobin hematocrit are adequate.
3. **Cultures.** Sputum, blood, urine, drains, and wounds as clinically indicated.
4. **Sputum exam.** Tenacious secretions are common in reactive airways disease. Purulent sputum indicates pneumonia, and frothy sputum pulmonary edema. Gram stain is a quick and useful evaluation of sputum.
5. **Mixed venous oxygen content.** Drawn from the pulmonary artery through a pulmonary artery catheter, oxygen should normally measure 40 mm Hg (approximately 70% saturated).

Lower levels indicate oxygen delivery to tissues is inadequate as would be found in major trauma and severe sepsis.

   6. Alveolar-arterial gradient.

C. Radiologic and Other Studies

   1. Chest radiograph. Critical to understanding the nature of the problem. Look for evidence of:

     a. ARDS.

     b. Pneumonia.

     c. Pulmonary edema.

     d. Atelectasis.

     e. Pneumothorax.

     f. Effusion.

     g. Endotracheal tube misplacement.

   2. Electrocardiogram. Look for dysrhythmias such as atrial fibrillation or flutter, which can be corrected; ischemic changes may indicate infarction.

   3. V/Q scan or pulmonary angiogram. If embolus suspected.

   4. CT scan of abdomen. If septic focus suspected.

   5. Bronchoscopy. Should be used aggressively to clear tenacious mucous plugs causing atelectasis, and with lavage, biopsy, and brushings as diagnostic aids.

   6. Open lung biopsy. Rarely indicated; used when hypoxemia and lung disease persist despite aggressive medical therapy and an unclear cause of lung disease.

V. Plan. The main objective is to provide adequate tissue oxygenation without subjecting the patient to the risks of oxygen toxicity. The goal is to keep F$_{IO_2}$ below 60%, especially with long-term oxygen use.

A. Correct Anemia. Keep Hct > 30% with transfusions.

B. Correct Pulmonary Disease

   1. Pneumothorax with a tube thoracostomy.

   2. Pneumonia. Antibiotics and pulmonary toilet, including nebulizer treatments and chest physiotherapy.

   3. Atelectasis. Ensure adequate tidal volume and frequent suctioning. Sigh's set at 2 times the tidal volume 6–10 times an hour will help reduce the incidence of atelectasis.

   4. Asthma. The use of bronchodilators, aminophylline, and steroids may help treat reactive airways.

   5. Effusion. Thoracentesis or tube thoracostomy.

   6. Pulmonary edema. Diuretics with careful attention to fluid management.

C. Pulmonary Toilet

   1. Frequent suctioning.

   2. Saline lavage into endotracheal tube.

   3. Provide an occasional large tidal volume ("sigh") by bagging before suctioning.

      4. Metaproterenol (Alupent) treatments.

      5. Chest physical therapy.

D. Treat Sepsis. Appropriate antibiotics and surgical drainage as required.

E. Optimize Ventilator Settings

      1. Place radial arterial catheter for frequent arterial blood gas measurements.

      2. Maintain normal Pco_2.

      3. Start with high Fio_2 (0.9–1.0) and wean down to avoid O_2 toxicity.

      4. Positive end expiratory pressure (PEEP) should be added slowly. Complications are rare below 10–15 mm Hg of PEEP, but may include barotrauma and decreased cardiac output (caused by decreased cardiac blood return). It may be necessary to increase PEEP to high levels to allow Fio_2 to be decreased to safe levels. This trade off results in higher mean and peak airway pressures. Consider Swan-Ganz catheter for higher PEEP settings (> 10 mm Hg).

      5. Sedation or paralysis. Consider these in the patient "fighting" the ventilator who still requires mechanically assisted ventilation. Agitation interferes with adequate function of the ventilator. Remember that agents such as pancuronium (Pavulon) should not routinely be used alone. Pavulon induces paralysis but does not cause sedation or relieve pain. Use it along with morphine or diazepam.

F. Maximize Hemodynamic State. Use of a pulmonary artery catheter may help in the management of the patient with respiratory failure.

      1. Maintain adequate filling pressures (15 mm Hg) with crystalloid or blood products. Give furosemide if the wedge pressure is above 20 mm Hg.

      2. Improve cardiac index as needed with dopamine or dobutamine.

G. Heparin. If pulmonary embolus suspected. Heparin 5000–10,000 U bolus followed by continuous drip at approximately 1000 U/hr to maintain activated partial thromboplastin time (PTT) between 2–2.5 times control. Some centers are using thrombolytic therapy with streptokinase.

73. VENTILATOR MANAGEMENT: HIGH PEAK PRESSURE

(Ventilators are discussed in Section VII, page 366)

  I. Problem. An intubated patient on the trauma service with multiple injuries from blunt trauma is continually setting off the peak pressure alarm.

II. Immediate Questions

A. What is the arterial blood gas? A change in peak pressure may represent a ventilator system malfunction, a decrease in sedation, or a new pulmonary event or condition. The most important issue is if the patient is being ventilated adequately. Send off an arterial blood sample for blood gas determination immediately.

B. Has the position of the endotracheal tube changed? If the endotracheal tube has migrated into the right mainstem bronchus the peak pressure will increase as the entire tidal volume is administered to one lung. Check the mark on the endotracheal tube at the lips and compare to previous positions. Chest x-ray is also indicated.

C. Are there increased secretions in the endotracheal tube? Find out if the nurse has been suctioning increased or thicker secretions from the endotracheal tube. The tube may become partially obstructed with secretions particularly in chronically intubated patients.

D. Is there any subcutaneous emphysema? An important cause for increased peak pressure in a patient on a ventilator with positive pressure is a tension pneumothorax, which can be associated with subcutaneous emphysema. The chest wall and neck can be palpated quickly for crepitus before a chest x-ray can be obtained.

E. Has there been any change in the ventilator or the control settings? Make sure that the peak pressure alarm is not due to resetting the control panel. Also troubleshoot the ventilator with the assistance of the respiratory therapist to look for circuit disconnections, etc.

III. Differential Diagnosis.

If the peak pressure alarm is sounded in a ventilated patient, the problem is either with the ventilator or an increased resistance to the delivered tidal volume in the patient. The increased resistance can be a result of intrinsic pulmonary pathology or to resistance to lung expansion from extrinsic compressive forces. Clinical situations can vary greatly, but in general, peak inspiratory pressures should be less than 20–30 cm H_2O.

A. Ventilator Problems
1. Lowered peak pressure setting.
2. Incorrect ventilator circuit set-up.
3. Shift in position of the endotracheal tube.

B. Intrinsic Pulmonary Problems
1. Obstruction of the endotracheal tube by secretions.
2. **Pulmonary edema.** ARDS, CHF can cause decreased compliance and high pressures will be required to ventilate the patient.

     3. Interstitial disease.
       a. Malignancy: Lymphangitic spread.
       b. Fibrosis: Such as bleomycin-induced.
     4. Reactive airway disease. Asthma.

  C. Extrinsic Pulmonary Compression
     1. Pneumothorax or tension pneumothorax.
     2. Pleural effusion including a hemothorax.
     3. Abdominal distention.
     4. Chest wall/respiratory muscle contraction
       a. Bucking the ventilator owing to anxiety, pain, or decreased sedation. However, agitation may be secondary to hypoventilation and hypoxia, so check the Pao_2
       b. Coughing spasm.

IV. Database
  A. Physical Exam Key Points
     1. Skin. Look for cyanosis, crepitus owing to subcutaneous emphysema.
     2. Lungs. Examine the secretions from the endotracheal tube noting amount and viscosity. Decreased or absent breath sounds, rales, wheezes.
     3. Cardiac. Elevated venous pressure, decreased heart sounds.
     4. Abdomen. Is there marked distention or ascites?

  B. Laboratory Data
     1. Arterial blood gas drawn immediately.
     2. Hemogram. For evidence of decreased hematocrit or leukocytosis.

  C. Radiologic and Other Studies
     1. Chest x-ray. Order portable film immediately if new problem with elevated pressure is not due to a technical problem with the ventilator. Look for pleural effusion, pulmonary edema, pneumothorax, or new infiltrate. Check the endotracheal tube position (tip should be 2 cm above the carina).

V. Plan
  A. Overall Plan. Initial therapy is to disconnect the patient from the ventilator and bag ventilate by hand. This maneuver allows for immediate hyperventilation, removes the ventilator as the source of the problem, allows manual assessment of pulmonary compliance, and allows the endotracheal tube to be irrigated and the patient to be suctioned of secretions. At the same time, draw an arterial blood gas, call for a portable chest x-ray, and check the ventilator. Decide whether the problem is the patient or the ventilator.

B. Specific Problems

1. **Hemo- or pneumothorax, effusion.** Treat with a tube thoracostomy. In urgent situations a tension pneumothorax can be treated with a 14 gauge IV catheter inserted into the anterior chest at the level of the second or third intercostal space (see page 307).

2. **Endotracheal tube malposition.** Adjust the tube, retape, and repeat the chest x-ray to document position.

3. Bucking the ventilator.

   a. Pain or sedation medications once hypoxia or mechanical problems have been ruled out (see page 225).

   b. Change pattern of ventilation to assist/control. Follow blood gases as patient may hyperventilate on this setting. Patients making small respiratory efforts will not do as well on assist/control as on IMV because the machine will overventilate them.

4. For cases of fibrosis, infiltrative disease, and ARDS being maximally treated, higher peak airway pressures may have to be tolerated to ventilate the patient. Adjust the alarm setting and follow closely for pneumothorax resulting from barotrauma.

74. VENTILATOR MANAGEMENT: LOW Po_2/HIGH Pco_2

(Ventilators are discussed in Section VII, page 366.)

I. **Problem.** An 83-year-old male has a Po_2 of 55 1 day after grafting of a ruptured abdominal aortic aneurysm.

II. **Immediate Questions**

A. **What are the current ventilator settings, and were there any recent changes in these settings?** Fio_2, rate (IMV or Assist Control), PEEP and tidal volume? Find out when the last ventilator changes were made, and what the blood gas results were before those changes.

B. **What are the most recent blood gas results? The prior set? On what ventilator settings?**

C. **What is the patient's respiratory rate?** Tachypnea is an important finding and suggests the ventilator settings may not be providing enough ventilatory support.

D. **What operation has the patient had? Type of incision?** Thoracotomy incisions, flank and large abdominal incisions are the most painful and limit the patient's ability to breathe on their own much more, than for example, a median sternotomy.

E. What are the patient's baseline blood gases (preop) on room air? Preop PFTs?

F. What is the peak pressure? This allows the clinician to calculate compliance (by tidal volume/peak pressure), thus following lung stiffness. A progressively stiffer lung may indicate ARDS as a cause for the low O_2 levels. Normal compliance is > 100 ml/cm H_2O.

G. When was the most recent chest x-ray? If not within a few hours, obtain a repeat chest film immediately.

III. Differential Diagnosis

A. Mucous Plugging.

B. Pulmonary Edema. Check fluid balance over the last several days. Is the patient ahead on fluids? This usually results in a lower Po_2.

C. Ventilator Leak. Usually because of a broken cuff. Be sure the patient is receiving all of the tidal volume delivered.

D. Pulmonary Parenchymal Disease. Such as COPD that existed preoperatively.

E. Inadequate Ventilatory Support. Such as low tidal volume. Assess by following Pco_2.

F. Pneumothorax. A simple pneumothorax can rapidly progress to a tension pneumothorax in a mechanically ventilated patient.

G. Endotracheal Tube Malposition. Evaluate on chest x-ray. Is the tube past the carina?

H. Aspiration.

I. Bronchospasm. Check for wheezing on physical exam.

J. ARDS.

K. Atelectasis/Pneumonia.

L. Pulmonary Embolus. No increase in saturation or Pao_2 may indicate acute V/Q mismatch.

M. Circulatory Problems. Including severe CHF.

N. Low hemoglobin.

IV. Database

A. Physical Exam Key Points

1. HEENT. Listen for an obvious air leak.

2. **Neck.** Look for distended neck veins with CHF, volume overload, or pneumothorax.
3. **Lungs.** Evaluate for bronchospasm or pulmonary edema. Check for subcutaneous emphysema, which can result from pneumothorax.
4. Look for equal expansion, tracheal deviation, and adequate breath sounds bilaterally.

B. **Laboratory Data**
   1. **Arterial blood gas.** Follow serial studies.

C. **Radiologic and Other Studies**
   1. **Chest x-ray.** Look for congestive heart failure, pneumothorax, endotracheal tube position, lobar infiltrate, collapse secondary to mucous plugging, or signs of ARDS.
   2. **Nuclear ventilation/Perfusion scan (V/Q scan).** If there is any question of a pulmonary embolus, then V/Q scan is indicated. An equivocal scan usually necessitates pulmonary angiography.

V. **Plan.** The goal of ventilatory support is to provide, in conjunction with alveolar exchange, adequate tissue oxygenation. Many times, sudden changes in Po$_2$ and Pco$_2$ in the absence of ventilatory changes are due to such phenomena as altered FIo$_2$, pneumothorax, mucous plugging, and so on. Consider bronchoscopy for severe mucous plugging if endotracheal tube suctioning is inadequate.

A. **Hypoxemia.** Keep the FIo$_2$ from about 0.4 to 0.5, because at this level, there is minimal oxygen toxicity. In general, a Pao$_2$ of 60 mm Hg or higher is the goal, because at this level, hemoglobin is about 90% saturated. An indicator of cardiac output is also needed, with direct measurement using a pulmonary artery balloon tipped catheter being most useful. Other indicators of cardiac output (eg, urine output) may be helpful in the absence of PA catheter. Hypoxemia may be treated by increasing oxygen delivery or by decreasing oxygen consumption.
   1. **Increased delivery**
      a. **Ventilatory**
         i. Increased FIo$_2$.
         ii. **Decreased Shunt:** By increasing PEEP. Remember that increasing PEEP can significantly affect cardiac output, so that a pulmonary artery catheter may be needed, especially with PEEP levels above 10–15 cm H$_2$O.
      b. **Circulatory**
         i. Improved cardiac output.
         ii. Treatment of physical obstruction to circulation such as pulmonary embolus. Treatment is anticoagulation after diagnosis by imaging studies as previously discussed.

    c. Hemoglobin
       i. Transfusion to acceptable range (usually to a Hct > 30%).
       ii. Decreased consumption: Sedation, paralysis, and hypothermia can be combined in critical situations.
B. Hypercarbia. The adequacy of ventilation is indicated by the Pco_2 and can be affected by changes in the ventilatory rate or by changes in the tidal volume set on the ventilator.
    1. Rule out mechanical problems such as leaks, plugging of the endotracheal tube, kinking, or malposition of the tube.
    2. Tidal volume should be 10–15 ml/kg body weight. Is the patient receiving the delivered volume? Hypoventilation (low minute volume) can raise Pco_2.
    3. Is the Pco_2 increased because of increased CO_2 production or excessive deadspace ventilation?
       a. Increased CO_2 production
          i. Sepsis: Treat appropriately (antibiotics, etc).
          ii. Excessive carbohydrate in hyperalimentation.
       b. Increased deadspace: Deadspace refers to the ventilation of areas such as the ventilator tubing, endotracheal tube, nonperfused alveoli, etc, where gas exchange cannot occur. Correct the following conditions when possible:
          i. Inadequate cardiac output.
          ii. PEEP causing overdistention.
          iii. Pulmonary emboli.
          iv. Vasoconstriction of pulmonary vessels by vasoactive medications.

75. WHEEZING

I. Problem. A 20-year-old has been admitted for laparoscopic appendectomy and begins wheezing in the anesthesia holding area.

II. Immediate Questions
    A. What are the vital signs? A respiratory rate > 40/min may indicate the need for immediate treatment. Associated hypotension may suggest an anaphylactic reaction or an acute myocardial infarction (MI). Fever may point to an underlying infection or new pulmonary embolism.
    B. Were any diagnostic tests recently performed or medicines administered? A ß-blocker given to a stable asthmatic may precipitate an acute attack of bronchospasm. Wheezing following the administration of a drug, such as penicillin or radiocontrast dye, suggests an anaphylactic reaction.

   C. For what condition was the patient admitted? A patient admitted to rule out MI may have developed acute pulmonary edema; whereas, a patient with a gastric ulcer may have gastric outlet obstruction and have aspirated.

   D. Is there any history of asthma? Childhood asthma may reactivate at any age given the right stimuli.

   E. Does the patient have any allergies to medications or other substances, such as shellfish? It is prudent to inquire about any known allergies.

III. Differential Diagnosis

   A. Diffuse Wheezing

      1. **Acute bronchospasm.** May be due to asthma, exacerbation of chronic obstructive pulmonary disease (COPD), or an anaphylactic reaction.

      2. **Aspiration.** This may trigger bronchospasm from mucosal irritation or from impacted foreign bodies.

      3. **Cardiogenic pulmonary edema.** The primary finding in "cardiac asthma" may be wheezing. Other findings of pulmonary edema should be present and the chest x-ray will be diagnostic.

      4. **Pulmonary embolism (PE).** Mediators may be released that not only cause hypoxemia, but may also cause transient bronchospasm.

   B. Stridor (Upper Airway) Wheezing

      1. **Laryngospasm.** This may be part of an anaphylactic reaction or secondary to aspiration.

      2. **Laryngeal or tracheal tumor.** History of dysphagia, hoarseness, cough, or weight loss and anorexia may be present.

      3. **Epiglottis.** The patient will often be unable to speak and will be unable to swallow secretions.

      4. Foreign body aspiration.

      5. **Vocal cord dysfunction.** Bilaterally paralyzed vocal cords may result in severe stridor and dyspnea. A subgroup of patients recently has been recognized to have "factitious asthma" in which they voluntarily adduct their vocal cords for psychogenic reasons.

   C. Localized Wheezing

      1. **Tumors.** May obstruct one bronchus leading to localized wheezing.

      2. Mucous plugging.

      3. Aspirated foreign body.

IV. Database

    A. Physical Exam Key Points. Localization of wheezing allows categorization as outlined in the differential diagnosis.

        1. Vital signs. A fever may indicate an infectious cause. A pulsus paradoxicus > 20 mm Hg indicates severe respiratory distress. Hypotension requires immediate assessment and action.

        2. HEENT. Check the mouth carefully. Examine the neck for angioneurotic edema. Palpate the sternocleidomastoid muscles for accessory muscle use. Auscultate over the mouth and larynx in an effort to localize the wheeze.

        3. Chest. Carefully auscultate for localized wheezing. Listen for bibasilar rales, which may be present in pulmonary edema. Rales, increased fremitus, and egophony suggest pneumonia.

        4. Cardiac. Check carefully for evidence of an S_3 or S_4 gallop or jugular venous distention, which points to pulmonary edema.

        5. Extremities. Clubbed fingers most likely indicate an underlying lung cancer or severe COPD. Cyanosis indicates underlying hypoxemia. Edema may signify chronic CHF.

        6. Skin. Urticaria probably indicates an acute allergic reaction. A malar rash may indicate acute systemic lupus erythematosus (SLE), which can present with acute pneumonitis.

    B. Laboratory Data

        1. Arterial blood gases. An elevated P_{CO_2} indicates significant ventilatory failure. Also check for hypoxemia.

        2. Complete blood count (CBC). An increased white blood cell (WBC) count may indicate an underlying infection; however, an increase in the WBCs without a left shift can be seen with an acute MI and PE. Eosinophilia suggests an allergic or asthmatic cause to the wheezing.

    C. Radiologic and Other Studies

        1. Electrocardiogram (ECG). An ECG may show an acute MI or ischemia. Occasionally, it will be suggestive of a PE, showing an S wave in I, Q wave in III and T wave inversion in III ($S_1Q_3T_3$), new right bundle branch block (RBBB) and right axis shift. It may also show a change in rhythm.

        2. Chest radiograph. PE severe enough to cause wheezing will always be evident on the chest film. Look for a pleural-based, wedge-shaped lesion. Also, Kerley B lines, bilateral pleural effusions, vascular redistribution, and cardiomegaly may suggest CHF or pulmonary edema. Look for localized infiltrates or masses suggesting other causes.

V. Plan. Treatment plans depend on the diagnosis. The above differential diagnoses and studies should enable the clinician to form a tentative categorization, on which to base initial therapy.

A. Bronchospasm (Asthma, COPD, Allergic Reaction)

1. Methylprednisolone (Solu-medrol) 200 mg IV stat dose.
2. Nebulized albuterol (Ventolin) 0.5 mL (2.5 mg) or metaproterenol (Alupent) 0.3 mL of 5% solution in 3.0 mL normal saline stat and then every 2–4 hours.
3. Aminophylline loading dose of 6 mg/kg (assuming the patient is not already on aminophylline) and then a maintenance IV of 0.2–0.6 mg/kg/hr (15–30 mg/hr). Aminophylline is now considered to be of only modest acute benefit and may cause considerable worsening of arrhythmias. Therefore, initial dosing should be on the "low side" and blood levels need to be monitored closely.

B. Stridor

1. Methylprednisolone 200 mg IV stat dose.
2. Nebulized racemic epinephrine (Micronephrine) 0.5 mL in 3 mL normal saline.
3. Consider intubation or tracheostomy.

C. Pulmonary Edema

1. Furosemide (Lasix) 20–80 mg IV.
2. Nitroglycerin 0.4 mg sl; or paste ½" on skin; or nitroglycerin drip 10–20 µg/min and increase by 5–10 µg every 10 minutes.
3. Afterload reduction with agents such as intravenous nitroprusside (Nipride) or oral agents such as captopril (Capoten) or enalapril (Vasotec).
4. IV morphine for venodilation and to relieve anxiety. Be prepared to intubate the patient.
5. **Oxygen.** Start with 2 L by nasal cannula.

D. Miscellaneous.
Treatment varies with the disease. Obviously, PE should be treated with anticoagulants. Suspected tumors require additional tests, such as bronchoscopy, before reasonable treatment can be initiated.

76. WOUND DEHISCENCE

I. **Problem.** A nurse notifies you that a laparotomy wound in a patient following a bilateral adrenalectomy has opened and there is a piece of fat poking out of the wound.

II. **Immediate Questions**

A. **Is there a wound dehiscence, and if so, to what extent?** Always evaluate the wound yourself as soon as possible. See how much of the wound has opened, how deep, and if there is an evisceration. Check the integrity of the fascia with a cotton-tipped applicator (an "open wound" is not a dehiscence unless the fascia opens).

B. Did any fluid leak from the wound? Look at the dressing and ask the nurse and the patient about the nature and amount of fluid. Serous/serosanguineous fluid is more ominous for a true fascial dehiscence. Grossly bloody or purulent fluid is indicative of a superficial wound infection, a liquefying hematoma, or active bleeding in the superficial tissues.

C. Are there any predisposing factors to dehiscence? Factors such as sepsis, poor nutrition, diabetes, and steroids predispose to poor wound healing and increase the likelihood of dehiscence.

III. Differential Diagnosis. A wound dehiscence is usually the result of a combination of factors including technical problems, local wound problems, poor wound healing, and increased stress on the wound. The following list is not so much a differential diagnosis as a list of contributing factors.

A. Technical Problems
   1. **Poorly placed sutures.** Failure to take a full-thickness bite or reapproximating muscle instead of fascia.
   2. **Inappropriate suture material.** Such as not using a heavy enough gauge suture for an abdominal closure.
   3. **Sutures tied too tightly.** This usually induces tissue ischemia causing the suture to pull out.

B. Local Wound Problems
   1. **Infection.** Either superficial wound infection or intraperitoneal abscess.
   2. **Hematoma.**

C. Poor Wound Healing
   1. Poor nutrition.
   2. Diabetes.
   3. **Steroids.** Endogenous or exogenous.
   4. Uremia.
   5. Chemotherapy.
   6. Advanced malignancy.

D. Decreased Tension On Wound
   1. **Abdominal distention**
      a. Ascites.
      b. Dilated bowel.
   2. Vomiting or coughing.
   3. **COPD.**

IV. Database

A. Physical Exam Key Points
   1. **Incision.** Use sterile gloves, take off all the dressings, and examine the entire wound. Look for the leakage of fluid when the

wound is palpated, and look for signs of infection. Examine for opening of the fascia with a cotton-tipped applicator.

B. Laboratory Data. Wound culture and gram stain if indicated.

V. Plan

A. Overall Plan. Determine by wound examination if there is an evisceration, fascial disruption without evisceration, or a superficial wound separation. In all cases, it is safe to make the patient NPO and start antibiotics (cephalosporins are used frequently) to cover at least skin organisms until a final plan is formulated.

B. Evisceration/Fascial Dehiscence. Cover the wound with saline soaked sterile gauze and cover with a large sterile dressing. Notify the senior staff and the operating room because evisceration requires operative repair.

C. Fascial Dehiscence Without Evisceration. If the overlying skin and subcutaneous tissues are intact but there is clearly a fascial defect, it may be treated by operative repair or observation with a resultant ventral hernia. Use an abdominal binder if senior staff opts for observation. Note, however, that a binder often compromises respiratory function, especially in the immediate postoperative period.

D. Superficial Wound Separation

1. Healing by secondary intention is mandatory when there is an associated superficial wound infection and is the safest management in any case. Open the wound to drain the pus or fluid, then treat with 2–4 wet to dry dressing changes per day (depending on the size of the defect saline soaked 4 × 4s are often used).

2. **Closure.** Some surgeons may attempt to re-close a superficial wound separation either immediately or following a period of wet-to-dry dressing changes. If this approach is used, realize that there is a substantial risk of developing a superficial infection or spread of the infection to the fascial layer.

77. WOUND DRAINAGE

I. Problem. A patient has new drainage from a midline laparotomy incision 5 days after small bowel resection for ischemic intestine.

II. Immediate Questions

A. How old is the wound, and what was the operative procedure? The diagnosis can be made partly on the basis of timing of the drainage as well as the type of surgery.

B. **Was there any prior drainage, and are drains present?** Increase in drainage from a wound may indicate that the suction or other drain may not be working.

C. **How was the wound closed? Sutures? Staples? Retention sutures? Packed open?**

D. **What is the character of the drainage? Bloody? Serosanguineous? Frankly purulent? Intestinal contents?**

E. **How much drainage is there?** Quantitation is essential especially to replace gastrointestinal tract losses in the presence of a fistula. Consider saving and weighing the dressings if volume determination is critical.

III. Differential Diagnosis

A. **Wound Infection.** Typically seen a few days postoperatively.
   1. **Wound tenderness and fluctuance.** This is most often due to *Staphylococcus* or *Streptococcus* species and seen 3–5 days postop.
   2. **Gas forming infections (*Clostridium,* necrotizing fasciitis). Severe pain is typical with crepitation present. This is a surgical emergency and must be promptly drained and débrided.** May be caused by *Clostridium,* or more commonly, a mixed gram-negative and microaerophilic gram-positive infection. Mixed infections are most often seen in diabetics.

B. **Impending Dehiscence.** Serosanguineous drainage after the first 24 postoperative hours is almost pathognomonic of wound dehiscence.

C. **Enterocutaneous Fistula.** Obvious as draining intestinal contents. Can be high output fistula or low output. Often caused by inadvertent suturing of a segment of intestine during fascial closure. This usually follows several days of abdominal pain and fevers.

D. **Hemorrhage.** Excessive bleeding usually exits through a fresh postoperative wound. DIC may manifest as bleeding through the wound as well as other sites (IV sites, etc).

E. **Pancreatic Fistula.** Postoperative or posttraumatic.

F. **Urinary Fistula.**

G. **Ascitic Leak.** Often avoided by closing one layer in a continuous running suture.

H. **Drain Malfunction.** If a surgically placed drain is not performing properly, the intended fluid may exit through the wound.

IV. Database

A. Physical Exam Key Points

1. **Vital signs.** Look for fever, tachycardia, and signs of sepsis.
2. **Abdomen.** Look for signs of peritonitis.
3. **Wound.** Examine with sterile gloves for surrounding inflammation, dehiscence, or crepitation.

B. Laboratory Data

1. **Hemogram.** May reveal infection or indicate severe anemia from bleeding. Platelets may be decreased in DIC or in other causes of thrombocytopenia.
2. **Coagulation profile.** PT, PTT, fibrin split products, if DIC is suspected.
3. Send drainage for culture, gram stain, and amylase. Amylase may be elevated in intestinal fistula but markedly elevated in pancreatic fistula.
4. **Drainage creatinine.** If the drainage is thought to be urine, the creatinine will be much higher than the serum level.

C. Radiologic and Other Studies.
Fistulogram may be helpful if there is no clue as to the origin of the drainage.

V. Plan

A. General Plan.
Immediately treat a life-threatening complication such as evisceration (see page 241) while performing a diagnostic workup in less acute situations. Effluent from a wound should be sent for gram stain, and culture. Chemistry determinations on clear fluid for creatinine or amylase may aid in diagnosis.

B. Specific Plans

1. **Wound infection.** The wound must be opened, which usually can be done at the bedside, and packed with saline moistened gauze after evacuating pus in the wound. Remove enough skin closure staples or sutures to fully drain the area. In the presence of advancing local cellulitis or systemic signs of infection, antibiotics are indicated.
   a. *Clostridium.* Early debridement along with high dose IV penicillin.
   b. Gas forming nonclostridial infections are treated with broad spectrum antibiotics.
2. **Dehiscence.** Fascial dehiscence indicated by serosanguineous wound drainage can be watched, if the skin closure remains intact. This results in a ventral hernia, which may require therapy at a later date. However, actual dehiscence with eviscerated abdominal contents (intestine in the bed) requires prompt operative intervention (see Problem 76, page 239).

3. **Enterocutaneous fistula.** Often needs a bag to capture the effluent and protect skin. Quantitate the drainage. This usually follows several days of abdominal pain and fevers. Oral administration of charcoal or dye may be used to confirm the diagnosis. Sump drains may be useful to help collect the material. Nasogastric suction and keeping the patient NPO is essential. Remember to institute early nutritional support by the parenteral route. Low output fistulas often close spontaneously, whereas fistulas that remain high-output will probably require surgical intervention.

4. **Pancreatic fistula.** Skin protection is essential. There can be serious nutritional deficits caused by pancreatic fistulae, especially by high losses of protein. Since the alkalinization of intestinal contents is prevented by the fistulous drainage of pancreatic juice, these patients are at high risk for peptic ulcer. A tube in the fistula opening may help to prevent early closure of the skin.

5. **Hemorrhage.** Evaluate the patient's volume status. Remember that a drop in hematocrit can be late. Replete volume with crystalloid, blood, or both. The decision whether to reoperate for bleeding depends on the clinical situation and overall status. It may be a vessel in the skin or subcutaneous fat. If a vessel is seen, it can be cauterized at the bedside with a battery powered cautery.

II. Laboratory Tests & Their Interpretation

If an increased or decreased value is not clinically useful, it is not listed. Because each laboratory has its own set of "normal" reference values, the values given should be used only as a rough guide. The range for common normal values is given in parentheses. Unless specified, values reflect normal adult levels.

ACTH (Adrenocorticotropic Hormone)

(8 AM 20–140 pg/mL [SI: 20–140 ng/L], midnight, approximately 50% of AM value).

Increased: Addison's disease (primary adrenal hypofunction), ectopic ACTH production (oat cell and large cell lung carcinoma, pancreatic islet-cell tumors, thymic tumors, renal cell carcinoma, bronchial carcinoid), Cushing's disease (pituitary adenoma), congenital adrenal hyperplasia (adrenogenital syndrome).

Decreased: Adrenal adenoma or carcinoma, nodular adrenal hyperplasia, pituitary insufficiency, corticosteroid use.

ACTH Stimulation Test (Cortrosyn Stimulation Test)

Used to help diagnose adrenal insufficiency. Cortrosyn (an ACTH analogue) is given at a dose of 0.25 mg IM or IV in adults or 0.125 mg in children younger than 2 years. Collect blood at time 0, 30, and 60 minutes for cortisol and aldosterone.

Normal Response: Three criteria are required: basal cortisol of at least 5 μg/dL, an incremental increase after Cortrosyn injection of at least 7 μg/dL, and a final serum cortisol of at least 16 μg/dL at 30 minutes or 18 μg/dL at 60 minutes or cortisol increase of >10 μg/dL. Aldosterone increases >5 ng/dL over baseline.

Addison's Disease (Primary Adrenal Insufficiency): Neither cortisol nor aldosterone increase over baseline.

Secondary Adrenal Insufficiency: Caused by pituitary insufficiency or suppression by exogenous steroids, cortisol does not increase, but aldosterone increases.

Acetone (Ketone Bodies, Acetoacetate)

(Normal = negative)

Positive: Diabetic ketoacidosis (DKA), starvation, emesis, stress, alcoholism, infantile organic acidemias, isopropanol ingestion.

Acid Phosphatase (Prostatic Acid Phosphatase, PAP)

(Less than 3.0 ng/mL by RIA or <0.8 IU/L by enzymatic)

Not a useful screening test for cancer; most useful as a marker of response to therapy. PSA is more sensitive in diagnosing cancer and is largely replacing PAP.

Increased: Carcinoma of the prostate (usually outside of prostate), prostatic surgery or trauma (including aggressive prostatic massage), rarely in infiltrative bone disease (Gaucher's disease, myeloid leukemia), prostatitis, or benign prostate hypertrophy.

Albumin

(Adult 3.5–5.0 g/dL [SI: 35–50 g/L], child 3.8–5.4 g/dL [SI: 38–54 g/L]).

Decreased: Malnutrition, over hydration, nephrotic syndrome, cystic fibrosis, multiple myeloma, Hodgkin's disease, leukemia, protein-losing enteropathies, chronic glomerulonephritis, alcoholic cirrhosis, inflammatory bowel disease, collagen-vascular diseases, hyperthyroidism.

Albumin/Globulin Ratio (A/G Ratio)

(Normal >1).

A calculated value [total protein minus albumin equals globulins. Albumin divided by globulins equals A/G ratio]. Serum protein electrophoresis is a more informative test.

Decreased: Cirrhosis, liver diseases, nephrotic syndrome, chronic glomerulonephritis, cachexia, burns, chronic infections and inflammatory states, and myeloma.

Aldosterone

(Serum: Supine 3–10 ng/dL [SI: 0.083–0.28 nmol/L] early AM, normal sodium intake [3 g sodium/d]; upright 5–30 ng/dL [SI: 0.138–0.83 nmol/L]; urinary 2-16 μg/24 hr [SI: 5.4–44.3 nmol/d]).

Discontinue antihypertensives and diuretics 2 weeks before test. Upright samples should be drawn after 2 hours. Primarily used to screen hypertensive patients for possible Conn's syndrome (adrenal adenoma producing excess aldosterone).

Increased: Primary hyperaldosteronism, secondary hyperaldosteronism (CHF, sodium depletion, nephrotic syndrome, cirrhosis with ascites, others), upright posture.

Decreased: Adrenal insufficiency, panhypopituitarism, supine posture.

Alkaline Phosphatase

(Adult 20–70 U/L, child 20–150 U/L)

A fractionated alkaline phosphatase often is useful to differentiate between bone and liver origin of the enzyme. The heat-stable fraction comes from the liver, and the heat-labile fraction comes from the bone ("bone burns"). On a fractionated sample, if the heat-stable fraction is <20%, suspect bone origin; if fraction is 25–55%, suspect liver origin. Largely replaced by the gamma-glutamyl transpeptidase (GGT) and 5′nucleotidase determinations.

Increased: Increased calcium deposition in bone (hyperparathyroidism), Paget's disease, osteoblastic bone tumors (metastatic or osteogenic sarcoma), osteomalacia, rickets, pregnancy, childhood, healing fracture, liver disease such as biliary obstruction (masses, drug therapy), hyperthyroidism.

Decreased: Malnutrition, excess vitamin D ingestion.

Alpha-Fetoprotein (AFP)

(Less than 16 ng/mL [SI: <16 μL]; third trimester of pregnancy maximum 550 ng/ml [SI: 550 μL]).

Increased: Hepatoma (hepatocellular carcinoma), testicular tumor (embryonal carcinoma, malignant teratoma, yolk sac tumor), neural tube defects (in mother's serum [spina bifida, anencephaly, myelomeningocoele]), fetal death, multiple gestations, ataxia-telangiectasia, some cases of benign hepatic diseases (alcoholic cirrhosis, hepatitis).

Decreased: Trisomy 21 (Down's syndrome) in maternal serum.

ALT (Alanine Aminotransferase, ALAT) (see SGPT)

(8–20 U/L)

Increased: Liver disease, liver metastasis, biliary obstruction, pancreatitis, liver congestion (ALT is more elevated than AST in viral hepatitis; AST elevated more than ALT in alcoholic hepatitis).

Ammonia

(Adult 10–80 μg/dL [SI: 5–50 μmol/L]). To convert μg/dL to μmol/L, multiply by 0.5872).

Increased: Liver failure, Reye's syndrome, inborn errors of metabolism, normal neonates (normalizes within 48 hours of birth).

Amylase

(50–150 Somogyi units/dL [SI: 100–300 U/L]).

Increased: Acute pancreatitis, pancreatic duct obstruction (stones, stricture, tumor, sphincter spasm secondary to drugs), pancreatic pseudocyst or abscess, alcohol ingestion, mumps, parotiditis, renal disease, macroamylasemia, cholecystitis, peptic ulcers, intestinal obstruction, mesenteric thrombosis, after surgery.

Decreased: Pancreatic destruction (pancreatitis, cystic fibrosis), liver damage (hepatitis, cirrhosis), normal newborns in the first year of life.

Autoantibodies

(Normal = negative)

Antinuclear Antibody (ANA, FANA): (Normal = negative)
A useful screening test in patients with symptoms suggesting collagen-vascular disease, especially if titer is ≥1 : 160.

Positive: Systemic lupus erythematosus (SLE), drug-induced lupuslike syndromes (procainamide, hydralazine, isoniazid, etc), scleroderma, mixed connective tissue disease (MCTD), rheumatoid arthritis, polymyositis, juvenile rheumatoid arthritis (5% to 20%). Low titers are also seen in noncollagen-vascular disease.

Anti-DNA (Anti-double stranded DNA): SLE, chronic active hepatitis, mononucleosis.

Antimitochondrial: Primary biliary cirrhosis, autoimmune diseases such as SLE.

Anti-Smooth Muscle: Low titers are seen in a variety of illnesses; high titers (>1 : 100) are suggestive of chronic active hepatitis.

Antimicrosomal: Hashimoto's thyroiditis.

ASO (Antistreptolysin O) Titer (Streptozyme)

(Less than 166 Todd units).

Increased: Streptococcal infections (pharyngitis, scarlet fever, rheumatic fever, poststreptococcal glomerulonephritis), rheumatoid arthritis, and other collagen diseases.

AST (Aspartate Aminotransferase, ASAT) (see SGOT)

(8–20 U/L)

Generally parallels changes in SGPT in liver disease.

Increased: Acute myocardial infarction, liver disease, Reye's syndrome, muscle trauma and injection, pancreatitis, intestinal injury or surgery, factitious increase (erythromycin, opiates), burns, cardiac catheterization, brain damage, renal infarction.

Decreased: Beriberi, severe diabetes with ketoacidosis, liver disease.

β₂ Microglobulin

(0.1–0.26 mg/dL [1–2.6 mg/L]).

A useful marker to follow the progression of HIV infections.

Increased: HIV infection, especially during periods of exacerbation, B-cell lymphomas, occasionally in renal insufficiency.

Base Excess/Deficit

(−2–+3 mEq/L [SI: −2–+3 mmol/L] (see Blood gases, page 250).

Increased: Metabolic alkalosis.

Decreased: Metabolic acidosis.

Bicarbonate (Total CO₂)

(23–29 mmol/L) (see Carbon dioxide, page 259).

Bilirubin

(Total, 0.3–1.0 mg/dL [SI: 3.4–17.1 μmol/L]; direct, <0.2 mg/dL [SI: <3.4 μmol/L]; indirect, <0.8 mg/dL [SI: <3.4 μmol/L]). To convert mg/dL to μmol/L, multiply by 17.10).

Increased Total: Hepatic damage (hepatitis, toxins, cirrhosis), biliary obstruction (stone or tumor), hemolysis, fasting.

Increased Direct (Conjugated): **Note:** Determination of the direct bilirubin is usually unnecessary with total bilirubin levels <1.2 mg/dL [SI: 21 μmol/L]. Biliary obstruction/cholestasis (gallstone, tumor, stricture), drug-induced cholestasis, Dubin-Johnson and Rotor's syndromes.

Increased Indirect (Unconjugated): **Note:** This is calculated as total minus direct bilirubin. So-called "hemolytic jaundice" caused by any type of hemolytic anemia (transfusion reaction, sickle cell, etc), Gilbert's disease, physiological jaundice of the newborn, Crigler-Najjar syndrome.

Bilirubin, Neonatal ("Baby Bilirubin")

(Normal levels dependent on prematurity and age in days; "panic levels" usually >15–20 mg/dL (SI: >257–342 μmol/L in term infants).

Increased: Erythroblastosis fetalis, physiologic jaundice (may be due to breastfeeding), resorption of hematoma or hemorrhage, obstructive jaundice, others.

Bleeding Time

(Duke, Ivy <6 min; Template <10 min)

Increased: Thrombocytopenia (disseminated intravascular coagulation [DIC], thrombotic thrombocytopenic purpura [TTP], idiopathic thrombocytopenic purpura [ITP]), von Willebrand's disease, defective platelet function including aspirin therapy.

Blood Gases, Capillary

When interpreting a CBG, apply the following rules:

pH: Same as arterial blood gas or slightly lower (N = 7.35–7.40).

Pco₂: Same as arterial blood gas or slightly higher (N = 40–45).

Po₂: Lower than arterial blood gas (N = 45–60).

O₂ Saturation: >70% is acceptable. Saturation is probably more useful than the Po₂ when interpreting a CBG.

Blood Gases, Arterial & Venous

There is little difference between arterial and venous pH and bicarbonate (except with congestive heart failure and shock); therefore, the venous blood gas may be used occasionally to assess acid-base status, but venous oxygen levels are significantly less than arterial levels (Table II–1).

See individual component for differential diagnosis. For acid-base disorders see the section below and Section I, Problems 3 and 4.

Metabolic Acidosis: A fall in plasma HCO_3 followed by a compensatory fall in Pco_2. Use the anion gap to help establish the diagnosis (Table II–2).

TABLE II–1. NORMAL BLOOD GAS VALUES.

Measurement	Arterial Blood	Mixed Venous[1]	Venous
pH	7.40	7.36	7.36
(range)	(7.36–7.44)	(7.31–7.41)	(7.31–7.41)
Po₂	80–100 mm Hg	35–40 mm Hg	30–50 mm Hg
(decreases with age)			
Pco₂	35–45 mm Hg	41–51 mm Hg	40–52 mm Hg
O₂ saturation (%)	> 95%	60–80%	60–85%
(decreases with age)			
[HCO₃⁻]	22–26 mEq/L	22–26 mEq/L	22–28 mEq/L
	(mmol/L)	(mmol/L)	(mmol/L)
Base deficit			
(deficit excess)	−2–+3	−2–+3	−2–+3

[1]Obtained from right atrium, usually through a pulmonary artery catheter.

TABLE II–2. SIMPLE ACID-BASE DISTURBANCES.

Acid-Base Disorder	Primary Abnormality	Secondary Abnormality	Expected Degree of Compensatory Response
Metabolic acidosis	$\downarrow\downarrow\downarrow[HCO_3^-]$	$\downarrow\downarrow Pco_2$	$Pco_2 = (1.5 \times [HCO_3^-]) + 8$
Metabolic alkalosis	$\uparrow\uparrow\uparrow[HCO_3^-]$	$\uparrow\uparrow Pco_2$	$\uparrow$ in $PCO_2 = \Delta\ HCO_3^- \times 0.6$
Acute respiratory acidosis	$\uparrow\uparrow\uparrow Pco_2$	$\uparrow[HCO_3^-]$	$\uparrow$ in $HCO_3^- = \Delta\ Pco_2/10$
Chronic respiratory acidosis	$\uparrow\uparrow\uparrow Pco_2$	$\uparrow\uparrow[HCO_3^-]$	$\uparrow$ in $HCO_3^- = 4 \times \Delta\ Pco_2/10$
Acute respiratory alkalosis	$\downarrow\downarrow\downarrow Pco_2$	$\downarrow[HCO_3^-]$	$\downarrow$ in $HCO_3^- = 2 \times \Delta\ Pco_2/10$
Chronic respiratory alkalosis	$\downarrow\downarrow\downarrow Pco_2$	$\downarrow\downarrow[HCO_3^-]$	$\downarrow$ in $HCO_3^- = 5 \times \Delta\ Pco_2/10$

$$\text{Anion Gap} = (Na) - (Cl + HCO_3)$$
$$\text{Normal Gap} = 8\text{–}12 \text{ mEq/L}$$

Differential Diagnosis: See also Section I, Problem 3.

Anion gap acidosis (Normochloremic acidosis): Gap >12 mEq/L; caused by a decrease in bicarbonate balanced by an increased in unmeasured acids. Lactic acidosis, ketoacidosis (diabetic, alcoholic, starvation), uremia, intoxication (salicylate, methanol, paraldehyde, ethylene glycol), hyperalimentation.

Nonanion gap acidosis (Hyperchloremic acidosis): Gap between 8 and 12 mEq/L; caused by a decrease in HCO_3 balanced by an increase in chloride. Renal bicarbonate losses (renal tubular acidosis, spironolactone, carbonic anhydrase inhibitors), gastrointestinal tract bicarbonate losses (diarrhea, pancreatic fistulas, biliary tract fistulas, ileal loop, ureterosigmoidostomy).

Low anion gap: Gap <8; not seen with acidosis, but can be seen with bromide ingestion, hyponatremia and multiple myeloma.

Metabolic Alkalosis: A rise in plasma HCO_3^- followed by a compensatory rise in the Pco_2. Spot urine for chloride helps establish the diagnosis (Table II–2).

Differential Diagnosis: See also Section I, Problem 4.

Urine chloride <10 mEq/L ("chloride responsive"): Diuretics, GI tract losses (NG suction, vomiting, diarrhea [villous adenoma, congenital chloride wasting diarrhea in children]), iatrogenic (inadequate chloride intake).

Urine chloride >10 mEq/L ("chloride resistant"): Adrenal diseases (Cushing's syndrome, hyperaldosteronism), exogenous steroid use, Bartter's syndrome, licorice ingestion.

Respiratory Acidosis: A primary rise in Pco_2 with a compensatory rise in plasma HCO_3^- not higher than 30 mEq/L if acute (Table II–2).

Differential Diagnosis: See also Section I, Problem 3.
   Acute: CNS depression (oversedation, narcotics, anesthetic), CNS trauma (CVA, head injury, spinal cord trauma), neuromuscular diseases (myasthenia gravis, Guillain-Barré disease), airway obstruction, laryngospasm, iatrogenic mechanical underventilation, pulmonary lesions (acute pulmonary edema, severe pneumonia), chest trauma (hemothorax, pneumothorax, flail chest).
   Chronic: Chronic asthma, emphysema or bronchitis, pickwickian syndrome.

Respiratory Alkalosis: A primary fall in Pco_2 (Table II–2).

Differential Diagnosis: See also Section I, Problem 4.
   Central nervous system causes: Anxiety, hyperventilation syndrome, pain, head trauma, CVA, encephalitis, CHS tumors, salicylates (early toxicity), fever, early sepsis.
   Peripheral stimulation: Pulmonary embolus, CHF, interstitial lung disease, pneumonia, altitude, hypoxemia of any cause.
   Miscellaneous: Delerium tremens, cirrhosis, thyrotoxicosis, pregnancy, iatrogenic overventilation.

Blood Urea Nitrogen (BUN)

(Birth–1 year: 4–16 mg/dL [SI: 1.4–5.7 mmol/L]; 1–40 years: 5–20 mg/dL [SI: 1.8–7.1 mmol/L]; gradual slight increase with increasing age. To convert mg/dL to mmol/L, multiply by 0.3570).

Increased: Renal failure, prerenal azotemia (decreased renal perfusion secondary to congestive heart failure [CHF], shock, volume depletion), postrenal (obstruction), gastrointestinal (GI) bleeding, stress, drugs (especially aminoglycosides).

Decreased: Starvation, liver failure (hepatitis, drugs), pregnancy, infancy, nephrotic syndrome, overhydration.

BUN/Creatinine Ratio (BUN/Cr)

(Mean 10, range 6–20)

Increased: Prerenal azotemia (renal hypoperfusion), GI bleeding, high protein diet, ileal conduit, drugs (steroids, tetracycline).

Decreased: Malnutrition, pregnancy, low protein diet, ketoacidosis, hemodialysis, SIADH, drugs (cimetidine).

CBC Differential Diagnosis

(See also Tables II–3 and II–4 for normal ranges)

Basophils: (0–1%)

Increased: Chronic myeloid leukemia, rarely in recovery from infection and from hypothyroidism.

Decreased: Acute rheumatic fever, lobar pneumonia, after steroid therapy, thyrotoxicosis, stress.

Eosinophils: (1–3%)

Increased: Allergy, parasites, skin diseases, malignancy, drugs, asthma, Addison's disease, collagen-vascular diseases (handy mnemonic: NAACP—Neoplasm, Allergy, Addison's disease, Collagen-vascular diseases, Parasites), pulmonary diseases including Löffler's syndrome and PIE (pulmonary infiltrates with eosinophilia).

Decreased: After steroids, adrenocorticotropic hormone (ACTH), after stress (infection, trauma, burns), Cushing's syndrome.

Hematocrit: (Male 40–54%; female 37–47%)

Decreased: Megaloblastic anemia (folate or B_{12} deficiency, iron deficiency anemia, sickle cell anemia, etc), acute or chronic blood loss, hemolysis, dilutional, alcohol, drugs.

Increased: Primary polycythemia (polycythemia vera), secondary polycythemia (reduced fluid intake or excess fluid loss, congenital and acquired heart disease, lung disease, high altitudes, heavy smokers, tumors [renal cell carcinoma, hepatoma], renal cysts).

Hemoglobin: (See Table II–3, page 254 for normal values)
(See also Section I, Problem 6.)

Increased: Polycythemia vera, secondary polycythemia, high altitude, vigorous exercise.

Decreased: See previous section, Hematocrit.

Lymphocytes: (24–44%)

Increased: Virtually any viral infection (AIDS, measles, German measles, mumps, whooping cough, smallpox, chickenpox, influenza, hepatitis, infectious mononucleosis), acute infectious lymphocytosis in children, acute and chronic lymphocytic leukemias.

Decreased: (Normal finding in 22% of population). Stress, burns, trauma, uremia, some viral infections, AIDS, AIDS related complex, bone marrow suppression after chemotherapy, steroids.

TABLE II–3. NORMAL COMPLETE BLOOD COUNT FOR SELECTED AGE RANGES.

Age	WBC Count (cells/cu mm) [SI: 10⁹/L]	RBC Count 10⁶/μL [SI: 10¹²/L]	Hemoglobin (gm/dL) [SI: g/L]	Hematocrit (%)	MCH (pg) [SI: pg]	MCHC (g/dL) [SI: g/L]¹	MCV (cu μm) [SI: fL]	RDW
Adult male	4500–11,000 [4.5–11.0]	4.73–5.49 [4.73–5.49]	14.40–16.60 [144–166]	42.9–49.1	27–31	33–37	76–100	11.5–14.5
Adult female	As above	4.15–4.87 [4.15–5.49]	12.2–14.7 [122–147]	37.9–43.9	As above	As above	As above	As above
11–15 years	4500–13,500	4.8	13.4	39	28	34	82	—
6–10 years	5000–14,500	4.7	12.9	37.5	27	34	80	—
4–6 years	5500–15,500	4.6	12.6	37.0	27	34	80	—
2–4 years	6000–17,000	4.5	12.5	35.5	25	32	77	—
4 months–2 years	6000–17,500	4.6	11.2	35.0	25	33	77	—
1 week–4 mo	5500–18,000	4.7 ± 0.9	14.0 ± 3.3	42.0 ± 7.0	30	33	90	—
24 hr–1 week	5000–21,000	5.1	18.3 ± 4.0	52.5	36	35	103	—
First day	9400–34,000	5.1 ± 1.0	19.5 ± 5.0	54.0 ± 10.0	38	36	106	—

¹To convert from standard reference value to SI units, multiply by 10.

TABLE II-4. NORMAL PLATELET AND WHITE BLOOD CELL DIFFERENTIAL FOR SELECTED AGES.

Age	Platelet Count (10³/µL) [SI: 10⁹/L]	Lymphocytes Total (% WBC count)	Neutrophils, Band (% WBC count)	Neutrophils, Segmented (% WBC count)	Eosinophils (% WBC count)	Basophils (% WBC count)	Monocytes (% WBC count)
Adult male	238 ± 49	34%	3.0%	56%	2.7%	0.5%	4.0%
Adult female	270 ± 58	As above	As above	As above	As above	As above	As above
11–15 years	282 ± 63	38%	3.0%	51%	2.4%	0.5%	4.3%
6–10 years	351 ± 85	39%	3.0%	50%	2.4%	0.6%	4.2%
4–6 years	357 ± 70	42%	3.0%	39%	2.8%	0.6%	5.0%
2–4 years	357 ± 70	59%	3.0%	30%	2.6%	0.5%	5.0%
4 month–2 years	As above	61%	3.1%	28%	2.6%	0.4%	4.8%
1 week–4 mo	As above	56%	4.5%	30%	2.8%	0.5%	6.5%
24 hr–1 week	240–380	24–41%	6.8–9.2%	39–52%	2.4–4.1%	0.5%	5.8–9.1%
First day	As above	24%	10.2%	58%	2.0%	0.6%	5.8%

Lymphocytes, atypical

Greater Than 20%: Infectious mononucleosis, cytomegalovirus (CMV) infection, infectious hepatitis, toxoplasmosis.

Less Than 20%: Viral infections (mumps, rubeola, varicella), rickettsial infections, TB.

MCH (Mean Cellular [Corpuscular] Hemoglobin): (27–31 pg [SI: pg]). The weight of hemoglobin of the average red cell. Calculated by:

$$MCH = \frac{\text{Hemoglobin (g/L)}}{\text{RBC } (10^6 \ \mu L)}$$

Increased: Macrocytosis (megaloblastic anemias, high reticulocyte counts).

Decreased: Microcytosis (iron deficiency, sideroblastic anemia, thalassemia).

MCHC (Mean Cellular [Corpuscular] Hemoglobin Concentration): (33–37 g/dL [SI: 330–370 g/L]).

The average concentration of hemoglobin in a given volume of red cells. Calculated by the formula:

$$MCHC = \frac{\text{Hemoglobin (g/dL)}}{\text{Hematocrit}}$$

Increased: Very severe, prolonged dehydration; spherocytosis.

Decreased: Iron deficiency anemia, overhydration, thalassemia, sideroblastic anemia.

MCV (Mean Cell [Corpuscular] Volume): (76–100 cu μm [SI: fL]). The average volume of red blood cells. Calculated by the formula:

$$MCV = \frac{\text{Hematocrit} \times 1000}{\text{RBC } (10^6/\mu L)}$$

Increased: Megaloblastic anemia (B_{12}, folate deficiency), macrocytic (normoblastic) anemia, reticulocytosis, Down syndrome, chronic liver disease.

Decreased: Iron deficiency, thalassemia, some cases of lead poisoning.

Monocytes: (3–7%)

Increased: Bacterial infection (TB, subacute bacterial endocarditis [SBE], brucellosis, typhoid, recovery from an acute infection), protozoal infections, infectious mononucleosis, leukemia, Hodgkin's disease, ulcerative colitis, regional enteritis.

Platelets: (150–450,000 μL)

Platelet counts may be normal in number, but abnormal in function as occurs in aspirin therapy. Abnormalities of platelet function are assessed by bleeding time.

Increased: Sudden exercise, after trauma, bone fracture, after asphyxia, after surgery (especially splenectomy), acute hemorrhage, polycythemia vera, primary thrombocythemia, leukemias, after childbirth, carcinoma, myeloproliferative disorders.

Decreased: Disseminated intravascular coagulation (DIC), idiopathic thrombocytopenic purpura (ITP), thrombotic thrombocytopenic purpura, congenital disease, marrow suppressants (chemotherapy, thiazide diuretics, alcohol, estrogens, x-rays), burns, snake and insect bites, leukemias, aplastic anemias, hypersplenism, infectious mononucleosis, viral infections, cirrhosis, massive transfusions, eclampsia and preeclampsia, more than 30 different drugs.

PMNs (Polymorphonuclear Neutrophils): (40–76%)

Increased:

- Physiologic (normal): Severe exercise, last months of pregnancy, labor, surgery, newborns, steroid therapy.
- Pathologic: Bacterial infections, noninfective tissue damage (myocardial infarction, pulmonary infarction, crush injury, burn injury), metabolic disorders (eclampsia, diabetic ketoacidosis, uremia, acute gout), leukemias.

Decreased: Pancytopenia, aplastic anemia, PMN depression (a mild decrease is referred to as neutropenia; severe is called agranulocytosis), marrow damage (x-rays, poisoning with benzene or antitumor drugs), severe overwhelming infections (disseminated TB, septicemia), acute malaria, severe osteomyelitis, infectious mononucleosis, atypical pneumonias, some viral infections, marrow obliteration (osteosclerosis, myelofibrosis, malignant infiltrate), more than 70 drugs (including chloramphenicol, phenylbutazone, chlorpromazine, and quinine), B_{12} and folate deficiencies, hypoadrenalism, hypopituitarism, dialysis, familial decrease, idiopathic causes.

Red Cell Distribution Width (RDW): (11.5–14.5)
A measure of the degree of anisocytosis (variation in RBC size) and measured by the automated hematology counters (eg, Coulter Counter).

Increased: Many anemias (concomitant macrocytic and microcytic anemia).

White blood cell count: (see Tables II–3 and II–4, pages 254 and 255)

Increased: Infections (especially bacterial), leukemia, leukemoid reactions, tissue necrosis, postsplenectomy, exercise, fever, pain, anesthesia, labor.

Decreased: Sepsis, overwhelming bacterial infections, certain nonbacterial infections (influenza, hepatitis, mononucleosis), aplastic anemia, pernicious anemia, hypersplenism, cachexia, chemotherapeutic agents, ionizing radiation.

C-Peptide

(Fasting, <4.0 ng/mL [SI: <4.0 µg/L]; male >60 years, 1.5–5.0 ng/mL [SI: 1.5–5.0 µg/L]; female 1.4–5.5 ng/mL [SI: 1.4–5.5 µg/L]).

Decreased: Diabetes (decreased endogenous insulin), insulin administration (factitious or therapeutic), hypoglycemia.

CA 19–9

(Less than 37 U/mL [SI: <37 kU/L]).

Increased: Gastrointestinal cancers such as pancreas, stomach, liver, colorectal, hepatobiliary; some cases of lung and prostate.

CA 125

(Less than 35 U/mL [SI: <35 kU/L]).

Not a useful screening test for ovarian cancer when used alone; used in conjunction with ultrasound and physical exam for detection. Rising levels after resection predictive for recurrence.

Increased: Ovarian, endometrial, and colon cancer, endometriosis, inflammatory bowel disease, pelvic inflammatory disease, pregnancy, breast lesions, and benign abdominal masses (teratomas).

Calcitonin (Thyrocalcitonin)

(Less than 19 pg/mL [SI: <19 ng/L]).

Increased: Medullary carcinoma of the thyroid, C-cell hyperplasia (precursor of medullary carcinoma), oat cell carcinoma of the lung, newborns, pregnancy, chronic renal insufficiency, Zollinger-Ellison syndrome, pernicious anemia.

Calcium, Serum

(Infants to 1 month 7–11.5 mg/dL [SI: 1.75–2.87 mmol/L]; 1 month to 1 year 8.6–11.2 mg/dL [SI: 2.15–2.79 mmol/L]; older than 1 year and adults 8.2–10.2 mg/dL [SI: 2.05–2.54 mmol/L]; ionized, 4.75–5.2 mg/dL [SI: 1.19–1.30 mmol/L]. To convert mg/dL to mmol/L, multiply by 0.2495).

When interpreting a total calcium value, the total protein and albumin must be known. If these are not within normal limits, a corrected calcium can be roughly calculated by the following formula:

Corrected total Ca = 0.8 (Normal albumin − measured albumin) + reported Ca

Values for ionized calcium need no special corrections.

Increased: **Note:** Levels >12 mg/dL [2.99 mmol/L] may lead to coma and death. Primary hyperthyroidism, parathyroid hormone (PTH) secreting tumors, vitamin D excess, metastatic bone tumors, osteoporosis, immobilization, milk-alkali syndrome, Paget's disease, idiopathic hypercalcemia of infants, infantile hypophosphatasia, thiazide drugs, chronic renal failure, sarcoidosis, multiple myeloma.

Decreased: **Note:** Levels <7 mg/dL [<1.75 mmol/L] may lead to tetany and death. Hypoparathyroidism (surgical, idiopathic), pseudohypoparathyroidism, insufficient vitamin D, calcium and phosphorus ingestion (pregnancy, osteomalacia, rickets), hypomagnesemia, renal tubular acidosis, hypoalbuminemia (cachexia, nephrotic syndrome, cystic fibrosis), chronic renal failure (phosphate retention), acute pancreatitis, factitious decrease because of low protein and albumin.

Calcium, Urine (24-hour Urine)

On a calcium-free diet <150 mg/24 hr [3.7 mmol/d], average calcium diet (600–800 mg/24 hr) 100–250 mg/24 hr [2.5–6.2 mmol/d].

Increased: Hyperparathyroidism, hyperthyroidism, hypervitaminosis D, distal renal tubular acidosis (type I), sarcoidosis, immobilization, osteolytic lesions (bony metastasis, multiple myeloma), Paget's disease, glucocorticoid excess.

Decreased: Thiazide diuretics, hypothyroidism, renal failure, steatorrhea, rickets, osteomalacia.

Carbon Dioxide (Total CO₂ or Bicarbonate)

(Adult 23–29 mmol/L, child 20–28 mmol/L; see also Pco₂ values)

Increased: Compensation for respiratory acidosis, metabolic alkalosis, emphysema, severe vomiting, primary aldosteronism, volume contraction, Bartter's syndrome.

Decreased: Compensation for respiratory alkalosis, metabolic acidosis, starvation, diabetic ketoacidosis, lactic acidosis, alcoholic ketoacidosis, toxins (methanol, ethylene glycol, paraldehyde), severe diarrhea, renal failure, drugs (salicylates, acetazolamide), dehydration, adrenal insufficiency.

Carbon Dioxide, Arterial (Pco$_2$)

See Table II–1.

Increased: Respiratory acidosis, compensatory increase in metabolic alkalosis.

Decreased: Respiratory alkalosis, compensatory in metabolic alkalosis.

Carboxyhemoglobin (Carbon Monoxide)

(Nonsmoker <2%; smoker <9%; toxic >15%)

Increased: Smokers, smoke inhalation, automobile exhaust inhalation, normal newborns.

Carcinoembryonic Antigen (CEA)

(Nonsmoker <3.0 ng/mL [SI: <3.0 μg/L]; smoker <5.0 ng/mL [SI: <5.0 μg]).

Not a screening test; useful for monitoring response to treatment and tumor recurrence of adenocarcinomas of the gastrointestinal tract especially colonic primaries.

Increased: Carcinoma (colon, pancreas, lung, stomach), smokers, non-neoplastic liver disease, Crohn's disease, and ulcerative colitis.

Catecholamines, Fractionated, Serum

(Values are variable and depend on the lab and method of assay used. Normal levels below are based on an HPLC technique.)

Catecholamine	Plasma (supine) levels
Norepinphrine	70–750 pg/mL [SI: 414–4435 pmol/L]
Epinephrine	0–100 pg/mL [SI: 0–546 pmol/L]
Dopamine	<30 pg/mL [SI: 196 pmol/L]

Increased: Pheochromocytoma, neural crest tumors (neuroblastoma), with extra-adrenal pheochromocytoma; norepinephrine may be markedly elevated compared with epinephrine.

Catecholamines, Fractionated (24-hour Urine)

(Values are variable and dependent on the assay method used. Norepinephrine 15–80 μg/24 hr [SI: 89–473 nmol/24 hr]; epinephrine

0–20 μg/24 hr [SI: 0–118 nmol/24 hr]; dopamine 65–400 μg/24 hr [SI: 384–2364 nmol/24 hr]).

Used to evaluate neuroendocrine tumors including pheochromocytoma and neuroblastoma. Avoid caffeine, and methyldopa (Aldomet) before test.

Increased: Pheochromocytoma, neuroblastoma, epinephrine administration, drugs (methyldopa and tetracyclines are false increases).

Chloride, Serum

(97–107 mEq/L [SI: 97–107 mmol/L]).

Increased: Diarrhea, renal tubular acidosis, mineralocorticoid deficiency, hyperalimentation, medications (acetazolamide, ammonium chloride).

Decreased: Vomiting, diabetes mellitus with ketoacidosis, mineralocorticoid excess, renal disease with sodium loss.

Cholesterol (Total)

(Normal–see Table II–5. To convert mg/dL to mmol/L, multiply by 0.02586).

Increased: Idiopathic hypercholesterolemia, biliary obstruction, nephrosis, hypothyroidism, pancreatic disease (diabetes), pregnancy, oral contraceptives, hyperlipoproteinemia (types IIb, III, V).

Decreased: Liver disease (hepatitis, etc), hyperthyroidism, malnutrition (cancer, starvation), chronic anemias, steroid therapy, lipoproteinemias.

Cholesterol, High Density Lipoprotein (HDL, HDL-C)

(Male fasting 30–70 mg/dL [SI: 0.8-1.80 mmol/L]; female 30–90 mg/dL [SI: 0.80–2.35]).

TABLE II–5. NORMAL TOTAL CHOLESTEROL LEVELS BY AGE.

Age	Standard Units	SI Units
Infant	<65–175 mg/dL	<1.68–4.52 mmol/L
1–19	<120–220 mg/dL	<3.10–5.68 mmol/L
20–29	<200 mg/dL	<5.20 mmol/L
30–39	<225 mg/dL	<5.85 mmol/L
40–49	<245 mg/dL	<6.35 mmol/L
>50	<265 mg/dL	<6.85 mmol/L

HDL-C has the best correlation with the development of coronary artery disease; decreased HDL-C in males leads to an increased risk. Levels <45 mg/dl associated with increased risk of coronary artery disease.

Increased: Estrogen (females), exercise, ethanol.

Decreased: Males, uremia, obesity, diabetes, liver disease, Tangier's disease.

Cholesterol, Low Density Lipoprotein (LDL, LDL-C)

(50–190 mg/dL [SI: 1.30–4.90 mmol/L]).

Increased: Excess dietary saturated fats, myocardial infarction (MI), hyperlipoproteinemia, biliary cirrhosis, endocrine disease (diabetes, hypothyroidism).

Decreased: Malabsorption, severe liver disease, abetalipoproteinemia, nicotinic acid.

Cold Agglutinins

(<1 : 32)

Increased: Atypical pneumonia (mycoplasmal pneumonia), other viral infections (especially mononucleosis, measles, mumps), cirrhosis, parasitic infections.

Complement C3

(85–155 mg/dL, [SI: 800–1500 ng/L]).

Increased: Rheumatoid arthritis (variable finding), rheumatic fever, various neoplasms (gastrointestinal, prostate, others).

Decreased: Erythematosus, glomerulonephritis (poststreptococcal and membranoproliferative), sepsis, subacute bacterial endocarditis (SBE), chronic active hepatitis.

Complement C4

(20–50 mg/dL [SI: 200–500 ng/L]).

Increased: Rheumatoid arthritis (variable finding), neoplasia (gastrointestinal, lung, others).

Decreased: SLE, chronic active hepatitis, cirrhosis, glomerulonephritis, hereditary angioedema.

Complement CH50 (Total)

(33–61 mg/mL [SI: 330–610 ng/L]).

Tests for complement deficiency in the classic pathway.

Increased: Acute phase reactants (tissue injury, infections, etc).

Decreased: Hereditary complement deficiencies.

Coombs' Test, Direct (Direct Antiglobulin Test)

(Normal = negative)

Uses patient's erythrocytes; tests for the presence of antibody on the patient's cells.

Positive: Autoimmune hemolytic anemia (leukemia, lymphoma, collagen-vascular diseases), hemolytic transfusion reaction, some drug sensitizations (methyldopa, levodopa, cephalothin), hemolytic disease of the newborn (erythroblastosis fetalis).

Coombs' Test, Indirect (Antibody Screening Test)

(Normal = negative)

Uses serum that contains antibody, usually from the patient.

Positive: Isoimmunization from previous transfusion, incompatible blood due to improper crossmatching.

Cortisol, Serum

(8 AM, 5.0–23.0 μg/dL [SI: 138–365 nmol/L]; 4 PM, 3.0–15.0 μg/dL [SI: 83–414 nmol/L]).

Increased: Adrenal adenoma, adrenal carcinoma, Cushing's disease, nonpituitary ACTH-producing tumor, steroid therapy, oral contraceptives.

Decreased: Primary adrenal insufficiency (Addison's disease), congenital adrenal hyperplasia, Waterhouse-Friderichsen syndrome, ACTH deficiency.

Cortisol, Free (24-hour Urine)

(30–100 μg/24 hr)

Used to evaluate adrenal cortical function; screening test of choice for Cushing's syndrome.

Increased: Cushing's syndrome (adrenal hyperfunction), stress during collection, oral contraceptives, pregnancy.

Counterimmunoelectrophoresis (CIEP, CEP)

(Normal = negative).

An immunologic technique that allows rapid identification of infecting organisms from fluids including serum, urine, cerebrospinal fluid (CSF), and other body fluids. Organisms identified include: *Neisseria meningitidis, Streptococcus pneumoniae, Haemophilus influenzae,* and group B streptococcus.

Creatine Phosphokinase (CPK)

(25–145 mU/mL [SI: 25–145 U/L]).

Increased: Muscle damage (acute myocardial infarction, myocarditis, muscular dystrophy, muscle trauma [injection]), after surgery, brain infarction, defibrillation, cardiac catheterization and surgery, rhabdomyolysis, polymyositis, hypothyroidism.

CPK Isoenzymes

MB: Normal <6%, heart origin. Increased by acute myocardial infarction (begins in 2–12 hours, peaks in 12–40 hours, returns to normal in 24–72 hours), pericarditis with myocarditis, rhabdomyolysis, crush injury, Duchenne's muscular dystrophy, polymyositis, malignant hyperthermia, and cardiac surgery.

MM: Normal 94–100%, skeletal muscle origin. Increased by crush injury, malignant hyperthermia, seizures, IM injections.

BB: Normal 0%, brain origin. Increased by brain injury (cerebrovascular accident [CVA], trauma), metastatic neoplasms (prostate), malignant hyperthermia, colonic infarction.

Creatinine, Serum

(Adult male <1.2 mg/dL [SI: 106 μmol/L]; adult female <1.1 mg/dL [SI: 97 μmol/L]; child 0.5–0.8 mg/dL [SI: 44–71 μmol/L]. To convert mg/dL to μmol/L, multiply by 88.40).

Increased: Renal failure (prerenal, renal, or postrenal obstruction), gigantism, acromegaly, ingestion of roasted meat, aminoglycosides and other drugs (cimetidine, some cephalosporins, ascorbic acid, others), false positive with DKA.

Decreased: Pregnancy, decreased muscle mass, severe liver disease.

Creatinine (Urine) & Creatinine Clearance

(Adult male: Total creatinine 1–2 g/24 hr [8.8–17.7 mmol/d]; clearance 85–125 mL/min/1.73 m^2; adult female: Total creatinine 0.8–1.8 g/24 hr [7.1–15.9 mmol/d]; clearance 75–115 mL/min 1.73 m^2 [1.25–1.92

ml/s/1.73 m^2]; child: Total creatinine (>3 years) 12–30 mg/kg/24 hr; clearance 70–140 mL/min/1.73 m^2 [1.17–2.33 mL/s/1.73 m^2]).

Increased: Early diabetes mellitus, pregnancy.

Decreased: A decreased creatinine clearance results in an increase in serum creatinine usually secondary to renal insufficiency.

Calculation of Creatinine Clearance: To determine a creatinine clearance, order a concurrent serum creatinine and a 24-hour urine creatinine. A shorter time interval can be used (eg, 12 hours), but remember that the formula must be corrected for this change and that a 24-hour sample is less prone to collection error.

Example: A quick formula is also found on page 503, "Aminoglycoside dosing".

Calculation of the creatinine clearance from a 24-hour urine sample with a volume of 1000 mL, a urine creatinine of 108 mg/100 mL, and a serum creatinine of 1 mg/100 mL (1 mg/dL).

$$\text{Clearance} = \frac{\text{Urine creatinine} \times \text{total urine volume}}{\text{plasma creatinine} \times \text{time (1440 min if 24-hour collection)}}$$

$$\text{Clearance} = \frac{(108 \text{ mg/100mL}) (1000 \text{ mL})}{(1 \text{ mg/100 mL}) (1440 \text{ min})} = 75 \text{ mL/min}$$

Some clinicians advocate a preliminary determination to see if the urine sample is valid by determining first if the sample contains at least 18–25 mg/kg/24 hr of creatinine for adult males or 12–20 mg/kg/24 hr for adult females. This preliminary test is not a requirement, but can help with the determination if a 24-hour sample was collected or if some of the sample was lost.

If the patient is an adult (150 lb = body surface area of 1.73 m^2), adjustment of the clearance for body size is not routinely done. Adjustment for pediatric patients is a necessity. If the values in the previous example were for a 10-year-old boy who weighed 70 lb (1.1 m^2; see page 505 for the conversion formula), then the clearance would be:

$$\frac{75 \text{ mL/min} \times 1.73 \text{ m}^2}{1.1 \text{ m}^2} = 118 \text{ mL/min}$$

Dehydroepiandrosterone (DHEA)

(Male 2.0–3.4 ng/mL [SI: 5.2–8.7 μmol/L]; female premenopausal 0.8–3.4 ng/mL [SI: 2.1–8.8 μmol/L], postmenopausal 0.1–0.6 ng/mL [SI: 0.3–1.6 μmol/L]).

Increased: Anovulation, polycystic ovaries, adrenal hyperplasia, adrenal tumors.

Decreased: Menopause.

Dehydroepiandrosterone Sulfate (DHEAS)

(Male 1.7–4.2 ng/mL [SI: 6–15 μmol/L]; female 2.0–5.2 ng/mL [SI: 7–18 μmol/L]).

Increased: Hyperprolactinemia, adrenal hyperplasia, adrenal tumor, polycystic ovaries, lipoid ovarian tumors.

Decreased: Menopause.

Dexamethasone Suppression Test

Used in the differential diagnosis of Cushing's syndrome (elevated cortisol).

Overnight Test: In the "rapid" version of this test, a patient takes 1 mg PO of dexamethasone at 11 PM and a fasting 8 AM plasma cortisol is obtained. Normally the cortisol level should be <5.0 μg/dL [138 nmol/L]. If the value is >5 μg/dL [138 nmol/L], this usually confirms the diagnosis of Cushing's syndrome; however, obesity, alcoholism, or depression may occasionally show the same result. In these patients, the best screening test is a 24-hour urine for free cortisol.

Low Dose Test: After collection of baseline serum cortisol and 24-hour urine free cortisol levels, dexamethasone 0.5 mg PO is administered every 6 hours for 8 doses. Serum and urine cortisol are repeated on the second day. Failure to suppress serum cortisol of <5.0 μg/dL [138 nmol/L] and a urine free cortisol of <30 μg/dL (82 nmol/L) confirms Cushing's syndrome.

High Dose Test: After the low dose test, dexamethasone, 2 mg PO every 6 hours for eight doses will cause a fall in urinary free cortisol to 50% of the baseline value in patients with bilateral adrenal hyperplasia (Cushing's disease), but not in patients with adrenal tumors or ectopic adrenocorticotropic hormone (ACTH) production.

Estradiol, Serum

Serial measurements useful to assess fetal well being, especially in high risk pregnancy.

Phase	Normal Values (Female)
Follicular	25–75 pg/mL
Midcycle Peak	200–600 pg/mL
Leuteal	100–300 pg/mL
Pregnancy 1st trimester	1–5 ng/mL
2nd trimester	5–15 ng/mL
3rd trimester	10–40 ng/mL
Postmenopause	5–25 pg/mL

Estrogen Receptors

(<3 fmol or negative)

These are typically determined on fresh surgical specimens. The presence of the receptors is associated with a longer disease-free interval and survival from breast cancer, and more likely to respond to endocrine therapy. Between 50 and 75% of breast cancers are estrogen receptor positive.

Fecal Fat

(2–6 g/d on a 80–100 g/d fat diet; 72-hour collection time)

Increased: Cystic fibrosis, pancreatic insufficiency, Crohn's disease, chronic pancreatitis, sprue.

Ferritin

(Male 15–200 ng/mL [SI: 15–200 μg/L]; female 12–150 ng/mL [SI: 12–150 μg/L]).

Increased: Hemochromatosis, hemosiderosis, sideroblastic anemia.

Decreased: Iron deficiency (earliest and most sensitive test before red cells show any morphologic change), severe liver disease.

Fibrin Degradation Products (FDP), Fibrin Split Products (FSP)

(<10 μg/mL)

Increased: Disseminated intravascular coagulation (DIC) (usually >40 μg/mL), any thromboembolic condition (deep venous thrombosis, myocardial infarction, pulmonary embolus), hepatic dysfunction.

Fibrinogen

(200–400 mg/dL [SI: 2.0–4.0 g/L]).

Increased: Inflammatory reactions, oral contraceptives, pregnancy, cancer (kidney, stomach, breast).

Decreased: DIC (sepsis, amniotic fluid embolism, abruptio placentae), surgery (prostate, open heart), neoplastic and hematologic conditions, acute severe bleeding, burns, venomous snake bite, congenital.

Folic Acid, Serum Folate

(>2.0 ng/mL [SI: >5 nmol/L]).

Folic Acid, RBC

(125–600 ng/mL [SI: 283–1360 nmol/L]).

Serum folate can fluctuate with diet. RBC levels are more indicative of tissue stores. B_{12} deficiency can result in the RBC unable to take up folate in spite of normal serum folate levels.

Increased: Folic acid administration.

Decreased: Malnutrition/malabsorption (folic acid deficiency), massive cellular growth (cancer), medications (trimethoprim, some anticonvulsants, oral contraceptives), vitamin B_{12} deficiency (low RBC levels), pregnancy.

Follicle Stimulating Hormone (FSH)

(Male <22 IU/L; female nonmid cycle <20 IU/L, midcycle surge <40 IU/L) (midcycle peak should be 2 times basal level; postmenopausal 40–160 IU/L).

Increased: Hypergonadotropic >40 IU/L, postmenopausal, surgical castration, gonadal failure, gonodotropin-secreting pituitary adenoma.

Decreased: Hypogonadotropic <5 IU/L prepubertal, hypothalamic and pituitary dysfunction, pregnancy.

FTA-ABS (Fluorescent Treponemal Antibody Absorbed)

(Normal = nonreactive)

Positive: Syphilis (test of choice to confirm diagnosis), other treponemal infections. **Note:** May be negative in early primary syphilis and remain positive despite adequate treatment.

Fungal Serologies

(Negative <1 : 8)

This is a complement-fixation fungal antibody screen that usually detects antibodies to *Histoplasma, Blastomyces, Aspergillus,* and *Coccidioides.*

Gastrin, Serum

(Fasting <100 pg/mL [SI: 47.7 pmol/L], postprandial 95–140 pg/mL [SI: 45.3–66.7 pmol/L]).

Increased: Zollinger-Ellison syndrome, pyloric stenosis, pernicious anemia, atrophic gastritis, ulcerative colitis, renal insufficiency, steroid and calcium administration.

GGT (See SGGT)

Glucose

(Fasting, 70–105 mg/dL [SI: 3.89–5.83 nmol/L]; 2 hours postprandial < 120 mg/dL [SI: <6.67 nmol/L]. To convert mg/dL to nmol/L, multiply by 0.05551).

Increased: Diabetes mellitus, Cushing's syndrome, acromegaly, increased epinephrine (injection, pheochromocytoma, stress, burns, etc), acute pancreatitis, ACTH administration, spurious increase caused by drawing blood from a site above an IV line containing dextrose, elderly patients, pancreatic glucagonoma, drugs (glucocorticoids, some diuretics).

Decreased: Pancreatic disorders (pancreatitis, islet-cell tumors), extra-pancreatic tumors (carcinoma of the adrenals, stomach), hepatic disease (hepatitis, cirrhosis, tumors), endocrine disorders (early diabetes, hypothyroidism, hypopituitarism), functional disorders (after gastrectomy), pediatric problems (prematurity, infant of a diabetic mother, ketotic hypoglycemia, enzyme diseases), exogenous insulin, oral hypoglycemic agents, malnutrition, sepsis.

Glucose Tolerance Test, Oral

Note: If fasting blood glucose is already elevated above 140 mg/dL, the GTT is usually unnecessary. Used to aid in the diagnosis of diabetes mellitus, especially when diagnosis cannot be made on the basis of fasting blood sugar levels. The test is unreliable in the presence of severe infection, prolonged fasting, or after the injection of insulin. After an overnight fast, a fasting blood glucose is drawn, and the patient is given a 75 g oral glucose load (100 g for gestational diabetes screening, 1.75 mg-kg ideal body weight in children up to 75 g). Plasma glucose is then drawn at 30, 60, 120, and 180 minutes.

Interpretation:

Adult onset diabetes: Any fasting blood sugar >140 or >200 at both 120 minutes and one other time interval measured.

Gestational diabetes: At least two of the following: any fasting blood sugar >105, at 60 minutes >190, at 120 minutes >165, or at 180 minutes >145.

Glycohemoglobin (Hemoglobin A$_{1c}$, Glycosylated Hemoglobin)

(4.6–7.1%)

Increased: Diabetes mellitus (uncontrolled; reflects levels over preceding 3–4 months).

Decreased: Chronic renal failure, hemolytic anemia, pregnancy, chronic blood loss.

Gram's Stain

Technique

1. The Gram's stain is used in the identification of gram-positive and gram-negative bacteria. Smear the specimen (sputum, peritoneal fluid, etc) on a glass slide in a fairly thin coat. If time permits, allow the specimen to air dry. The smear may also be fixed under very low heat (excessive heat can cause artifacts). If a Bunsen burner is not available, other heat sources include a hot light bulb, or an alcohol swab set on fire. Heat the slide until it is warm, but not hot, when touched to the back of the hand.
2. Timing for the stain is not critical, but at least 10 seconds should be allowed for each set of reagents.
3. Apply the crystal violet (Gram's stain), rinse the slide with tap water, apply iodine solution, and rinse with water.
4. Decolorize the slide carefully with the acetone-alcohol solution until the blue color is barely visible in the runoff. (This is the step where most Gram's stains are ruined.)
5. Counterstain with a few drops of safranin, rinse the slide with water, and blot it dry with lint-free bibulous or filter paper.
6. Use the high dry and oil immersion lenses on the microscope to examine the slide. If the Gram's stain is satisfactory, any polys on the slide should be pink with light blue nuclei. On a Gram's stain of sputum, an excessive number of epithelial cells means the sample was more saliva than sputum.

Gram's Stain Characteristics Of Common Pathogens

Gram-Positive Cocci: *Staphylococcus, Streptococcus, Diplococcus, Micrococcus, Peptococcus* (anaerobic), and *Peptostreptococcus* (anaerobic) species. (If *Staphylococcus* initially reported as coagulase positive, suspect *S aureus,* if coagulase negative, suspect *S epidermidis*).

Gram-Positive Rods: *Clostridium* (anaerobic), *Cornebacterium, Listeria,* and *Bacillus* species.

Gram-Negative Cocci: *Neisseria* (*Branhamella*) species.

Gram-Negative Coccoid Rods: *Haemophilus, Pasteurella, Brucella,* and *Bordetella* species.

Gram-Negative Straight Rods: *Escherichia, Salmonella, Shigella, Proteus, Enterobacter, Klebsiella, Serratia, Pseudomonas, Providencia, Yersinia, Acinetobacter* (Mima polymorpha, Herellea), *Eikenella, Legionella, Bacteroides* (anaerobic), *Fusobacterium* (anaerobic), and *Campylobacter* (comma-shaped) species.

5-Hydroxyindoleacetic Acid (5-HIAA) (24-hour urine)

(2–8 mg [SI: 10.4–41.6] μmol/24-h urine collection).

5-HIAA is a serotonin metabolite and is useful to diagnose carcinoid syndrome.

Increased: Carcinoid tumors, certain foods (banana, pineapple, tomato), phenothiazine derivatives.

Haptoglobin

(40–180 mg/dL [SI: 0.4–1.8 g/L]).

Increased: Obstructive liver disease, any cause if increased erythrocyte sedimentation rate (ESR) (inflammation, collagen-vascular diseases).

Decreased: Any type of hemolysis (transfusion reaction, etc), liver disease, anemia, oral contraceptives.

Hepatitis Testing

Recommended hepatitis panel tests based on clinical settings are shown in Table II–6. Interpretation of testing patterns is shown in Table II–7.

Hepatitis Tests

HBsAg	Hepatitis B surface antigen (formerly Australia antigen—HAA). Indicates either chronic or acute infection with hepatitis B. Used by blood banks to screen donors.
Total Anti-HBc	IgG and IgM antibody to hepatitis B core antigen; confirms either previous exposure to hepatitis B virus (HBV) or ongoing infection. Used by blood banks to screen donors.
Anti-HBc IgM	IgM antibody to hepatitis B core antigen. Early and best indicator of acute infection with hepatitis B.
HBeAg	Hepatitis Be antigen; when present, indicates high degree of infectivity. Order only when evaluating a patient with chronic HBV infection.
Anti-HBe	Antibody to hepatitis Be antigen; presence associated with resolution of active inflammation, but often signifies virus is integrated into host DNA, especially if the host remains HBsAg positive.
Anti-HBs	Antibody to hepatitis B surface antigen; when present, typically indicates immunity associated with clinical recovery from HBV infection or previous immunization with hepatitis B vaccine. Order only to assess effectiveness of vaccine and request titer levels.

TABLE II–6. HEPATITIS PANEL TESTING TO GUIDE IN THE ORDERING OF HEPATITIS PROFILES FOR GIVEN CLINICAL SETTINGS.

Medical Setting	Test	Purpose
Screening tests		
Pregnancy	• HBsAg	All expectant mothers should be screened during 3rd trimester.
High risk patients on admission (homosexuals, dialysis patients	• HBsAg	To screen for chronic or active infection.
Percutaneous inoculation (donor)	• HBsAg • Anti-HBc IgM • Anti-Hepatitis C	To test patients blood (especially dialysis patients and HIV-infected individuals) for infectivity with HBV and HCV if health care worker exposed.
Percutaneous inoculation (victim)	• HBsAg • Anti-HBc • Anti-hepatitis C	To test exposed health care worker for immunity or chronic infection.
Pre-HBV Vaccine	• Anti-HBc • Anti-HBs	To determine if an individual is infected or has antibodies to HBV.
Screening blood donors	• HBsAg • Anti-HBc • Anti-hepatitis C	Used by blood banks to screen donors for hepatitis B and C.
Diagnostic tests		
Differential diagnosis of acute jaundice, hepatitis, or fulminant liver failure	• HBsAg • Anti-HBc IgM • Anti-HAV IgM • Anti-hepatitis C	To differentiate between HBV, HAV, and HCV in acutely jaundiced patient with hepatitis or fulminant liver failure.
Chronic hepatitis	• HBsAg + HBeAg + Anti-HBe + Anti-hepatitis D (total + Igm)	To diagnose HBV infection + If positive for HBsAg to determine infectivity. + If HBsAg patient worsens or is very ill, to diagnose concomitant infection with hepatitis delta virus.
Monitor		
Infant follow-up	• HBsAg • Anti-HBc • Anti-HBs	To monitor the success of vaccination and passive immunization for perinatal transmission of HBV 12–15 months after birth.
Postvaccination screening	• Anti-HBs	To ensure immunity has been achieved after vaccination (CDC recommends titer determination, but usually qualitative assay adequate).
Sexual contact	• HBsAg • Anti-HBc • Anti-hepatitis C	To monitor sexual partners of patient with chronic HBV or HCV.

(Reproduced, with permission, from Gomella LG (editor): Diagnosis: Chemistry, Immunology, and Serology. In: Clinician's Pocket Reference, 7/e. *Appleton & Lange, 1993.)*

TABLE II–7. INTERPRETATION OF VIRAL HEPATITIS SEROLOGIC TESTING PATTERNS.

Anti-HAV (IgM)	HBsAg	Anti-HBc (IgM)	Anti-HBc (Total)	Anti-HCV (Elisa)	Interpretation
+	—	—	—	—	Acute hepatitis A
+	+	—	+	—	Acute hepatitis A in hepatitis B carrier
—	+	—	+	—	Chronic hepatitis B[1]
—	—	+	+	—	Acute hepatitis B
—	+	+	+	—	Acute hepatitis B
—	—	—	+	—	Past hepatitis B infection
—	—	—	—	+	Hepatitis C[2]
—	—	—	—	—	Early hepatitis C or other cause (other virus, toxic, etc.)

[1]Patients with chronic hepatitis B (either active hepatitis or carrier state) should have HBeAg and Anti-HBe checked to determine activity of infection and relative infectivity. Anti-HBs is used to determine response to hepatitis B vaccination.
[2]Anti-HCV often takes 3–6 months before being positive. Will soon be replaced by more sensitive tests, eg, polymerase chain reaction (PCR).

Anti-HAV	Total antibody to hepatitis A virus; confirms previous exposure to hepatitis A virus.
Anti-HAV IgM	IgM antibody to hepatitis A virus; indicative of recent infection with hepatitis A virus.
Anti-HDV	Total antibody to delta hepatitis; confirms previous exposure. Order only in patients with known acute or chronic HBV infection.
Anti-HDV IgM	IgM antibody to delta hepatitis; indicates recent infection. Order only in patients with known acute or chronic HBV infection.
Anti-HCV	Antibody against hepatitis C (formerly known as non-A, non-B hepatitis) and is the major cause of posttransfusion hepatitis. Used by blood banks to screen donors. Many false positives.

High Density Lipoprotein Cholesterol

(See Cholesterol, page 261)

Human Leukocyte Antigens (HLA; HLA Typing)

This test identifies a group of antigens on the cell surface that are the primary determinants of histocompatability and useful in assessing transplantation compatibility. Some are associated with specific diseases, but are not diagnostic of these diseases.

HLA-B27: Ankylosing spondylitis, psoriatic arthritis, Reiter's syndrome, juvenile rheumatoid arthritis.

HLA-DR4/HLA DR2: Chronic Lyme disease arthritis.

HLA-DRw2: Multiple sclerosis.

HLA-B8: Addison's disease, juvenile onset diabetes, Graves' disease, gluten sensitive enteropathy.

Human Immunodeficiency Virus (HIV) Antibody

(Normal = negative)

Used in the diagnosis of acquired immunodeficiency syndrome (AIDS) and to screen blood for use in transfusion. **Note:** New CDC guidelines released in 1993 indicate that any HIV positive person over 13 years of age with a CD4+ T-cell level <200/ul or an HIV positive with a series of indicator conditions (eg, pulmonary candidiasis, disseminated histoplasmosis, HIV wasting, Kaposi's sarcoma, TB, various lymphomas, *Pneumocystis carinii* pneumonia) is considered to have AIDS.

ELISA: Enzyme-linked immunosorbent assay to detect HIV antibody; a positive test should be confirmed by Western blot.

Positive: AIDS, asymptomatic HIV infection, false-positive.

Western Blot

(Normal = negative)

The technique used as the reference procedure for confirming the presence or absence of HIV antibody, usually after a positive HIV antibody by ELISA determination. In the future, polymerase chain reaction (PCR) may become the confirmatory test for HIV.

Positive: AIDS, asymptomatic HIV infection (If indeterminate, repeat in one month).

Human Chorionic Gonadotropin, Serum (HCG, Beta Subunit)

(Normal, <3.0 mIU/mL; 10 days postconception, >3 mIU/mL; 30 days, 100–5000 mIU/mL; 10 weeks, 50,000–140,000 mIU/mL; >16 weeks, 10,000–50,000 mIU/mL; thereafter, levels slowly decline [SI: IU/L equivalent to mIU/mL]. See also Urinary HCG, page 292).

Increased: Pregnancy, testicular tumors, trophoblastic disease (hydatidiform mole, choriocarcinoma levels usually >100,000 mIU/mL).

Iron

(Male 65–175 μg/dL [SI: 11.64–31.33 μmol/L]; female 50–170 μg/dL [SI: 8.95–30.43 μmol/L]. To convert μg/dL to μmol/L, multiply by 0.1791).

Increased: Hemochromatosis, hemosiderosis caused by excessive iron intake, excess destruction or decreased production of erythrocytes, liver necrosis.

Decreased: Iron deficiency anemia, nephrosis (loss of iron-binding proteins), normochromic anemia of chronic diseases and infections.

Iron-Binding Capacity (Total) (TIBC)

(250–450 μg/dL [SI: 44.75–80.55 μmol/L]).

The normal iron/TIBC ratio is 20–50%. Less than 15% is almost diagnostic of iron deficiency anemia. Increased ratio is seen with hemochromatosis.

Increased: Acute and chronic blood loss, iron deficiency anemia, hepatitis, oral contraceptives.

Decreased: Anemia of infection and chronic diseases, cirrhosis, nephrosis, hemochromatosis.

17-Ketogenic Steroids (17-KGS, Corticosteroids) (24-hour urine)

(Male 5–24 mg/24 hr [SI: 17–83 μmol/24 hr]; female 4–15 mg/24 hr [SI: 14–52 μmol/24 hr]).

Overall adrenal function test, largely replaced by serum or urine cortisol levels.

Increased: Adrenal hyperplasia (Cushing's syndrome), adrenogenital syndrome.

Decreased: Panhypopituitarism, Addison's disease, acute steroid withdrawal.

17-Ketosteroids, Total (17-KS) (24-hour urine) (Adult males 8–20 mg/24 hr [SI: 28–69 μmol/L]; adult female 6–15 mg/dL [SI: 21–52 μmol/L]. Note: Low values in prepubertal children).

Measures dehydroepiandrosterone (DHEA), androstenedione (adrenal androgens); largely replaced by assay of individual elements.

Increased: Adrenal cortex abnormalities (hyperplasia [Cushing's disease], adenoma, carcinoma, adrenogenital syndrome), severe stress, adrenocorticotropic hormone (ACTH) or pituitary tumor, testicular interstitial tumor, and arrhenoblastoma (both produce testosterone).

Decreased: Panhypopituitarism, Addison's disease, castration in men.

KOH Preparation (Potassium Hydroxide Wet Mount)

Technique

1. KOH preps are used for diagnosis of fungal infections. Apply the specimen (vaginal secretion, sputum, skin scrapings) to a slide.
2. Add 1–2 drops of 10% KOH solution and mix. Gentle heating may help.
3. Put a coverslip over the specimen and examine the slide for branching hyphae and blastospores that indicate the presence of a fungus. KOH should destroy most elements other than fungus. If there is dense keratin and debris, allow the slide to sit for several hours and then repeat the microscopic examination. Lowering the substage condenser will give better contrast between organisms and the background.

Positive: Filaments, hyphae, spores, budding yeast suggest fungal infection. Note that false-positives can be seen with cotton or cellulose fibers that may be mistaken for hyphae.

Lactate Dehydrogenase (LDH)

(Adults <200 U/L, higher levels in childhood)

Increased: Acute myocardial infarction, cardiac surgery, prosthetic valve, hepatitis, pernicious anemia, malignant tumors, pulmonary embolus, hemolysis (anemias or factitious), renal infarction, muscle injury, megaloblastic anemia, liver disease.

LDH Isoenzymes (LDH 1 to LDH 5): Normally, the ratio LDH 1/LDH 2 is <0.6–0.7. If the ratio becomes >1 (also termed "flipped"), suspect a recent myocardial infarction (change in ratio can also be seen in pernicious or hemolytic anemia). With an acute myocardial infarction, the LDH will begin to rise in 12–48 hours, peak in 3–6 days and return to normal in 8–14 days. LDH 5 is >LHD 4 in liver diseases.

Lactic Acid (Lactate)

(4.5–19.8 mg/dL [SI: 0.5–2.2 mmol/L]).

Increased: Lactic acidosis is due to hypoxia, hemorrhage, shock, sepsis, cirrhosis, exercise.

LAP Score (Leukocyte Alkaline Phosphatase Score)

(70–140)

Increased: Leukemoid reaction, acute inflammation, Hodgkin's disease, pregnancy, liver disease.

Decreased: Chronic myelogenous leukemia, nephrotic syndrome.

LE (Lupus Erythematosus) Preparation

(Normal = no cells seen)

Positive: Systemic lupus erythematosus (SLE), scleroderma, rheumatoid arthritis, drug-induced lupus (procainamide, others).

Lee White Clotting Time

(5–15 minutes)

Increased: Heparin therapy, plasma-clotting factor deficiency (except factors VII and XIII). **Note:** This is not a good screening test because it is not sensitive.

Luteinizing Hormone, Serum (LH)

(Male 7–24 IU/L; female 6–30 IU/L, midcycle peak increase 2–3-fold over baseline).

Increased: Hypergonadotropic >40 IU/L, postmenopausal, surgical or radiation castration, ovarian or testicular failure, polycystic ovaries.

Decreased: Hypogonodotropic <40 IU/L, prepubertal hypothalamic, and pituitary dysfunction, Kallmann's syndrome.

Lipase

(0–1.5 U/mL [SI: 10–150 U/L] by turbidmetric method).

Increased: Acute pancreatitis, pancreatic duct obstruction (stone, stricture, tumor, drug-induced spasm), fat embolus syndrome, renal failure, dialysis (usually normal in mumps).

Low Density Lipoprotein-Cholesterol (LDL, LDL-C)

(See Cholesterol, page 261)

Lyme Disease Serology

(Normal varies with assay)

Most useful when comparing acute and convalescent serum levels to compare titers. Marked interlaboratory variability is present.

Positive: Infection with *Borrelia burgdorferi* (some cross-reactivity with antibodies to Epstein-Barr, syphilis, *Rickettsia*).

Lymphocyte Subsets

Specific monoclonal antibodies are used to identify specific T- and B-cells. Lymphocyte subsets (also called lymphocyte marker assays, or T- and B-cell assay) are useful in the diagnosis of AIDS and various leukemias and lymphomas. The newer designation CD (clusters of differentiation) has largely replaced the older antibody designations (such as Leu 3a or OKT3). Results are most reliable when reported as an absolute number of cells/μL rather than a percentage of cells. CD4/CD8 ratio <1 is seen in patients with AIDS. Absolute CD4 count is used to follow therapy with ZDV.

Normal lymphocyte subsets

- Total lymphocytes 0.66–4.60 thousand/μL.
- T-cell 644–2201 μL (60–88%).
- B-cell 82–392 μL (3–20%).
- T-helper/inducer cell (CD4, Leu 3a, OKT4) 493–1191 μL (34–67%).
- Suppressor/cytotoxic T-cell (CD8, Leu 2, OKT8) 182–785 μL (10–42%).
- CD4/CD8 ratio >1.

Magnesium

(1.6–2.6 mg/dL [SI: 0.80–1.20 mmol/L]).

Increased: Renal failure, hypothyroidism, magnesium-containing antacids, Addison's disease, diabetic coma, severe dehydration, lithium intoxication.

Decreased: Malabsorption, steatorrhea, alcoholism and cirrhosis, hyperthyroidism, aldosteronism, diuretics, acute pancreatitis, hyperparathyroidism, hyperalimentation, nasogastric suctioning, chronic dialysis, renal tubular acidosis, drugs (eg, cis-platinum, amphotericin B, aminoglycosides), hungry bone syndrome, hypophosphatemia, intracellular shifts with respiratory or metabolic acidosis.

Metanephrines (24-hour urine)

(<1.3 mg/24 hr [SI: 7.1 μmol/L] for adults, but variable in children).

These are metabolic products of epinephrine and norepinephrine, a primary screening test for pheochromocytoma.

Increased: Pheochromocytoma, neuroblastoma (neural crest tumors), false-positive with drugs (eg, phenobarbital, guanethidine, hydrocortisone).

MHA-TP (Microhemagglutination, Treponema Pallium)

(Normal <1 : 160)

Confirmatory test for syphilis, similar to FTA-ABS. Once a patient tests positive, will remain so; therefore, test cannot be used to judge effect of treatment. False-positives with other tremonemal infections (pinta, yaws, etc), mononucleosis, and systemic lupus.

Monospot

(Normal = negative)

Positive: Mononucleosis, rarely in leukemia, serum sickness, Burkitt's lymphoma, viral hepatitis, rheumatoid arthritis.

5' Nucleotidase

(2–15 U/L)

Used in the workup of increased alkaline phosphatase and biliary obstruction.

Increased: Obstructive/cholestatic liver disease, liver metastasis, biliary cirrhosis.

Osmolality, Serum

(278–298 mosm/kg [SI: 278–298 mmol/kg]).

A rough estimation of osmolality is [2 (sodium) + BUN/2.8 + glucose/18]. Measured value is usually greater than calculated value. If measured value is 15 mosm/kg > calculated value, consider methanol, ethanol, or ethylene glycol ingestion.

Increased: Hyperglycemia, alcohol ingestion, increased sodium because of water loss (diabetes, hypercalcemia, diuresis), ethylene glycol ingestion, mannitol.

Decreased: Low serum sodium, diuretics, Addison's disease, inappropriate antidiuretic hormone (ADH) (syndrome of inappropriate ADH [SIADH], seen in bronchogenic carcinoma, hypothyroidism), iatrogenic causes (poor fluid balance).

Oxygen, Arterial (Po$_2$)

See Section I, Problems 48 and 74, pages 166 and 233, respectively. See also Table II–1.

Decreased: Ventilation-perfusion (V/Q) abnormalities, COPD (asthma, emphysema), atelectasis, pneumonia, pulmonary embolus, respiratory distress syndrome, pneumothorax, TB, cystic fibrosis, obstructed airway.

Alveolar hypoventilation: Skeletal abnormalities, neuromuscular disorders, Pickwickian syndrome.

Decreased pulmonary diffusing capacity: Pneumoconiosis, pulmonary edema, pulmonary fibrosis (bleomycin).

Right to left shunt: Congenital heart disease (tetrology of Fallot, transposition, etc).

pH, Arterial

(See Table II–1)

Increased: Metabolic and respiratory alkalosis (see Section I, Problem 3, page 13).

Decreased: Metabolic and respiratory acidosis (see Section I, Problem 4, page 17).

P-24 Antigen (HIV Core Antigen)

(Normal = negative)

Used to diagnose recent acute HIV infection; can be positive as early as 2–4 weeks, but becomes undetectable during antibody seroconversion (periods of latency). With progression of disease, P-24 usually becomes evident again.

Parathyroid Hormone (PTH)

(Normal based on relationship to serum calcium, usually provided on the lab report; also, reference values will vary depending on the laboratory and whether the n-terminal, c-terminal or mid-molecule is measured. PTH mid-molecule 0.29–0.85 ng/mL [SI: 29–85 pmol/L] with calcium 8.4–10.2 mg/dL [SI: 2.1–2.55 mmol/L]).

Increased: Primary hyperparathyroidism, secondary hyperparathyroidism (hypocalcemic states such as chronic renal failure).

Decreased: Hypercalcemia is not due to hyperparathyroidism or hypoparathyroidism.

Partial Thromboplastin Time (Activated Partial Thromboplastin Time, PTT, APTT)

(27–38 seconds)

Increased: Heparin and any defect in the intrinsic coagulation system (includes factors I, II, V, VIII, IX, X, XI, and XII), prolonged use of a tourniquet before drawing a blood sample, hemophilia A and B.

Phosphorus

(Adult 2.5–4.5 mg/dL [SI: 0.81–1.45 mmol/L]; child 4.0–6.0 mg/dL [SI: 1.29–1.95 mmol/L]. To convert mg/dL to mmol/L, multiply by 0.3229).

Increased: Hypoparathyroidism (surgical, pseudohypoparathyroidism), excess vitamin D, secondary hyperparathyroidism, renal failure, bone disease (healing fractures), Addison's disease, childhood, factitious increase (hemolysis of specimen).

Decreased: Hyperparathyroidism, alcoholism, diabetes, hyperalimentation, acidosis, alkalosis, gout, salicylate poisoning, IV steroid, glucose and/or insulin administration, hyperparathyroidism, hypokalemia, hypomagnesemia, diuretics, vitamin D deficiency, phosphate-binding antacids.

Potassium, Serum

(3.5–5 mEq/L [SI: 3.5–5 mmol/L]).

Increased: Factitious increase (hemolysis of specimen, thrombocytosis), renal failure, Addison's disease, acidosis, spironolactone, triamterene, dehydration, hemolysis, massive tissue damage, excess intake (oral or IV), potassium-containing medications, acidosis.

Decreased: Diuretics, decreased intake, vomiting, nasogastric suctioning, villous adenoma, diarrhea, Zollinger-Ellison syndrome, chronic pyelonephritis, renal tubular acidosis, metabolic alkalosis (primary aldosteronism, Cushing's syndrome).

Potassium, Urine

(see Urine, Spot, page 292)

Progesterone

Used to confirm ovulation and corpus luteum function.

Phase	Normal values (female)
Follicular	<1 ng/mL
Leuteal	5–20 ng/mL
Pregnancy 1st trimester	10–30 ng/mL
2nd trimester	50–100 ng/mL
3rd trimester	100–400 ng/mL
Postmenopause	<1 ng/mL

Prolactin

(Male 1–20 ng/mL [SI: 1–20 µg/L]; female 1–25 ng/mL [SI: 1–25 µg/L]).

Increased: Pregnancy, breast-feeding, prolactinoma, hypothalamic tumors, sarcoidosis or granulomatous disease of the hypothalmus, hypothyroidism, renal failure, Addison's disease, phenothiazines, haloperidol.

Prostate-Specific Antigen (PSA)

(<4 ng/dL by monoclonal, [eg, Hybritech assay]).

Most useful as a measure of response to therapy of prostate cancer; approved to be used in screening for prostate cancer. Although any elevation increases suspicion of prostate cancer, levels >10.0 ng/dL are associated with carcinoma at the 90% confidence level. Age corrected levels gaining popularity (40–50 years 2.5 ng/dL; 50–60 years 3.5 ng/dL; 60–70 years 4.5 ng/dL; >70 years 6.5 ng/dL.)

Increased: Prostate cancer, acute prostatitis, some cases of benign prostatic hypertrophy (BPH), prostatic infarction, prostate surgery (biopsy, resection), vigorous prostatic massage (routine rectal exam does not elevate levels).

Decreased: Total (radical) prostatectomy (should be <0.2), response to therapy of prostatic carcinoma (radiation or hormonal therapy).

Protein, Serum

(6.0–8.0 g/dL)

Increased: Multiple myeloma, Waldenström's macroglobulinemia, benign monoclonal gammopathy, lymphoma, chronic inflammatory disease, sarcoidosis.

Decreased: Malnutrition, inflammatory bowel disease, Hodgkin's disease, leukemias, any cause of decreased albumin.

Protein, Urine (24-hour urine)

(<150 mg/24 hr [SI: <0.15 g/d]).

Increased: See Differential Diagnosis under Urinalysis, page 289. Nephrotic syndrome usually associated with >4 g/24 hr.

Prothrombin Time (PT)

(11.5–13.5 seconds)

Some labs report the International Normalized Ratio [INR] instead of the patient/control ratio to guide Coumadin therapy.

	PT Patient/control ratio	INR
Normal	0.9–1.1	0.75–1.30
Therapeutic	1.5–2.5	2.0–4.5

PT evaluates the extrinsic clotting mechanism that includes factors I, II, V, VII, and X.

Increased: Drugs (eg, sodium warfarin [Coumadin]), vitamin K deficiency, fat malabsorption, liver disease, prolonged use of a tourniquet before drawing a blood sample, disseminated intravascular coagulation (DIC).

RBC Morphology

The below list is some erythrocyte abnormalities and the associated conditions. General terms include poikilocytosis (irregular RBC shape, eg, sickle and Burr) and anisocytosis (irregular RBC size, eg, microcytes and macrocytes).

Basophilic Stippling: Lead or heavy metal poisoning, thalassemia, severe anemia.

Howell-Jolly Bodies: After splenectomy, some severe hemolytic anemias, eg, pernicious anemia, leukemia, thalassemia, may present more frequently.

Sickling: Sickle cell disease and trait.

Nucleated RBCs: Severe bone marrow stress (hemorrhage, hemolysis, etc), marrow replacement by tumor, extramedullary hematopoiesis.

Target Cells (Leptocytes): Thalassemia, hemoglobinopathies, obstructive jaundice, any hypochromic anemia, after splenectomy.

Spherocytes: Hereditary spherocytosis, immune or microangiopathic hemolysis, severe burns, ABO transfusion reactions.

Helmet Cells (Schistocytes): Microangiopathic hemolysis, hemolytic transfusion reaction, transplant rejection, other severe anemias, TTP.

Burr Cells (Acanthocytes): Severe liver disease; high levels of bile, fatty acids, or toxins.

Polychromasia (Basophilia): The appearance of a bluish-gray red cell on routine Wright's stain suggests reticulocytes.

Reticulocyte Count

(Normal corrected reticulocyte count is <1.5%).

The result is reported as a percentage; the clinician should calculate the corrected reticulocyte count for interpretation of the results (corrected reticulocyte count = reported count × patient's Hct % normal Hct). This corrected count is an excellent indicator of erythropoietic activity. The normal bone marrow responds to a decrease in erythrocytes (shown by a decreased hematocrit) with an increase in the production of reticulocytes. Lack of increase in a reticulocyte count in an anemic patient suggests a chronic disease, a deficiency disease, marrow replacement, or marrow failure.

Retinol-Binding Protein (RBP)

(Adults 3–6 mg/dL; children 1.5–3.0 mg/dL).

Decreased: Malnutrition, vitamin A deficiency, intestinal malabsorption of fats, chronic liver disease.

Rheumatoid Factor (RA Latex Test)

(<15 IU by Microscan kit or <1 : 40).

Increased: Rheumatoid arthritis, systemic lupus erythematosis (SLE), syphilis, chronic inflammation, subacute bacterial endocorditis (SBE), some lung diseases.

Sedimentation Rate (Erythrocyte Sedimentation Rate [ESR])

Wintrobe Scale: Male 0–9 mm/hr; female 0–20 mm/hr.

ZETA Scale: 40–54% normal; 55–59% mildly elevated; 60–64% moderately elevated; >65% markedly elevated.

Westergren Scale: Male <50 years 15 mm/hr, >50 years 20 mm/hr; female <50 years 20 mm/hr, >50 years 30 mm/hr.

ESR is a nonspecific test. ZETA rate is not affected by anemia.

Increased: Any type of infection, inflammation, rheumatic fever, endocarditis, neoplasm, acute myocardial infarction.

Serum Gamma-Glutamyl Transpeptidase (SGGT, GGT)

(Male 9–50 U/L; female 8–40 U/L).

Generally parallels changes in serum alkaline phosphatase and 5′ nucleotidase in liver disease.

Increased: Liver disease (hepatitis, cirrhosis, obstructive jaundice), pancreatitis.

Serum Glutamic-Oxaloacetic Transaminase (SGOT)

(See Aspartate Aminotransaminase [AST], page 248)

Serum Glutamic-Pyruvic Transaminase (SGPT)

(See Alanine Aminotransaminase [ALT], page 247)

Sodium, Serum

(136–145 mmol/L)

Increased: Associated with low total body sodium (glycosuria, mannitol, urea, excess sweating), normal total body sodium (diabetes insipidus—central and nephrogenic, respiratory losses, and sweating), and total body sodium (administration of hypertonic sodium bicarbonate, Cushing's syndrome, hyperaldosteronism).

Decreased: Associated with excess total body sodium and water (nephrotic syndrome, congestive heart failure [CHF], cirrhosis, renal failure), excess body water (syndrome of inappropriate antidiuretic hormone [SIADH], hypothyroidism, adrenal insufficiency). Also associated with decreased total body water and sodium (diuretic use, renal tubular acidosis, use of mannitol or urea, mineralocorticoid deficiency, vomiting, diarrhea, pancreatitis) and pseudohyponatremia (hyperlipidemia, hyperglycemia, and multiple myeloma).

Note: For every 100 mmol/L blood glucose above normal, serum sodium decreases 1.6 in factitious hyponatremia resulting from hyperglycemia. For example, a patient presents with a blood glucose of 800 and a sodium of 129. This would factitiously lower sodium by about (7×1.6) or 11.6. Corrected serum sodium would therefore be $129 + 11 = 140$.

Sodium, Urine

(See Urine, Spot, page 292).

Stool for Occult Blood (Hemoccult Test)

(Negative).

Positive: Swallowed blood, ingestion of rare red meat, any gastrointestinal tract ulcerated lesion (ulcer, carcinoma, polyp), large doses of vitamin C (>500 mg/d).

Stool for White Blood Count (WBC)

(Occasional WBC is normal).

Increased: Usually polymorphonuclear leukocytes, *Shigella, Salmonella,* enteropathogenic *Escherichia coli,* ulcerative colitis, pseudomembranous colitis.

Sweat Chloride

(5–40 mEq/L [SI: 5–40 mmol/L]).

Increased: Cystic fibrosis (not valid on children younger than 3 weeks).

T_3 RIA (Triiodothyronine)

(120–195 ng/dL [SI: 1.85–3.00 nmol/L]).

Increased: Hyperthyroidism, T_3 thyrotoxicosis, oral estrogen, pregnancy, exogenous T_4.

Decreased: Hypothyroidism and euthyroid sick state, any cause of decreased thyroid-binding globulin.

T_3 RU (Resin Uptake)

(24–34%)

Increased: Hyperthyroidism, medications (eg, phenytoin [Dilantin], steroids, heparin, aspirin), nephrotic syndrome.

Decreased: Hypothyroidism, pregnancy, medications (eg, estrogens, iodine, propylthiouracil).

T_4 Total (Thyroxine)

(5–12 μg/dL [SI: 65–155 nmol/L]; males >60 years 5–10 μg/dL [SI: 65–129 nmol]; females: 5.5–10.5 μg/dL [SI: 71–135 nmol/L]).

Good screening test for hyperthyroidism.

Increased: Hyperthyroidism, exogenous thyroid hormone, estrogens, pregnancy, severe illness, euthyroid sick syndrome.

Decreased: Euthyroid sick syndrome.

Testosterone

(Male free 9–30 ng/dL, total 300–1200 ng/dL; female see below).

Phase	Normal values (female)
Follicular	20–80 ng/dL
Midcycle Peak	20–80 ng/dL
Luteal	20–80 ng/dL
Postmenopause	10–40 ng/dL

Increased: Adrenogenital syndrome, ovarian stromal hyperthecosis, polycystic ovaries, menopause, ovarian tumors.

Decreased: Some cases of impotence, hypogonadism, hypopituitarism, Klinefelter's syndrome.

Thrombin Time

(10–14 seconds)

Increased: Systemic heparin, disseminated intravascular coagulation (DIC), fibrinogen deficiency, congenitally abnormal fibrinogen molecules.

Thyroxine Binding Globulin (TBG)

(21–52 μg/dL [SI: 270–669 nmol/L]).

Increased: Hypothyroidism, pregnancy, oral contraceptives, estrogens, hepatic disease, acute porphyria.

Decreased: Hyperthyroidism, androgens, anabolic steroids, prednisone, nephrotic syndrome, severe illness, surgical stress, phenytoin, hepatic disease.

Thyroglobulin

(1–20 ng/mL)

Increased: Differentiated thyroid carcinomas (papillary, follicular), Graves' disease, nontoxic goiter.

Decreased: Hypothyroidism, testosterone, steroids, phenytoin.

Thyroid-Stimulating Hormone (TSH)

(0.7–5.3 mU/mL).

Newer sensitive assay is an excellent screening test for hyperthyroidism as well as hypothyroidism. Allows the clinician to distinguish between a low normal and a decreased TSH.

Increased: Hypothyroidism.

Decreased: Hyperthyroidism. Less than 1% of hypothyroidism is from pituitary or hypothalamic disease resulting in a decreased TSH.

Transferrin

(220–400 mg/dL [SI: 2.20–4.0 g/L)

Increased: Acute and chronic blood loss, iron deficiency.

Decreased: Anemia of chronic disease, cirrhosis, nephrosis, hemochromatosis.

Triglycerides

(Male 40–160 mg/dL [SI: 0.45–1.81 mmol/L]; female 35–135 mg/dL [SI: 0.40–1.53 mmol/L]. Can vary with age).

Increased: Hyperlipoproteinemias (types I, IIb, III, IV, V), hypothyroidism, liver diseases, alcoholism, pancreatitis, acute myocardial infarction, nephrotic syndrome, familial increase.

Decreased: Malnutrition, congenital abetalipoproteinemia.

Uric Acid

(Male 3.4–7 mg/dL [SI: 202–416 μmol/L]; female 2.4–6 mg/dL [SI: 143–357 μmol/L]. To convert mg/dL to mmol/L, multiply by 59.48).

Increased: Gout, renal failure, destruction of massive amounts of nucleoproteins (leukemia, anemia, chemotherapy, toxemia of pregnancy), drugs (especially diuretics), lactic acidosis, hypothyroidism, polycystic kidney disease, parathyroid diseases.

Decreased: Uricosuric drugs (salicylates, probenecid, allopurinol), Wilson's disease, Fanconi's syndrome.

Urinalysis

Normal Values

Appearance: "yellow, clear" or "straw-colored, clear."

Specific Gravity: Neonate 1.012; infant 1.002–1.006; child and adult 1.001–1.035 (with normal fluid intake 1.016–1.022).

pH: Newborn/neonate 5–7; child and adult 4.6–8.0.

Negative for: Bilirubin, blood, acetone, glucose, protein, nitrite, leukocyte esterase, reducing substances.

Trace: Urobilinogen.

Sediment:

Red Blood Count (RBC): Male 0–3/high power field (HPF); female 0–5/HPF.

White Blood Count (WBC): 0–4/HPF.

Epithelial cells: Occasional.

Hyaline casts: Occasional.

Bacteria: None.

Crystals: Warm, fresh urine none.

Note: Refrigeration or urine left standing at room temperature may precipitate various crystals.

Differential Diagnosis for Routine Urinalysis

A. Appearance
1. **Colorless.** Diabetes insipidus, diuretics, excess fluid intake.
2. **Dark.** Acute intermittant porphyria, malignant melanoma.
3. **Cloudy.** Urinary tract infection (pyuria), amorphous phosphate salts (normal in alkaline urine), blood, mucus, bilirubin.
4. **Pink/red.** Blood, hemoglobin, myoglobin, food coloring, beets, ibuprofen.
5. **Orange/yellow.** Phenazopyridine (Pyridium), bile pigments.
6. **Brown/black.** Myoglobin, bile pigments, melanin, cascara, iron, macrodantin, alkaptonuria.
7. **Green.** Urinary bile pigments, indigo carmine, methylene blue, Urised.
8. **Foamy.** Proteinuria, bile salts.
9. **Acid.** High protein (meat) diet, ammonium chloride, mandelic acid and other medications, acidosis, ketoacidosis (starvation, diabetic), chronic obstructive pulmonary disease (COPD).
10. **Basic.** Urinary tract infections (UTI), renal tubular acidosis, diet (high vegetable, milk, immediately after meals), sodium bicarbonate therapy, vomiting, metabolic alkalosis.

B. Specific Gravity
Usually corresponds with osmolarity except with osmotic diuresis. Value >1.023 indicates normal renal concentrating ability.

Increased: Volume depletion; congestive heart failure (CHF); adrenal insufficiency; diabetes mellitus; inappropriate antidiuretic hormone (ADH); increased proteins (nephrosis); if markedly increased (1.040–1.050), suspect artifact or excretion of radiographic contrast media.

Decreased: Diabetes insipidus, pyelonephritis, glomerulonephritis, waterload with normal renal function.

C. Bilirubin

Positive: Obstructive jaundice (intra- and extrahepatic), hepatitis.

D. Blood

Positive: Stones, trauma, tumors (benign and malignant, anywhere in the urinary tract), urethral strictures, coagulopathy, infection, menses (contamination), polycystic kidneys, interstitial nephritis, hemolytic anemia, transfusion reaction, instrumentation (Foley catheter, etc).

Note: If the dipstick is positive for blood, but no red cells are seen, there may be free hemoglobin from trauma or a transfusion reaction or from lysis of RBCs. RBCs will lyse if the pH is < 5 or >8, or if there is myoglobin present because of a crush injury, burn, or tissue ischemia.

E. Glucose

Positive: Diabetes mellitus, pancreatitis, pancreatic carcinoma, pheochromocytoma, Cushing's disease, shock, burns, pain, steroids, hyperthyroidism, renal tubular disease, iatrogenic causes. **Note:** Glucose oxidase technique in many kits is specific for glucose and will not react with lactose, fructose, or galactose.

F. Ketones. Detects primarily acetone and acetoacetic acid and not beta-hydroxybutyric acid.

Positive: Starvation, high-fat diet, diabetic ketoacidosis, vomiting, diarrhea, hyperthyroidism, pregnancy, febrile states (especially in children).

G. Nitrite. Many bacteria will convert nitrates to nitrite (see also Leukocyte Esterase, following).

Positive: Infection. A negative test does not rule out infection because some organisms such as *Streptococcus faecalis* and other gram-positive cocci will not produce nitrite, and the urine must also be retained in the bladder for several hours to allow the reaction to take place.

H. Protein. Persistent proteinuria by dipstick should be quantified by 24-hour urine studies.

Positive: Pyelonephritis, glomerulonephritis, Kimmelstiel-Wilson syndrome (diabetes), nephrotic syndrome, myeloma, postural causes, preeclampsia, inflammation and malignancies of the lower tract, functional causes (fever, stress, heavy exercise), malignant hypertension, congestive heart failure (CHF).

I. Leukocyte Esterase

Positive: Infection (false-positive with vaginal contamination).

J. Reducing Substance

Positive: Glucose, fructose, galactose, false-positives (vitamin C, salicylates, antibiotics, etc).

K. Urobilinogen

Positive: Cirrhosis, CHF with hepatic congestion, hepatitis, hyperthyroidism, suppression of gut flora with antibiotics.

Urine Sediment

Red Blood Cells (RBCs): Trauma, pyelonephritis, genitourinary TB, cystitis, prostatitis, stones, tumors (malignant and benign), coagulopathy, and any cause of blood on dipstick (see above).

White Blood Cells (WBCs): Infection anywhere in the urinary tract, TB, renal tumors, acute glomerulonephritis, radiation, interstitial nephritis (analgesic abuse).

Epithelial Cells: Acute tubular necrosis, necrotizing papillitis (most epithelial cells are from an otherwise unremarkable urethra).

Parasites: *Trichomonas vaginalis, Schistosoma haematobium.*

Yeast: *Candida albicans* (especially in diabetics, immunosuppressed patients or if a vaginal yeast infection is present).

Spermatozoa: Normal in males immediately after intercourse or nocturnal emission.

Crystals:

Abnormal: Any of the following types: cystine, sulfonamide, leucine, tyrosine, cholesterol.

Normal (if present in small numbers):

Acid urine: Oxalate (small square crystals with a central cross), uric acid.

Alkaline urine: Calcium carbonate, triple phosphate (resemble coffin lids).

Contaminants: Cotton threads, hair, wood fibers, amorphous substances (all usually unimportant).

Mucus: Large amounts suggest urethral disease (normal from ileal conduit or other forms of urinary diversion).

Glitter cells: White blood cells (WBCs) lysed in hypotonic solution.

Casts: The presence of casts in urine localizes some or all of the disease process to the kidney.

Hyaline cast: Acceptable unless they are numerous, benign hypertension, nephrotic syndrome, after exercise.

Red Blood Cell (RBC) cast: Acute glomerulonephritis, lupus nephritis, subacute bacterial endocarditis (SBE), Goodpasture's disease, after a streptococcal infection, vasculitis, malignant hypertension.

White Blood Cell (WBC) cast: Pyelonephritis.

Epithelial (tubular) cast: Tubular damage, nephrotoxin, virus.

Granular cast: Breakdown of cellular casts, lead to waxy casts. "Dirty brown granular casts" typical for acute tubular necrosis.

Waxy cast: End-stage of granular cast. Severe chronic renal disease, amyloidosis.

Fatty cast: Nephrotic syndrome, diabetes mellitus, damaged renal tubular epithelial cells.

Broad cast: Chronic renal disease.

Urine, Human Chorionic Gonadotropin (HCG)

(See also serum HCG, page 274)

(Negative).

Positive: Pregnancy (may be positive by day 4, most positive by 14 days postexpected menstrual date), testicular carcinoma (choriocarcinoma) hydatidiform mole.

Urine, Indices

Urinary indices useful in the differential diagnosis of oliguria. They help differentiate between prerenal and intrinsic renal causes.

Index	Prerenal	Renal (ATN)[1]
Urine osmolality (mosm/kg)	>500	<350
Urinary sodium (mEq/L)	<20	>40
Urine/serum creatinine	>40	<20
Urine/serum osmolarity	>1.2	<1.2
Fractional excreted sodium[2]	<1	>1
Renal Failure Index (RFI)[3]	<1	>1

[1] Acute tubular necrosis (intrinsic renal failure).
[2] Fractional excreted sodium = Urine/serum sodium × 100 % Urine/serum creatinine.
[3] Renal Failure Index = Urine sodium × serum creatinine % Urine creatinine.

Urine, Spot (Random) Studies

The so-called "spot urine" is often ordered to aid in diagnosing various conditions. The test relies on only a small sample (10–20 mL) of urine.

Spot Urine for Electrolytes

The usefulness of this assay is limited because of large variations in daily fluid and salt intake, and the results are usually indeterminate if a diuretic has been given.

1. **Sodium <10 mEq/L [mmol/L]:** Volume depletion, hyponatremic states, prerenal azotemia (CHF, shock, etc), hepatorenal syndrome.
2. **Sodium >20 mEq/L [mmol/L]:** SIADH, acute tubular necrosis (usually >40 mEq/L).

3. **Chloride <10 mEq/L [mmol/L]:** Chloride-sensitive metabolic alkalosis (vomiting, excessive diuretic use), volume depletion.
4. **Potassium <10 mEq/L [mmol/L]:** Hypokalemia, potassium depletion, extrarenal loss.

Spot Urine for Protein

(Normal <10 mg/dL [0.1 g/L] or <20 mg/dL [0.2 g/L] for a sample taken in the early AM [see page 290 for the differential diagnosis of protein in the urine]).

Spot Urine for Osmolality

(250–900 mosm/kg [mmol/kg] (varies with water intake). Patients with normal renal function should concentrate >800 mosm/kg [mmol/kg] after a 14-hour fluid restriction; <400 mosm/kg [mmol/kg] is a sign of renal impairment.)

Increased: Dehydration, syndrome of inappropriate antidiuretic hormone (SIADH), adrenal insufficiency, glycosuria, high-protein diet.

Decreased: Excessive fluid intake, diabetes insipidus, acute renal failure.

Spot Urine for Myoglobin

(Qualitative negative)

Positive: Skeletal muscle conditions (crush injury, electrical burns, carbon monoxide poisioning, delirium tremens, surgical procedures, malignant hyperthermia), polymyositis.

Vanillylmandelic Acid (VMA) (24-hour urine)

(<7–9 mg/24 hr [SI: 35–45 μmol/L]).

VMA is the urinary product of both epinephrine and norepinephrine; good screening test for pheochromocytoma also used to diagnose and follow-up neuroblastoma and ganglioneuroma.

Increased: Pheochromocytoma, other neural crest tumors (ganglioneuroma), factitious (chocolate, coffee, tea, monoamine oxidase [MAO] inhibitors, methyldopa).

VDRL (Venereal Disease Research Laboratory) Test or Rapid Plasma Reagin (RPR)

(Normal = nonreactive).

Good for screening syphilis. Almost always positive in secondary syphilis, but frequently becomes negative in late syphilis. Also, in some patients with HIV infection, the VDRL can be negative in primary and secondary syphilis.

Positive (reactive): Syphilis, systemic lupus erythematosus, pregnancy and drug addicts. If reactive, confirm with FTA-ABS (false-positives with bacterial or viral illnesses).

Vitamin B$_{12}$ (Extrinsic Factor, Cyanocobalamin)

(>100–700 pg/mL [SI: 74–516 pmol/L]).

Increased: Excessive intake, myeloproliferative disorders.

Decreased: Inadequate intake (especially strict vegetarians), malabsorption, hyperthyroidism, pregnancy.

White Blood Count (WBC)

(See CBC, page 253).

WBC Morphology

Conditions associated with certain changes in the normal morphology of WBCs:

- **Auer's bodies:** Acute myelogenous leukemias.
- **Döhle's inclusion bodies:** Severe infection, burns, malignancy, pregnancy.
- **Hypersegmentation:** Megaloblastic anemias.
- **Toxic granulation:** Severe illness (sepsis, burn, high temperature).

Zinc

(60–130 µg/dL [SI: 9–20 µmol/L]).

Increased: Atherosclerosis, coronary artery disease.

Decreased: Inadequate dietary intake (parenteral nutrition, alcoholism), malabsorption, increased needs such as pregnancy or wound healing, acrodermatitis enteropathica.

III. Bedside Procedures

Universal precautions should be used for any invasive procedure during which the operator can be exposed to potentially infectious body fluids. Not all patients infected with transmissible pathogens can be identified at the time of hospital admission or even later in their course. Because blood and body fluid-transmissible pathogens pose a hazard to personnel caring for these patients, primarily at the time of invasive procedures, certain precautions are now **required** for **routine** care of all patients whether or not they have been placed on isolation precautions of any type. The CDC defines universal precautions as follows:

1. Hands must be washed before and after all patient contact.
2. Hands must be washed before and after all invasive procedures.
3. Gloves must be worn in every instance in which contact with blood is certain or likely. For example, gloves must be worn for all venipunctures, IV starts, IV manipulation, wound care, etc.
4. Gloves must be worn once and discarded. They may not be worn to perform tasks on two different patients or two different tasks at different sites on the same patient.
5. Gloves must be worn in every instance in which contact with any body fluid is likely, including urine, feces, wound secretions, respiratory tract care, thoracenteses, paracenteses, etc.
6. Gown must be worn when splatter of blood or of body fluids on clothing seems likely.
7. Additional barrier precautions may be necessary for certain invasive procedures in which significant splatter or aerosol generation seems likely. This will not occur during most routine patient care activities. It may occur in certain instances in the operating room, emergency room, the ICUs, and during invasive procedures or cardiopulmonary resuscitation. Masks are always worn when goggles are worn and vice versa.

Patients should be counseled before any procedure concerning its necessity as well as the potential risks and benefits. Explaining the various steps can often make the patient more cooperative and the procedure easier on both parties. In general, procedures (eg, bladder catheterization, nasogastric intubation, or venipuncture) do not require a written informed consent beyond normal hospital sign-in protocols. More invasive procedures (eg, thoracentesis or lumbar puncture) require the patient's written consent.

1. Arterial Line Placement

(See also Section I, Problem 7, page 26)

Indications:

1. Frequent sampling of arterial blood.
2. Hemodynamic monitoring when continuous blood pressure readings are needed (eg, patient on pressors).

Materials: Prepackaged arterial line set (eg, Arrow) or 20 gauge (or smaller) 1¼–2 inch IV catheter over needle assembly (Angiocath TM), arterial line setup per ICU routine (transducer, tubing and pressure bag with heparinized saline), armboard, sterile dressing, lidocaine).

Procedure:

1. The radial artery is most frequently used. Other sites, in decreasing order of preference, are the dorsalis pedis, femoral, axillary, and brachial arteries; these are used infrequently. Never puncture the radial and ulnar arteries in the same hand because this may compromise blood supply to the hand and fingers.
2. Verify the patency of the radial artery using the Allen test (see page 297).
3. Place the extremity on an armboard with a gauze roll behind the wrist to hyperextend the joint. Prepare with povidone-iodine and drape with towels. The operator should wear gloves and mask, if possible.
4. Raise a very small skin wheal at the puncture site with 1% lidocaine using a 25 gauge needle. Carefully palpate the artery and choose the puncture site where it appears most superficial.

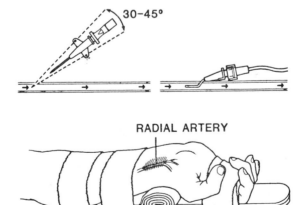

RADIAL ARTERY

Figure III–1. Technique of radial artery catheterization. *(Reproduced, with permission, from Gomella TL (editor): Arterial Access. In: Neonatology, 3/e. Appleton & Lange, 1994.)*

5. Standard technique: See Figure III–1. While palpating the path of the artery with the left hand, advance the 20 gauge catheter over needle assembly into the artery at a 30 degree angle to the skin. Once a "flash" of blood is seen in the hub, hold the needle steady and advance the catheter into the artery. Briefly occlude the artery with manual pressure while the pressure tubing is being connected.

   Prepackaged technique: Kits are available with a needle and guidewire that allow the Seldinger technique to be used. The entry needle is placed at a 30 degree angle to the skin site and is inserted until there is a flash of blood that rises in the catheter. The guidewire (orange handle in some kits) is inserted in the vessel and the catheter is advanced. The wire is removed and connected to the pressure tubing.

6. Suture in place with 3-0 silk and apply a sterile dressing. Flush systems are necessary to assure patency and transducers allow continuous blood pressure monitoring.

Complications: Infection, hemorrhage, thrombosis of the artery, emboli, pseudoaneurysm formation.

2. Arterial Puncture

Indications:

1. Blood gas determinations.
2. When arterial blood is needed for chemistry determinations (eg, ammonia levels).

Materials: Blood gas sampling kit **or** 3–5 mL syringe, 23–25 gauge needle (20–22 if femoral artery), 1 mL heparin (1000 u/mL), alcohol **or** povidone-iodine swabs, and cup of ice.

Procedure

1. Use a "heparinized" syringe for blood gas and a nonheparinized syringe for chemistry determinations. "Heparinize" the syringe by drawing up about 0.5–1 mL of heparin, pulling the plunger all the way back, and discarding the heparin. Obtain a blood gas kit (contains a preheparinized syringe) or a small syringe (3–5 mL) with a small gauge needle (23–25 gauge for radial, 20–22 acceptable for femoral artery).

2. Arteries in the order of preference are radial, femoral, and brachial. If using the radial artery, perform the modified Allen test to verify collateral flow in the ulnar artery. Have the patient make a tight fist with the hand slightly flexed. Occlude both the radial and ulnar arteries at the wrist and have the patient open his hand. While maintaining pressure on the radial artery, release the ulnar artery. If the ulnar artery is patent, the hand should flush red within 6 seconds. If the Allen test is positive (no radial flow) the artery should probably not be used.

3. If using the femoral artery, the mnemonic NAVEL aids in locating the important structures in the groin. Palpate the femoral artery just be-

low the inguinal ligament. From lateral to medial the structures are **N**erve, **A**rtery, **V**ein, **E**mpty space, **L**ymphatic. The clinician may inject 1% lidocaine subcutaneously for anesthesia. Palpate the artery proximally and distally with two fingers or trap the artery between two fingers placed on either side of the vessel. If using the upper extremity, hyperextension of the joint will often bring the radial and brachial arteries closer to the surface.

4. Prepare the area with either a povidone-iodine solution or alcohol swab. Hold the syringe like a pencil with the needle bevel up and enter the skin at a 60–90 degree angle. Maintain a slight negative pressure on the syringe.

5. Obtain blood on the downstroke or upon slow withdrawal. Aspirate very slowly. A good arterial sample should require only minimal back pressure. If a glass or special blood-gas syringe is used, the barrel may rise spontaneously.

6. If the vessel cannot be located, redirect the needle without coming out of the skin. A portable Doppler probe can also be used to help locate the vessel.

7. Withdraw the needle quickly and apply firm pressure at the site for at least 5 minutes, even if the sample was not obtained to avoid a hematoma. Longer time may be needed in patients with elevated coagulation parameters.

8. If the sample is for a blood gas, expel any air from the syringe, mix the contents thoroughly by twirling the syringe between your fingers and make the syringe airtight with a cap. Place the syringe in an ice bath if more than a few minutes will pass before the sample is processed.

3. Bladder Catheterization

(See also Section I, Problem 32, page 113)

Indications:

1. Relieve urinary retention.
2. Collect an uncontaminated urine sample.
3. Monitor urinary output accurately.
4. Perform bladder tests (cystogram, cystometrogram).

Contraindications: Urethral disruption associated with pelvic fracture, acute prostatitis (relative).

Materials: Prepackaged Foley catheter tray (may need to add a catheter), drainage bag (often not part of the kit), catheter of choice (16–20 Fr Foley in adults, 8–15 Fr in children; elbowed (coudé) catheters have a bend to allow easier passage in males; three-way catheters are usually larger 22–30 Fr to allow irrigation of fluid and clots.) See Figure III–2 for catheter description.

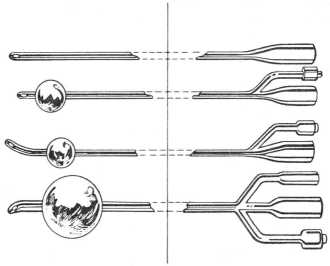

Figure III–2. Types of bladder catheters (from the top): straight Robinson catheter ("red rubber"), Foley catheter with standard 5 mL balloon, coudé ("elbow") catheter, and irrigating ("three-way") Foley catheter with 30 mL balloon. *(Reproduced, with permission, from Gomella LG (editor):* Clinician's Pocket Reference, *7/e. Appleton & Lange, 1993.)*

Procedure:

1. Have the patient in a well-lighted area in a supine position. With females, knees are flexed wide and heels placed together to get adequate exposure of the meatus.
2. Open the kit and put on the gloves. Get all the materials ready before attempting to insert the catheter. Open the prep solution and soak the cotton balls. Apply the sterile drapes.
3. Inflate and deflate the balloon of the Foley catheter with 5–10 mL of sterile water to assure its proper function. Coat the end of the catheter with lubricant jelly.
4. In females, use one gloved hand to prep the urethral meatus in a pubis toward anus direction; hold the labia apart with the other, gloved hand. With uncircumcised males, retract the foreskin to prep the glands; use a gloved hand to hold the penis still.
5. The hand used to hold the penis or labia should not touch the catheter to insert it. Disposable forceps in the kit can be used to insert the catheter, or the forceps can be used to prep, then the gloved hand can insert the catheter.

6. In the male, stretch the penis upwards perpendicular to the body to eliminate any folds in the urethra that might lead to a false passage. **Gentle** pressure should be used to advance the catheter. Any significant resistance that is encountered may represent a stricture and requires urologic consultation. In males with benign prostatic hypertrophy (BPH), a coudé tip catheter may facilitate passage. Other helpful tricks to get a catheter to pass in a male are to make sure that the penis is well stretched and to instill 30–50 mL of sterile surgical lubricant into the urethra with a catheter-tipped syringe or 2% lidocaine jelly with a urethral instillation nozzle.

7. In both males and females, insert the catheter to the hilt of the drainage end. Compress the penis towards the pubis. These maneuvers help ensure that the balloon will be inflated in the bladder and not in the urethra. The balloon is inflated with 5–10 mL of sterile water or, occasionally, air. After inflation, pull the catheter back until the balloon rests on the bladder neck. There should be good urine return when the catheter is in place. **Note:** In an uncircumcised male, after the catheter is inserted, the clinician should reposition the foreskin to prevent massive edema of the glans penis.

8. If no urine returns, attempt to irrigate with sterile saline and a catheter tipped syringe. **A catheter that will not irrigate is in the urethra, not the bladder.**

9. Catheters in females can be taped to the leg. In males, the catheter should be taped to the abdominal wall to decrease urethral stricture formation.

10. If blood or clots are present, the bladder should be gently irrigated with a catheter tipped syringe and normal saline. Urology should be consulted because there may have been insertion trauma (false passage) or the patient may need a three-way catheter placed to allow continuous bladder irrigation.

11. For sample collection or determination of residual urine, a straight red rubber catheter without a balloon (Robinson catheter) can be used according to the previously noted technique.

Complications: Infection, bleeding, false passage.

4. Central Venous Catheterization

(See also Section I, Problem 20, page 78)

Indications:

1. Administration of fluids and medications, especially when there is no peripheral access.
2. Administration of hyperalimentation solutions.
3. Measurement of central venous pressure (CVP).
4. Adjunct to placement of a pulmonary artery catheter or transvenous pacemaker.
5. Acute dialysis or plasmapheresis (Shiley catheter).

Materials: Minor procedure tray and instrument tray (see Table III–8, page 334), gloves, hat, mask, gown (especially for hyperalimentation lines), central venous catheter of choice (Intracath, subclavian line, triple lumen catheters, Shiley for dialysis), IV fluid, and tubing.

Procedures: There are several different sites for inserting a "deep line," including the subclavian, internal jugular, supraclavicular, external jugular, antecubital, and femoral. The first two are most commonly used. Shiley catheters for dialysis are typically placed in the subclavian or femoral veins. Additional hints for catheter insertion can be found on page 115. Informed consent is usually needed for elective line placement. Coagulation studies should be available for review.

A. Subclavian Technique (Figure III–3):

1. Use sterile technique (povidone-iodine prep, gloves, mask, and a sterile field) whenever possible.
2. Place the patient head down in the Trendelenburg position with his head straight up or turned to the opposite side. The right side is preferred for deep line placement because the dome of the pleura is lower, the thoracic duct is on the left, and there is more of a direct path to the right atrium. It may be helpful to place a towel roll along the patient's spine.
3. Use a 25 gauge needle to make a small skin wheal with 1% lidocaine 1 cm below the midclavicle. At this point, a larger needle (eg, 22 gauge) can be used to anesthetize the deeper tissues as well as locate the vein.
4. Attach a large-bore, deep-line needle (a 14 gauge needle with a 16 gauge catheter at least 8–12 inches long) to a 10–20 mL syringe and introduce it into the site of the skin wheal.
5. Place a finger in the suprasternal notch and direct the needle toward this finger. Keep the needle parallel to the lateral border of the clavicle and parallel to the skin.
6. Apply constant back pressure as the needle is advanced deep to the clavicle, but above the first rib.
7. Free return of blood indicates entry into the subclavian vein. Bright red blood that forcibly enters the syringe indicates that the subclavian artery has been entered. If the arterial entry occurs, remove the needle and apply firm pressure for 10 minutes.
8a. If an **Intracath** is being used, remove the syringe, place a finger over the needle hub, and advance the catheter an appropriate distance through the needle. Then withdraw the needle to just outside the skin and snap the protective cap over the tip of the needle.
8b. If the **Seldinger** wire technique is to be used, advance the wire through the needle and then withdraw the needle. Nick the skin with an 11 blade and advance the dilator approximately 5 cm; remove the dilator and advance catheter in over the guidewire (use the brown port on the triple lumen catheter). Maintain a firm grip on

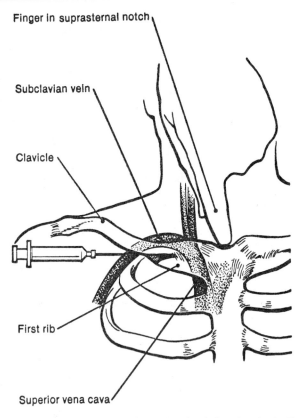

Finger in suprasternal notch

Subclavian vein

Clavicle

First rib

Superior vena cava

Figure III-3. The technique for subclavian vein catheterization. *(Reproduced, with permission, from Gomella LG (editor):* Clinician's Pocket Reference, *7/e. Appleton & Lange, 1993.)*

the end of the guidewire. Remove the wire and attach the IV tubing. Note that the wire used to insert a single lumen catheter is shorter than the wire supplied with the triple lumen catheter. This is most critical when exchanging a triple lumen for a single lumen catheter; the clinician must use the longer triple lumen wire and insert the wire into the brown port. Shiley catheters are placed using the Seldinger wire technique.

9. Attach the catheter to the appropriate IV solution and place the IV bottle below the level of the deep-line site to ensure a good back-

flow of blood into the tubing. If there is no backflow, the catheter may be kinked or not in the proper position.

10. Securely suture the assembly in place with 2-0 or 3-0 silk. Apply an occlusive dressing with povidone-iodine ointment.

11. Obtain a chest x-ray film to verify placement of the catheter tip and to rule out pneumothorax. The catheter tip should lie in the superior vena cava in the vicinity of the right atrium, at about the fifth thoracic vertebra. Catheters that go into the neck may be only used for saline infusion and not for monitoring or TPN infusion. Catheters that cannot be manipulated at the bedside into the chest usually can be placed properly in the interventional radiology department with the aid of fluoroscopy.

B. Internal Jugular Technique (Central Approach) (Figure III–4):

1. & 2. Follow steps 1 and 2 for the subclavian technique.

3. Locate the triangle formed by the clavicle and the two heads of the sternocleidomastoid muscle. Use a 25 gauge needle and 1% lidocaine to raise a small skin wheal at the apex of this triangle. Change to a 22 gauge needle to anesthetize the deeper layers, and then use gentle aspiration, with the same needle, to initially locate the internal jugular vein.

4. Attach a large-bore, deep-line needle (14 gauge needle with a 16 gauge catheter at least 12 inches long) to a 10–20 mL syringe. Direct the needle through the skin wheal caudally, directed toward the ipsilateral nipple and at a 30 degree angle to the frontal plane. If the vein is not entered, withdraw the needle slightly and redirect it 5–10 degrees more laterally. Apply constant back pressure.

5. If bright red blood forcibly fills the syringe, the carotid artery has been punctured. Remove the needle and apply firm pressure for 10 minutes.

6. Follow steps 8 through 11 as described for the subclavian technique.

C. Femoral Vein Approach:
There are several advantages to this procedure: it is safer because arterial and venous sites are easily compressible and it is impossible to cause pneumothorax from this site. Placement can be accomplished without interrupting cardiopulmonary resuscitation. This site can be used to place a variety of intravascular appliances, including temporary pacemakers, pulmonary artery catheters (expertise with fluoroscopy is needed), and triple-lumen catheters. The major disadvantage is the high risk of sepsis and the immobilization it causes and that fluoroscopy is required for placement of pulmonary artery catheters or transvenous pacemakers.

1. Place the patient in the supine position.

2. Use sterile preparation and appropriate draping. Administer local anesthesia in the area to be explored.

3. Palpate the femoral artery. Use the NAVEL technique to locate the vein.

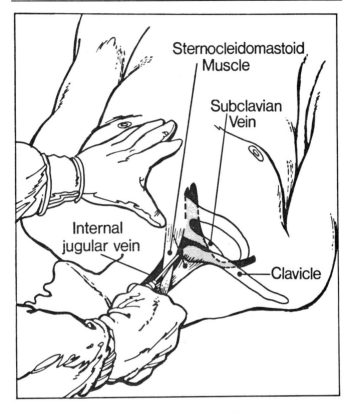

Figure III–4. The technique for internal jugular vein catheterization, central approach. *(Reproduced, with permission, from Gomella LG (editor):* Clinician's Pocket Reference, *7/e. Appleton & Lange, 1993.)*

4. Guard the artery with the fingers of one hand.
5. Explore for the vein just medial to the operator's fingers with a needle and syringe.
6. It may be helpful to have a small amount of anesthetic in the syringe ready for injection during the exploration.
7. The needle is directed cephalad at about a 30 degree angle and should be inserted below the femoral crease.
8. Puncture is heralded by the return of venous, nonpulsatile blood on application of negative pressure to the syringe.

9. Advance the guidewire through the needle.
10. The guidewire should pass with ease into the vein to a depth at which the distal tip of the guidewire is always under the operator's control even when the sheath/dilator or catheter is placed over the guidewire.
11. Remove the needle once the guidewire has advanced into the femoral vein.
12. If the catheter is 6 Fr or larger, a skin incision with a scalpel blade generally is needed. The catheter can then be advanced in unison with the guidewire into the femoral vein. Be sure always to control the distal end of the guidewire.
13. Follow steps 1 through 6 for the internal jugular technique.

Complications: Pneumothorax, hemothorax, hydrothorax, arterial puncture with hematoma, catheter tip embolus, air embolus. If you suspect that has occurred, place the patient head down and turned on his left side to keep the air in the right atrium; attempt to aspirate the air through the catheter. Obtain an immediate portable chest film to see if air is present in the heart.

5. Chest Tube Insertion

(See also Section I, Problem 13, page 57)

Indications:

1. Pneumothorax (simple or tension).
2. Hemothorax.
3. Hydrothorax.
4. Empyema.

Materials: Chest tube (28–36 Fr for adults; 18–28 Fr for children), water-seal drainage system (Pleurovac, etc) with connecting tubing, minor procedure tray and instrument tray (see page 000), silk suture (0 or 2-0), Vaseline gauze.

Procedure:

1. For a pneumothorax, choose a high anterior site, such as the second or third intercostal space, midclavicular line, or subaxillary position (more cosmetic). Place a low lateral chest tube in the fifth or sixth intercostal space in the midaxillary line and directed posteriorly for fluid removal. For a traumatic pneumothorax, use a low lateral tube because this condition usually is associated with bleeding. Use a 24–28 Fr tube for pneumothorax and 36 Fr for fluid removal.
2. If the procedure is elective, sedation may be helpful. Prep the area with antiseptic and drape it with towels. Use 1% lidocaine (with or without epinephrine) to anesthetize the skin and periosteum of the

rib; start at the center of the rib and gently work over the top. Remember, the neurovascular bundle runs under the rib (Figure III–5).

3. Make a 2–3 cm transverse incision over the center of the rib. Use a hemostat to bluntly dissect over the top of the rib and create a subcutaneous tunnel. Injection of additional lidocaine into the muscle will help ease the discomfort.

4. Puncture the parietal pleura with the hemostat and spread the opening. Insert a gloved finger into the pleural cavity to gently clear any clots or adhesions and to make certain the lung is not accidentally punctured by the tube.

5. Carefully insert the tube superiorly into the desired position with a hemostat or gloved finger. Make sure all the holes in the tube are in the chest cavity. Attach the end of the tube to a water-seal or Pleurovac suction system.

6. Suture the tube in place. Place a heavy silk (0 or 2-0) suture through the incision next to the tube. Tie the incision together, then tie the ends around the chest tube. Alternatively, a purse string suture can be placed. Make sure all of the suction holes are beneath

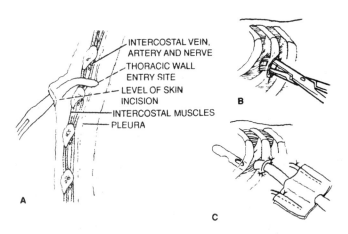

Figure III–5. Chest tube technique, demonstrating the location of the neurovascular bundle and the creation of the subcutaneous tunnel. *(Reproduced, with permission, from Gomella TL (editor): Chest Tube Placement. In: Neonatology, 3/e. Appleton & Lange, 1994.)*

the skin before the tube is secured. An alternative technique is to secure the tube with tape and suture the tape to the skin. This is most useful for smaller chest tubes used in infants and children (Figure III–6).

7. Wrap the tube with Vaseline gauze and cover with plain gauze. Make the dressing as airtight as possible with tape.

8. Start suction (usually −20 cm in adult; −16 cm in children) and take a chest x-ray film immediately to check the placement of the tube and to evaluate for residual pneumothorax or fluid.

9. If a patient manifests signs of a tension pneumothorax (acute shortness of breath, hypotension, distended neck veins, tachypnea, tracheal deviation) before a chest tube is placed, urgent treatment is needed. Insert a 14 gauge needle into the chest in the second intercostal space in the midclavicular line to rapidly decompress the tension pneumothorax and proceed with chest tube insertion.

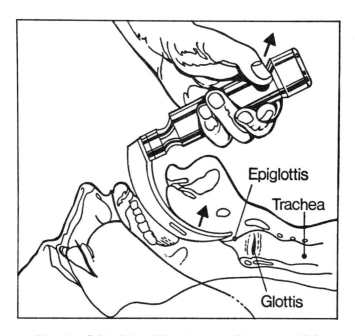

Figure III–6. Endotracheal intubation using a curved laryngoscope blade. *(Reproduced, with permission, from Gomella LG (editor):* Clinician's Pocket Reference, *7/e. Appleton & Lange, 1993.)*

10. To remove a chest tube, make sure the pneumothorax or hemo-thorax is cleared. Check for an air leak by having the patient cough; observe the water-seal system for bubbling that indicates either a system (tubing leak) or persistent pleural air leak.

11. Take the tube off suction **but not off water seal** and cut the retention suture. (Some clinicians advocate clamping the tube before pulling it). Have the patient perform the Valsalva maneuver while the clinician applies pressure with Vaseline gauze and 4 × 4 gauze squares or Tegaderm. Pull the tube rapidly and make an airtight seal with tape. Check an upright chest x-ray film for pneumothorax.

Complications: Infection, bleeding, lung damage, subcutaneous emphysema, persistent pneumothorax or fluid collection, poor tube placement.

6. Cricothyrotomy (Needle and Surgical)

Indications: Mechanical ventilation is indicated, but an endotracheal tube cannot be placed (eg, severe maxillofacial trauma, excessive oropharyngeal hemorrhage).

Contraindications: Surgical cricothyrotomy is contraindicated in children younger than 12 years.

Materials:

Needle Cricothyrotomy: 12–14 gauge catheter over needle (Angiocath or Jelco), 6–12 mL syringe, 3 mm pediatric endotracheal tube adapter, oxygen connecting tubing, high flow oxygen source (tank or wall).

Surgical Cricothyrotomy (Minimum Requirements): Povidone-iodine solution, sterile gauze pads, scalpel handle and blade (No. 10 preferred), hemostat (optional), No. 5 to No. 7 tracheostomy tube, tracheostomy tube adapter to connect to bag-mask ventilator.

Procedures:

A. Needle Cricothyrotomy:

1. Palpate the cricothyroid membrane, which resembles a notch located between the caudal end of the thyroid cartilage and the first tracheal ring (also called the cricoid cartilage).

2. Prep the area with povidone-iodine solution. Local anesthesia can be used if the patient is awake.

3. Mount the syringe on the 12 or 14 gauge catheter over needle assembly, and advance through the cricothyroid membrane at a 45 degree angle, applying back pressure on the syringe until air is aspirated.

4. Advance the catheter and remove the needle. Attach the hub to a 3 mm endotracheal tube adapter, which is connected to the oxygen tubing. Allow the oxygen to flow at 15 L/min for 1–2 seconds on, then 4 seconds off by using a "Y-connector" or a hole in the side of the tubing to turn the flow on and off.

5. The needle technique is only useful for about 45 minutes because the exhalation of CO_2 is suboptimal.

B. Surgical Cricothyrotomy:

1. & 2. Follow steps 1 and 2 for needle cricothyrotomy.

3. Make a horizontal skin incision over the cricothyroid membrane and then through the membrane itself. Insert the knife handle and rotate it 90 degrees to open the hole in the membrane. Alternatively, a hemostat can be used to dilate the opening.

4. Insert a small (5–7 mm) tracheostomy tube, inflate the balloon (if present), and secure in position with the attached cotton tapes.

5. A surgical cricothyrotomy should be replaced in the operating room with a formal tracheostomy within 24 hours.

Complications: Bleeding, esophageal perforation, subcutaneous emphysema, pneumomediastinum and thorax, CO_2 retention (especially with the needle procedure).

7. Endotracheal Intubation

Indications:

1. Airway management during cardiopulmonary resuscitation.
2. Any indication for using mechanical ventilation (coma, surgery, etc).

Contraindications: Massive maxillofacial trauma, fractured larynx, suspected cervical spinal cord injury.

Materials: Endotracheal tube (see Table III–1), laryngoscope handle and blade (straight or curved, No. 3 for adults, No. 1–1.5 for small children), 10 mL syringe, adhesive tape, suction equipment, malleable stylet (optional).

Procedure:

1. Orotracheal intubation is most commonly used. The use of orotracheal intubation should be strongly discouraged when cervical spine injuries are suspected, in which case, nasotracheal intubation is preferred.

2. Any patient who is hypoxic or apneic must be ventilated before attempting endotracheal intubation (bag-mask or mouth-to-mask). Remember to avoid prolonged periods of no ventilation if the intubation is difficult.

TABLE III–1. RECOMMENDED ENDOTRACHEAL TUBE SIZES.

Patient	Internal Diameter (mm)
Premature infant	2.5–3.0 (uncuffed)
Newborn infant	3.5 (uncuffed)
3–12 months	4.0 (uncuffed)
1–8 years	4.0–6.0 (uncuffed)[1]
8–16 years	6.0–7.0 (cuffed)
Adult	7.0–9.0 (cuffed)

[1]Rough estimate is to measure the little finger.

3. Extend the laryngoscope blade to 90 degrees to verify the light is working and check the balloon on the tube (if present) for leaks.
4. Place the patients head in the "sniffing position" (neck extended anteriorly and the head extended posteriorly). Use suction to clear the upper airway if needed.
5. Hold the laryngoscope in the left hand, hold the mouth open with the right hand, and use the blade to push the tongue to the patient's left and make certain the tongue remains anterior to the blade. Advance carefully towards the midline until the epiglottis is seen.
6. If straight laryngoscope blade is passed under the epiglottis, the blade is then lifted upward and the vocal cords should be visualized. If using a curved blade, it is placed anterior to the epiglottis and gently lifted anteriorly. The handle should not be used to pry the epiglottis open, but rather gently lifted in both cases (Figure III–6).
7. While maintaining visualization of the cords, the tube is grasped in the right hand and passed through the cords. With more difficult intubations, the malleable stylet can be used to direct the tube.
8. When using a cuffed tube (adult and older children), gently inflate with a 10 mL syringe until there is an adequate seal (about 5 mL). Ventilate the patient while auscultating and visualizing both sides of the chest to verify positioning. If the left side does not seem to be ventilating, it may signify that the tube has been advanced down the right mainstem bronchus. Withdraw the tube 1–2 cm and recheck the breath sounds. Confirm positioning with an immediate chest x-ray. The end of the endotracheal tube should lie approximately 3 cm below the cords and 3 cm above the carina.
9. Tape the tube in position and insert an oropharyngeal airway to prevent the patient from biting the tube.

Complications: Bleeding, oral or pharyngeal trauma, improper tube positioning (esophageal intubation, right mainstem bronchus), aspiration, tube obstruction or kinking.

8. Gastrointestinal Tubes

(See also Section I, Problems 54 and 55, pages 183, 185, respectively)

Indications:

1. Gastrointestinal decompression (ileus, obstruction, pancreatitis, postoperatively).
2. Lavage of the stomach with gastrointestinal bleeding or drug overdose.
3. Prevention aspiration in an obtunded patient.
4. Feeding a patient who is unable to swallow.

Materials: Gastrointestinal tube of choice (see below), lubricant jelly, catheter tip syringe, glass of water with a straw, stethoscope.

Types of Gastrointestinal Tubes:

A. Nasogastric Tubes:
1. **Levin tube:** Single lumen tube that must be placed on intermittent suction to evacuate gastric contents.
2. **Salem-sump tube:** A double lumen tube, with the smaller tube acting as an air intake vent. Use 14–18 Fr size in adults—the best tube for continuous suction.
3. **Ewald tube:** Large (18–36 Fr) double lumen tube, especially suited for gastric lavage of drug overdose, more often inserted by the orogastric route.

B. Intestinal Tubes: These are usually used to decompress the small bowel and are normally not taped in position so that they can migrate through the small bowel to the point of obstruction.
1. **Cantor tube:** A long single lumen tube with a rubber balloon at the tip. The balloon is partially filled with mercury (3–5 mL), which allows it to gravitate into the small bowel with the aid of peristalsis.
2. **Miller-Abbott tube:** A long double lumen tube with a rubber balloon at the tip. One lumen is used for aspiration; the other connects to the balloon. After the tube is in the stomach, inflate it with 5–10 mL of air, inject 2–3 mL of mercury, and then aspirate the air.
3. **Dennis, Baker, Leonard tubes:** These are used for intraoperative decompression of the bowel and are manually passed into the bowel at the time of laparotomy.

C. Feeding Tubes: Although any small bore nasogastric tube can be used as a feeding tube, certain weighted tubes are designed to pass into the duodenum and decrease the risk of aspiration of gastric contents.
1. **Dobbhoff, Entriflex, Keogh tubes:** Weighted mercury tip with stylet.
2. **Vivonex:** Tungsten tipped.

D. Sengstaken-Blakemore tube: A triple lumen tube used exclusively for the control of bleeding esophageal varices by tamponade. One lumen is for aspiration, one is for the gastric balloon, and the third is for the esophageal balloon.

Procedure (General outline for most tubes):

1. Inform the patient about the procedure and encourage cooperation, if the patient is able. Choose the nasal passage that appears most open.
2. Lubricate the distal 3–4 inches of the tube with a water-soluble jelly (K-Y jelly or viscous 2% lidocaine) and insert the tube gently along the floor of the nasal passageway. Maintain gentle pressure that will allow the tube to pass into the nasopharynx.
3. When the patient can feel the tube in the back of the throat, ask the patient to swallow small amounts of water through a straw as you advance the tube 2–3 inches at a time.
4. To be sure that the tube is in the stomach, aspirate gastric contents or blow air into the tube and listen over the stomach with a stethoscope for a "pop" or "gurgle."
5. Attach sump tubes (Salem-sump) to continuous low wall suction and the single lumen tube (Levin) to intermittent suction.
6. Feeding tubes and pediatric feeding tubes in adults are more difficult to insert because they are more flexible. A stylet or guidewire can be used or the smaller tube can be attached to a larger, stiffer tube by wedging both into a gelatin capsule. Pass the tube in the usual fashion and allow it to remain in the stomach for 10–15 minutes. After this time, the capsule dissolves and the larger tube can be removed.
7. Tape the tube securely in place but do not allow it to apply pressure to the ala of the nose. Patients have been disfigured because of ischemic necrosis of the nose caused by a poorly positioned tube.
8. For Cantor and Miller-Abbott tubes a loop should be left outside the patient to allow the tube to pass down the genitourinary tract, and therefore these should not be as securely fastened to the nose. When inserting a Cantor tube, a cotton tipped swab is useful to aid in passing the mercury-filled balloon through the nose.
9. A flat plate should be obtained before starting any feeding through a tube or to follow the progress of the weighted intestinal tubes.

Complications: Inadvertent passage into the trachea, coiling of the tube in the mouth or pharynx, bleeding in the mucosa of the nose, pharynx, or stomach.

9. IV Techniques

(See Section I, Problem 52, page 177)

Indications: To establish an intravenous access for the administration of fluids, blood, or medications.

Materials: IV fluid, connecting tubing, tourniquet, alcohol swab, intravenous cannulas (a catheter over a needle, such as Angiocath, Jelco, or a butterfly needle), antiseptic ointment, dressing, and tape. **Note:** It helps to rip the tape into strips and to flush the air out of the tubing before beginning.

Procedure:

1. Verify there are no relative contraindications for using an extremity for an IV before starting. These include recent axillary node dissection and planned or recently placed AV-fistula or graft.

   The upper, nondominant extremity is the site of choice for an IV. Choose a distal vein so that if the vein is lost, you can reposition the IV more proximally. Avoid veins that cross a joint space. Also avoid inserting an IV into the leg because of the high incidence of thrombophlebitis. If no extremity vein can be found, try the external jugular. If all these fail, the only alternatives are a deep line or a cutdown (see page 332).

2. Apply a tourniquet above the proposed IV site. Techniques to help expose difficult to locate veins include wrapping the extremity in a warm towel, leaving the arm in a dependent position for a few minutes after the tourniquet is applied or using a blood pressure cuff as a tourniquet inflated as much as possible so that arterial flow is maintained. See Section I, Problem 52 for a more complete discussion of the difficult IV access patient. Carefully clean the site with an alcohol or povidone-iodine swab. If a large bore IV is to be used (16 or 14 Fr), local anesthesia with 1% lidocaine is helpful.

3. Stabilize the vein distally with the thumb of your free hand. Using the catheter over needle assembly (Intracath or Angiocath), either enter the vein directly or enter the skin alongside the vein first and then stick the vein along the side at about a 20 degree angle. Once the vein is punctured, blood should appear in the "flash chamber." Advance a few more millimeters to be sure that both the needle and the tip of the catheter have entered the vein. Carefully withdraw the needle as you advance the catheter into the vein. **Caution: Never withdraw the catheter over the needle because the plastic tip can be sheared off and cause a catheter embolus.** Apply pressure with your thumb over the vein just proximal to the site to prevent significant blood loss while you connect the IV line to the catheter.

4. Observe the site with the IV fluid running for signs of induration or swelling that indicate improper placement or damage to the vein.

5. Tape IV securely in place, apply a drop of povidone-iodine or antibiotic ointment and sterile dressing. Ideally, the dressing should be changed every 24–48 hours to help reduce infections. Armboards are also useful to help maintain an IV site.

6. If the veins are deep and difficult to locate, a small 3–5 mL syringe can be mounted on the catheter assembly. Proper position inside the vein is determined by aspiration of blood.
7. If venous access is limited, a "butterfly" needle can sometimes be used or the external jugular may be considered as a site.

10. Joint Aspiration (Arthrocentesis)

Indications:

1. **Diagnostic:** Arthrocentesis is helpful in the diagnosis of new-onset arthritis; to rule out infection in acute or chronic, unremitting joint effusion.
2. **Therapeutic:** To instill steroids and maintain drainage of septic arthritis.

Materials: Minor procedure tray (Table III–8, page 334) 18 or 20 gauge needle (smaller for finger or toe); ethyl chloride spray can be substituted for lidocaine; two heparinized tubes for cell count and crystal examination; discuss with colleagues in your microbiology lab their preference for transporting fluid for bacterial, fungal, acid-fast bacillus (AFB) culture, and Gram's stain. A Thayer-Martin plate is needed if *Neisseria gonorrhoeae* is suspected. A small syringe containing a long-acting corticosteroid, eg, Depo-Medrol or triamcinolone, is optional for therapeutic arthrocentesis.

Procedures:

A. General:
1. Obtain consent form describing the procedure and review possible complications.
2. Determine the optimal site for aspiration and mark with indelible ink.
3. When aspiration is to be followed by corticosteroid injection, maintaining a sterile field with sterile implements minimizes the risk of infection to the patient.
4. Clean the area with Betadine, dry, and wipe over the aspiration site with alcohol. Betadine can render cultures negative. Let the alcohol dry before beginning the procedure.
5. Anesthetize the area with lidocaine using a 25 gauge needle, taking care not to inject into the joint space. Lidocaine is bactericidal. Avoid preparations containing epinephrine especially in a small digit. Alternatively, spray the area with ethyl chloride just before needle aspiration.
6. Insert the aspirating needle applying a small amount of vacuum to the syringe. Remove as much fluid as possible, repositioning the syringe if necessary.
7. If corticosteroid is to be injected, remove the aspirating syringe from the needle that is still in the joint space. It is helpful to ensure that the syringe can be removed easily from the needle before step 6. Attach the syringe containing corticosteroid, pull back on

plunger to ensure the syringe is not in a vein and inject contents. Never inject steroids when there is any possibility of an infected joint. Remove the needle and apply pressure to the area. Generally, the equivalent of 40 mg of methylprednisolone is injected into large joints such as the knee and 20 mg into medium-sized joints such as the ankle or wrist.

8. Joint fluid is sent for cell count and differential, crystal exam, Gram's stain, and cultures for bacteria, fungi and AFB as indicated.

B. Specific:

1. Arthrocentesis of the knee:

a. The knee should be fully extended with the patient supine. Wait until the patient has a relaxed quadriceps muscle because its contraction plants the patella against the femur, making aspiration painful.

b. The needle is inserted posterior to the medial portion of the patella into the patellar-femoral groove. The advancing needle is directed slightly posteriorly and inferiorly (Figure III–7A).

2. Arthrocentesis of the wrist:

a. The easiest site for aspiration is between the navicular bone and radius on the dorsal wrist. Locate the distal radius between the tendons of the extensor pollicus longus and the extensor carpi radialis longus to the second finger. This site is just ulnar to the anatomic snuff box. The needle is directed perpendicular to the mark (Figure III–7B).

3. Arthrocentesis of the ankle:

a. The most accessible site is between the tibia and the talus. The angle of the foot to leg is positioned at 90 degrees. A mark is made lateral and anterior to the medial malleolus and medial and posterior to the tibialis anterior tendon. The advancing needle is directed posteriorly towards the heel.

b. The subtalar ankle joint does not communicate with the ankle joint and is difficult to aspirate even by an expert. One should be aware that "ankle pain" may originate in the subtalar joint rather than in the ankle (Figure III–7C).

Synovial Fluid Interpretation

A. Noninflammatory Arthritis: Traumatic, lupus, rheumatic fever.

B. Inflammatory Arthritis: Osteoarthritis, gout, pseudogout, rheumatoid arthritis.

C. Septic Arthritis: *Staphylococcus aureus* and *Neisseria gonorrhoeae* most common.

D. WBC: Normal 0–300 µL; 300–2000 noninflammatory; 2000–75,000 inflammatory; >100,000 septic arthritis.

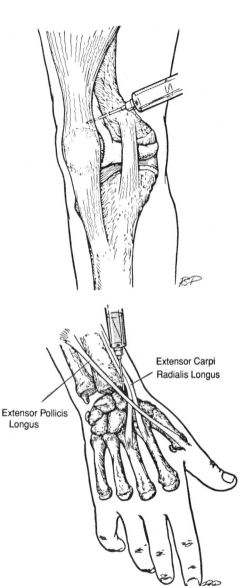

A

Extensor Carpi
Radialis Longus

Extensor Pollicis
Longus

B

Figure III–7. *A:* Arthrocentesis of the knee. *B:* Arthrocentesis of the wrist.
C: Arthrocentesis of the ankle. *(Reproduced, with permission, from Haist SA et al (editors):* Internal Medicine On-Call. *Appleton & Lange, 1991.)*

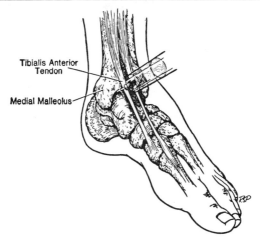

Tibialis Anterior Tendon

Medial Malleolus

C

Figure III–7. *(continued)*

E. WBC Differential: Normal <25% neutrophils; >50% neutrophils inflammatory; >90% neutrophils septic; 2% eosinophils suggests Lyme disease.

F. Uric Acid: Normal <8 mg/dL [mol/L].

G. Microscopic: Normal no debris, crystals or bacteria; urate, gout; calcium pyrophosphate, pseudogout; bacteria, septic (33% of cases of septic arthritis may be initially negative).

Complications: Infection, bleeding, pain. Postinjection flare of joint pain and swelling can occur after steroid injection and persist up to 24 hours. This complication is believed to be a crystal-induced synovitis resulting from the crystalline suspension used in long-acting steroids.

11. Lumbar Puncture

Indications:
1. Diagnostic purposes (analysis of cerebrospinal fluid [CSF]).
2. Measurement of CSF pressure.
3. Injection of various agents (contrast media, chemotherapy).

Contraindications: Increased intracranial pressure, (papilledema, mass lesion), infection near the puncture site, planned myelography or pneumoencephalography, coagulopathy.

Materials: A sterile, disposable LP kit **or** minor procedure tray (see Table III–8, page 334), spinal needles (20–21 gauge for adults, 22 gauge for children), sterile specimen tubes.

Procedure:

1. Examine the visual fields for evidence of papilledema, and review the CT scan of the head if available. Discuss the procedure with the patient to dispel any myths. Some prefer to call the procedure a "subarachnoid analysis" rather than a spinal tap. Obtain informed consent from the patient or legal representative.

2. Place the patient in the lateral decubitus position close to the edge of the bed or table. The patient (held by an assistant, if possible) should be positioned with his knees pulled up towards his stomach and his head flexed onto his chest. This enhances flexion of the vertebral spine and widens the interspaces between the spinous processes. Place a pillow beneath the patient's side to prevent sagging and ensure alignment of the spinal column. In an obese patient or a patient with arthritis or scoliosis, the sitting position or leaning forward may be preferred.

3. Draw an imaginary line between the iliac crests. This should cross the spine at the L4 vertebral body and assist in locating the L4–L5 interspace.

4. Open the kit, put on sterile gloves, and prep the area with povidone-iodine solution in a circular fashion, covering several interspaces. Next, drape the patient.

5. With a 25 gauge needle and 1% lidocaine, raise a skin wheal over the L4–L5 interspace. Anesthetize the deeper structures with a 22 gauge needle.

6. Examine the spinal needle with stylet for defects and then insert it into the skin wheal and into the spinous ligament. Hold the needle between your index and middle fingers, with your thumb holding the stylet in place. Direct the needle cephalad at a 30–45 degree angle in the midline and parallel to the bed.

7. Advance through the major structures and "pop" into the subarachnoid space through the dura. An experienced operator can feel these layers, but an inexperienced one may need to periodically remove the obturator to look for return of fluid. Direct the bevel of the needle parallel to the long axis of the body so that the dural fibers are separated rather than sheared; this method helps cut down on "spinal headaches."

8. If no fluid returns, it is sometimes helpful to rotate the needle slightly. If still no fluid appears, and you think that you are within the subarachnoid space, 1 mL of air can be injected since it is not uncommon for a piece of tissue to clog the needle. **Never** inject saline or distilled water. If no air returns and if spinal fluid cannot be aspirated, the bevel of the needle probably lies in the epidural space; advance it with the stylet into place.

9. When fluid returns, attach a manometer and stopcock and measure the pressure. Normal opening pressure is 70–180 mm water. Increased pressure may be a result of a tense patient, CHF, ascites, subarachnoid hemorrhage, infection, or a space-occupying lesion. Decreased pressure may result from needle position or obstructed flow (you may need to leave the needle in for a myelogram because if it is moved, the subarachnoid space may be lost).

10. Collect 0.5–2.0 mL samples in serial, labeled containers. Send them to the lab in the following order:

   1st tube for bacteriology: Gram's stain, routine culture and sensitivity (C&S), acid-fast bacilli (AFB), and fungal cultures and stains.

   2nd tube for glucose and protein.

   3rd tube for cell count: CBC with differential.

   4th tube for special studies: VDRL test, CIEP, etc.

Note: Some prefer to send the first and last tubes for CBC because this procedure permits a better differentiation between a subarachnoid hemorrhage and a traumatic tap. In a traumatic tap, the number of red blood cells in the first tube should be much higher than in the last tube. In a subarachnoid hemorrhage, the cell counts should be equal, and xanthochromia of the fluid should be present, indicating the presence of old blood.

11. Withdraw the needle and place a sterile dressing over the site.

12. Instruct the patient to remain recumbent for 6–12 hours and encourage an increased fluid intake to help prevent spinal headaches. Interpret the results based on Table III–2.

Complications: Spinal headache is the most common complication seen about 20% of the time. It typically goes away when the patient is lying down and is aggravated when sitting up. To help prevent spinal headaches, keep the patient recumbent for 6–12 hours, encourage the intake of fluids, use the smallest needle possible, and keep the bevel of the needle parallel to the long axis of the body to help prevent a persistent CSF leak. Other complications include trauma to nerve roots, herniation of either the cerebellum or the medulla, meningitis.

12. Nasal Packing

(See page 102).

13. Paracentesis (Peritoneal)

Indications:

1. To determine the cause of ascites.
2. To determine if intra-abdominal bleeding is present, or if a viscus has ruptured. Diagnostic peritoneal lavage is considered a more accurate test.
3. Therapeutic removal of fluid (eg, respiratory distress).

TABLE III–2. DIFFERENTIAL DIAGNOSIS OF CEREBROSINAL FLUID.

Condition	Color	Opening Pressure (mm H_2O)	Protein (mg/100 mL)	Glucose (mg/100 mL)	Cells (#/µL)
Adult (normal)	Clear	70–180	15–45	45–80	0–5 lymphs
Newborn (normal)	Clear	70–180	20–120	2/3 serum glucose	40–60 lymphs
Viral infection	Clear or opalescent	Normal or slightly increased	Normal or slightly increased	Normal	10–500 lymphs (polys early)
Bacterial infection	Opalescent or yellow, may clot	Increased	50–1500	<, usually < 20	25–10,000 polys
Granulomatous (TB, fungal)	Clear or opalescent	Often >	>, but usually < 500	<, usually 20–40	10–500 lymphs
Subarachnoid hemorrhage	Bloody or xanthochromic after 2–8 hr	Usually >	>	Normal	WBC/RBC[1] ratio same as blood

[1]WBC = white blood cell; RBC = red blood cell.

Contraindications: Abnormal coagulation factors, uncertainty if distention is due to peritoneal fluid or to a cystic structure (ultrasound can often differentiate these).

Materials: Minor procedure tray (see Table III–8, page 334), catheter over needle IV needle (18–20 gauge with a 1½ inch needle), 20–60 mL syringe, sterile specimen containers.

Procedure:

1. Informed consent is obtained. Have the patient empty his bladder.
2. The entry site is usually the midline 3–4 cm below the umbilicus. Avoid old surgical scars because the bowel may be clinging to the abdominal wall. Alternatively, the entry site can be in the left or right lower quadrant midway between the umbilicus and the anterior superior iliac spine or in the patient's flank, depending on the percussion of the fluid wave.
3. Raise a skin wheal with the 1% lidocaine over the proposed entry site. Prep and drape the patient.
4. With the Angiocath mounted on the syringe, go through the anesthetized area carefully while gently aspirating. You will meet some resistance as you enter the fascia. When you get free return of fluid, leave the catheter in place, remove the needle, and begin to aspirate. Sometimes it is necessary to reposition the catheter because of abutting bowel.

TABLE III–3. DIFFERENTIAL DIAGNOSIS OF ASCITIC FLUID.
TRANSUDATIVE ASCITES: CIRRHOSIS, NEPHROSIS, CONGESTIVE HEART FAILURE.
EXUDATIVE ASCITES: MALIGNANCY, PERITONITIS (TB, PERFORATED VISCUS), HYPOALBUMINEMIA.

Lab Value	Transudate	Exudate
Specific gravity	<1.016	>1.016
Protein (Ascitic fluid)	<3 gm/100 mL	>3 gm/100 mL
Protein (Ascitic to serum ratio)	<0.5	>0.5
LDH (Ascitic to serum ratio)	<0.6	>0.6
Ascitic fluid LDH	<200 IU	>200 IU
Glucose (Serum to ascitic ratio)	<1	>1
Fibrinogen (Clot)	No	Yes
White blood cells	<500/μL	>1000/μL
Red blood cells		>100 RBC/μL

Food fibers: Found in most causes of a perforated viscus.
Cytology: Bizarre cells with large nuclei may represent reactive mesothelial cells and not a
malignancy; malignant cells suggest a tumor.

5. Aspirate the amount needed for tests (20–30 mL). For a therapeutic
   tap, do not remove more than 500 mL in 10 minutes. A liter is the
   maximum that should be removed at one time.
6. Quickly remove the needle, apply a sterile 4 × 4 gauze square, and
   apply pressure with tape.
7. Depending on the clinical picture of the patient, send samples for total protein, specific gravity, lactate dehydrogenase (LDH), amylase,
   cytology, culture, stains, CBC, or food fibers. See Table III–3 for the
   differential diagnosis of the fluid obtained.
8. Complications: Peritonitis, perforated viscus, hemorrhage, precipita-
   tion of hepatic coma if patient has severe liver disease, oliguria, hypotension

14. Pericardiocentesis

Indications: Emergency treatment of cardiac tamponade (see Figure
I–6, pages 44 and 45), diagnose pericardial effusion.

Materials: Electrocardiogram machine, procedure and instrument tray
(see Table III–8, page 334), pericardiocentesis needle or 16–18 gauge
needle 10 cm long.

Procedure:

1. If time permits, use sterile prep and draping with gown, mask and
   gloves.

2. The approach to drainage of pericardiocentesis can be either left paraxiphoid or through a left parasternal fourth intercostal approach. The paraxiphoid is more commonly used (see Figure III–8).
3. The insertion site is anesthetized with lidocaine. The needle is connected with an alligator clip to lead V on the ECG machine. The limb leads are attached and the machine is monitored.
4. Insert the pericardiocentesis needle just to the left of the xiphoid and directed upwards 45 degrees towards the left shoulder.
5. Aspirate while advancing the needle until the pericardium is punctured and the effusion is tapped. If the ventricular wall is felt, with-

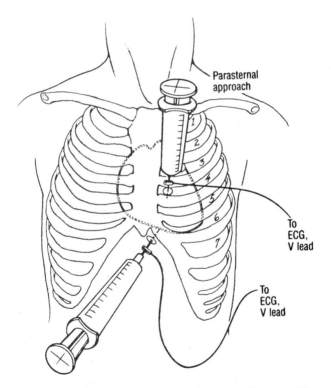

Parasternal approach

To ECG, V lead

To ECG, V lead

Figure III–8. Techniques for pericardiocentesis. The paraxiphoid approach is the most popular. *(Reproduced, with permission, from Stillman RM (editor): Surgery, Diagnosis, and Therapy. Appleton & Lange, 1989.)*

draw the needle slightly. Additionally, if the needle contacts the myocardium, pronounced ST segment elevation will be noted on the ECG.

6. If performed for cardiac tamponade, removal of as little as 50 mL of fluid will dramatically improve blood pressure.

7. Blood from a bloody pericardial effusion is usually defibrinated and will not clot whereas blood from the ventricle will clot.

8. Send fluid for hematocrit, cell count, or cytology if indicated. Serous fluid is consistent with CHF, bacterial, tuberculous, hypoalbuminemia or viral pericarditis. Bloody fluid (HCT >10%) may be traumatic, iatrogenic, MI, uremia, or due to coagulopathy or malignancy (lymphoma, leukemia, breast, and lung most common).

Complications: Arrhythmia, ventricular puncture, lung injury.

15. Peritoneal Lavage (Diagnostic Peritoneal Lavage)

Indications:

1. Evaluation of intra-abdominal trauma (bleeding, perforation).

2. Acute peritoneal dialysis.

Contraindications: None are absolute. Relative contraindications include multiple abdominal procedures, pregnancy, and any coagulopathy.

Materials: Prepackaged diagnostic peritoneal lavage or peritoneal dialysis tray.

Procedure:

1. For a diagnostic peritoneal lavage (DPL), a Foley catheter and NG tube must be in place. Prep the abdomen from above the umbilicus to the pubis. Wear gloves and mask.

2. The site of choice is in the midline 1–2 cm below the umbilicus. Avoid the site of old surgical scars (danger of adherent bowel). If a subumbilical scar or pelvic fracture is present, a supraumbilical approach is acceptable.

3. Infiltrate the skin with 1% lidocaine with epinephrine. Incise the skin in the midline vertically and expose the fascia.

4. Either pick up the fascia and incise it or puncture it with the trocar and peritoneal catheter. Caution is needed to avoid puncturing any viscera. Use one hand to hold the catheter near the skin and to control the insertion while the other hand applies pressure to the end of the catheter. After entering the peritoneal cavity, remove the trocar and direct the catheter inferiorly into the pelvis.

5. For a diagnostic lavage, gross blood indicates a positive tap. If no blood is encountered, instill 10 mL/kg (about 1 L in adults) of lactated Ringer's solution or normal saline into the abdominal cavity.

TABLE III–4. DIAGNOSTIC PERITONEAL LAVAGE FINDINGS THAT SUGGEST
INTRA-ABDOMINAL TRAUMA.

Positive	20 mL gross blood on free aspiration (10 mL in children)
	>100,000 RBC/μL
	>500 WBC/μL (if obtained >3 hours after the injury)
	>175 units amylase/dL
	Bacteria on Gram stain
	Bile (by inspection or chemical determination of bilirubin contents)
	Food particles (microscopic analysis of strained or spun specimen)
Intermediate	Pink fluid on free aspiration
	50,000–100,000 RBC/μL in blunt trauma
	100–500 WBC/μL
	75–175 units amylase/dL
Negative	Clear aspirate
	<100 WBC/μL
	<75 units amylase/dL

(Reproduced, with permission, from Macho JR, Lewis FR Jr, Krupski WC: Management of the Injured Patient. In: Current Surgical Diagnosis & Treatment, 10/e. Way LW (editor). Appleton & Lange, 1994.)

6. Gently agitate the abdomen to distribute the fluid and after 5 minutes, drain off as much fluid as possible into a bag on the floor (minimum fluid for a valid analysis is 200 mL in an adult). Send the fluid for analysis (amylase, bile, bacteria, food fibers, hematocrit, cell count). See Table III–4 for the diagnosis of the fluid.
7. Remove the catheter and suture the skin. If the catheter is inserted for pancreatitis or peritoneal dialysis, suture it in place.
8. A negative DPL does not rule out retroperitoneal trauma. A false-positive DPL can be caused by a pelvic fracture.

Complications: Infection, bleeding, perforated viscus.

16. Pulmonary Artery Catheterization

(See also Section I, Problem 61, page 199)

Indications:

1. Acute heart failure.
2. Complex circulatory and fluid conditions (burn patients, patients in shock).
3. Diagnosis of cardiac tamponade.
4. Perioperative management (elderly or debilitated patients, patients with severe cardiac or pulmonary diseases).

Materials: Central venous catheter equipment (see page 301); flow directed balloon tipped catheter (eg, Swan-Ganz catheter); 7F with thermistor or pulse oximetry port is most frequently used in adults (Figure III–9A); sheath; dilator; 11 blade and guidewires for catheter insertion (usually supplied as a kit such as Cordis or Arrow Introducer Kit); connecting tubing; transducer and oscilloscope; heparin flush solution (1 U heparin/mL normal saline); pressure bags; ECG monitor; crash cart; and rapid access to 100 mg lidocaine bolus for IV use.

Procedure:

1. Informed consent is needed. The patient must be on an ECG monitor, have a working IV in place and the crash cart should be nearby because arrhythmias are a frequent complication. Coagulation profile should ideally be normal.
2. Gown, gloves, mask, and cap along with a wide sterile field are needed.
3. Remove the pulmonary artery catheter from the package, place on a sterile field and flush all the lumens with heparinized saline. The transducer should be balanced at the reference point of the midaxillary line with the patient supine. All ports should be connected to the monitoring lines. Check the function of the transducer by gently flicking the tip and observing oscillation on the monitor.
4. Check the flow balloon at the end of the catheter by gently inflating with 1.5 mL of air (for a 7F catheter). Some operators check the balloon in a cup of sterile water for leaks. If there is the possibility of a left-right shunt, carbon dioxide is suggested for inflation. Liquid should **not** be used to inflate the balloon.
5. Obtain access to a central vein as described in "Central venous catheter placement," page 301 using a guidewire. The subclavian access is usually preferred because of the ease of securing the catheter to the relatively flat upper chest wall. The internal jugular, antecubital routes are also acceptable. The femoral vein should be avoided, if possible, because of the increased risk of infection and embolism.
6. The guidewire in the introducer set should be placed at least halfway into the vein. The patient must be monitored continuously during the procedure because arrhythmia, most frequently ventricular, may occur.
7. The dilator is then mounted inside the introducer, the skin is nicked with an 11 blade, and the assembly is slowly advanced over the guidewire.
8. The pulmonary artery catheter ports are flushed with heparinized saline one more time to remove air bubbles. The guidewire and dilator are removed and the introducer left in position. A finger should be placed over the end of the introducer to prevent excessive bleeding or an air embolus. A telescoping clear plastic contamination guard, if used, should be mounted to the hub of the introducer and a rubber gasket assembly usually prevents excessive bleeding before the time the catheter is threaded into the intro-

ducer. This guard allows the catheter to be adjusted over a range of approximately 20 cm under sterile conditions after the catheter has been positioned.

9. Slowly advance the catheter to approximately the right atrium. Follow the characteristic patterns as the catheter is advanced (Figure III–9B). Most catheters have markings every 10 cm. The reference lengths to the right atrium are as follows: right internal jugular or subclavian 10–20 cm, left internal jugular or subclavian 20–30 cm, left or right antecubital vein 40–50 cm, left or right femoral vein 30 cm.

10. While at the approximate level of the right atrium, slowly inflate the balloon of the 7 F catheter with 1.5 mL air (.8 mL for the 5 Fr catheter). Advance the catheter and observe the pressure tracing (Figure III–10) on the oscilloscope from the distal port to follow the catheter tip as it flows through the right ventricle and out the pulmonary artery. Do not hesitate if ventricular ectopy is seen. Rapidly

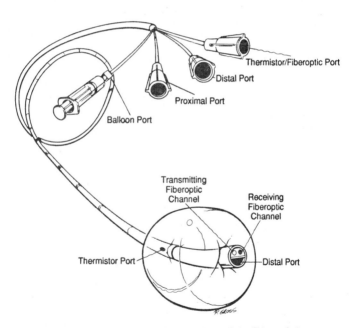

Figure III–9. A: An example of a pulmonary artery catheter. This one features an oximetric measuring feature. (Reproduced, with permission, from Gomella LG (editor): Clinician's Pocket Reference, 7/e. Appleton & Lange, 1993.) B: Positioning and pressure waveforms seen as the pulmonary artery catheter is advanced. (Reproduced, with permission, from Stillman RM (editor): Surgery, Diagnosis, and Therapy. Appleton & Lange, 1989.)

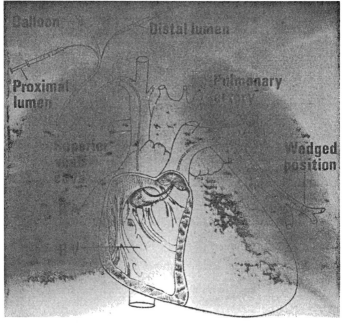

A

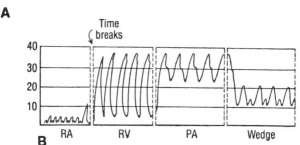

B

Figure III–9. (*continued*)

pass the catheter through the ventricle and use IV lidocaine (50–100 mg IV bolus) if the ectopy persists. Once at the pulmonary artery, advance the catheter 10–20 cm further to obtain the wedge pressure. If multiple attempts fail to successfully pass the catheter out the pulmonary artery, fluoroscopy may be needed.

TABLE III–5. NORMAL PULMONARY ARTERY CATHETER MEASUREMENTS.

Parameter	Range
Right atrial pressure	1–7 mm Hg
Right ventricular systolic pressure	15–25 mm Hg
Right ventricular diastolic pressure	0–8 mm Hg
Pulmonary artery systolic pressure	15–25 mm Hg
Pulmonary artery diastolic pressure	8–15 mm Hg
Pulmonary artery mean pressure	10–20 mm Hg
Pulmonary capillary wedge pressure	6–12 mm Hg
SVR (systemic vascular resistance)[1]	900–1200 dynes/sec/cm^5
Cardiac output	3.5–5.5 L/min
Cardiac index	2.8–3.2 L/min

[1]$SVR = \dfrac{(\text{mean arterial pressure} - \text{central venous pressure}) \times 80}{\text{Cardiac output}}$

11. Deflate the balloon and the pulmonary artery tracing should reappear. Adjust the catheter as needed so that this pattern is reproduced. **Never** leave the balloon inflated continuously or pulmonary infarction or arterial rupture may occur. Never leave the balloon inflated while pulling the catheter back. The pulmonary artery tracing should be observed at all times unless the balloon is inflated.

12. Suture the introducer and pulmonary artery catheter in position with 2-0 silk. If there is a contamination shield, extend it about half way to allow the catheter to be moved, should repositioning be needed.

13. Dress the site with povidone-iodine and gauze or transparent shield dressing (Op-Site).

14. Obtain an immediate portable chest x-ray to verify proper catheter position and to rule out a pneumothorax. A properly positioned pulmonary artery catheter should follow a smooth curve and the tip of the catheter should not be further than 5 cm from the midline, and most often in the right pulmonary artery.

15. Normal pulmonary artery parameters are listed in Table III–5 and diagnosis of conditions associated with certain readings are listed in Table III–6.

Complications: All complications associated with central venous catheter placement (see page 305), arrhythmia, pulmonary artery rupture or pulmonary infarction, knotting of catheter or rupture of the balloon, sepsis, complete heart block.

TABLE III–6. DIFFERENTIAL DIAGNOSIS OF COMMON PULMONARY ARTERY
CATHETER READINGS.

Low right atrial pressure: Volume depletion

High right atrial pressure: Volume overload, congestive heart failure, cardiogenic shock,
increased pulmonary vascular resistance (hypoxia, ventilator effects of PEEP, pulmonary
disease, primary pulmonary hypertension)

Low right ventricular pressures: Volume depletion

High right ventricular pressures: Volume overload, congestive heart failure, cardiogenic
shock, increased pulmonary vascular resistance (see above)

High pulmonary artery pressure: Congestive heart failure, increased pulmonary vascular
resistance (hypoxia, ventilator effect of PEEP, pulmonary disease), cardiac tamponade

Low wedge pressure: Volume depletion

High wedge pressure: Cardiogenic shock, left ventricular failure, ventricular septal defect,
mitral regurgitation and stenosis, severe hypertension, volume overload, cardiac
tamponade

17. Sigmoidoscopy

Indications:

1. Workup of gastrointestinal tract bleeding or lower gastrointestinal
   tract symptoms.
2. Evaluation of trauma.

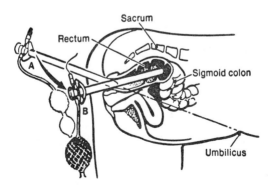

Figure III–10. The sigmoidoscope is advanced under direct vision as shown.
(Reproduced, with permission, from Gomella LG (editor): Clinician's Pocket Reference,
7/e. Appleton & Lange, 1993.)

Materials: Gloves, lubricant, hemoccult paper and developer, sigmoido-scope and light source, insufflation bag, tissues, long (rectal) swabs and a suction catheter, proctologic examination table (not essential).

Procedure:

1. Enemas and cathartics are not given routinely before sigmoi-doscopy, although some clinicians prefer to give a mild prep, such as a Fleet's Enema, just before the exam. Have the patient sign a consent form.

2. Sigmoidoscopy can be performed with the patient in bed lying on his side in the knee-chest position, but the best results are obtained with the patient in the "jackknife" position on the proctologic table. Do not position the patient until all materials are at hand and you are ready to start.

3. Converse with the patient to create distraction and to relieve appre-hension. Announce each maneuver in advance. Put on gloves be-fore proceeding.

4. Observe the anal region for skin tags, hemorrhoids, fissures, etc. Do a careful rectal exam and Hemoccult test with a gloved finger and plenty of lubricant.

5. Lubricate the sigmoidoscope well and insert it with the obturator in place. Aim towards the patient's umbilicus initially. Advance 2–3 cm past the internal sphincter and remove the obturator.

6. Always advance under direct vision and make sure that the lumen is always visible (Figure III–10). Insufflation (introducing air) may be used to help visualize the lumen, but remember this may be painful to the patient. It is necessary to follow the curve of the sigmoid to-wards the sacrum by directing the scope more posteriorly towards the back. A change from a smooth mucosa to concentric rings sig-nifies entry into the sigmoid colon. The scope should reach 15 cm with ease. Use suction and the rectal swabs as needed to clear the way.

7. At this point, the sigmoid curves to the patient's left. Warn the patient that he may feel a cramping sensation. If you ever have difficulty ne-gotiating a curve, do not force the scope.

8. After advancing as far as possible, slowly remove the scope; use a small rotary motion to view all surfaces. Observation here is critical. Remember to release the air from the colon before withdrawing the scope.

9. Inform the patient that he may experience mild cramping after the procedure.

Complications: Bleeding, perforation, abdominal cramping.

18. Thoracentesis

Indications:

1. Diagnosis of pleural effusion,
2. Therapeutic removal of pleural fluid,

3. Instillation of sclerosing compounds (such as tetracycline) to obliterate the pleural space

Contraindications: Pneumothorax, hemothorax, or respiratory impairment in the contralateral side, coagulopathy (relative).

Materials: Prepackaged thoracentesis kit or minor procedure tray (see page 000) plus 20–60 mL syringe, 20 or 22 gauge needle 1½ inch needle, three-way stopcock, specimen containers.

Procedure:

1. It takes at least 300 mL of fluid to visualize a pleural effusion on a standard chest x-ray.
2. Discuss the procedure with the patient and obtain informed consent. Teach the patient the Valsalva maneuver or make sure the patient can hum. Some recommend oxygen supplementation by mask while performing thoracentesis.
3. The usual site for the thoracentesis is the posterolateral back over the diaphragm but under the fluid level. Percuss out the fluid level or use the chest x-ray and count out the ribs. The site will be above the rib to avoid the neurovascular bundle that travels below the rib.
4. Prep the area with povidone-iodine and drape. The patient should be sitting up comfortably, leaning slightly forward. The bed stand is helpful for this.
5. Make a skin wheal over the proposed site with a 25 gauge needle and 1% lidocaine. Change to a 22 gauge, 1½ inch needle and infiltrate up and over the rib; try to anesthetize the deeper structures and the pleura. During this time you should be aspirating back for pleural fluid. Once fluid returns, note the depth of the needle and mark it with a hemostat. This gives you an approximate depth. Remove the needle.
6. Measure the 15–18 gauge thoracentesis needle to the same depth as the first needle with a hemostat. Penetrate through the anesthetized area with the thoracentesis needle. You may also use a catheter over needle assembly (Angiocath) and leave the plastic catheter in position to remove the fluid. Always go over the top of the rib to avoid the neurovascular bundle that runs below the rib. Never pull the catheter back over the needle to prevent shearing. Attach the three-way stopcock and tubing and aspirate the amount needed. Turn the stopcock and evacuate the fluid through the tubing. **Never remove more than 1000 mL per tap!**
7. Have the patient hum or do the Valsalva maneuver as you withdraw the needle. This maneuver increases intrathoracic pressure and decreases the chances of a pneumothorax. Bandage the site.
8. Obtain a chest x-ray to evaluate the fluid level and to rule out a pneumothorax. An expiratory film may be best because it helps reveal a small pneumothorax.

TABLE III–7. DIFFERENTIAL DIAGNOSIS OF PLEURAL FLUID.
TRANSUDATE: NEPHROSIS, CONGESTIVE HEART FAILURE (CHF), CIRRHOSIS.
EXUDATE: INFECTION (PNEUMONIA, TB), MALIGNANCY, EMPYEMA, PERITONEAL DIALYSIS,
PANCREATITIS, CHYLOTHORAX.

Lab Value	Transudate	Exudate
Specific gravity	<1.016	>1.016
Protein (Pleural fluid)	<2.5 gm/100 mL	>3 gm/100 mL
Protein ratio (Pleural fluid to serum ratio)	<0.5	>0.5
LDH ratio (Pleural fluid to serum ratio)	<0.5	>0.6
Pleural fluid LDH	<200 IU	>200 IU
Fibrinogen (Clot)	No	Yes
Cell count and differential	Very low WBC	WBC >2500/μL
		Suspect an inflammatory exudate (early polys, later monos)

Grossly bloody tap: Trauma, pulmonary infarction, tumor, and iatrogenic causes.

pH: The pH of pleural fluid is usually >7.3. If between 7.2 and 7.3, suspect TB or malignancy or both. If <7.2, suspect an empyema.

Glucose: Normal pleural fluid glucose is ⅔ serum glucose pleural fluid glucose is **much** lower than serum glucose in effusions due to rheumatoid arthritis (0–16 mg/100 mL).

Triglycerides and postive sudan stain: Chylothorax.

9. Distribute specimens in containers, label slips, and send them to the lab. Always order pH, specific gravity, protein, LDH, cell count and differential, glucose, Gram's stain and cultures, acid-fast and fungal cultures, and smears. Optional lab studies are cytology if you suspect a malignancy, amylase if you suspect an effusion secondary to pancreatitis (usually on the left), and a Sudan stain and triglycerides if a chylothorax is suspected. See Table III–7 for the differential diagnosis.

Complications: Pneumothorax, hemothorax, infection, pulmonary laceration, hypotension.

19. Venous Cutdown

Indication: Venous access when percutaneous puncture is not practical.

Materials: Prepackaged cutdown tray **or** minor procedure tray and instrument tray (Table III–8) (see page 334) with silk suture (3-0, 4-0), catheter of choice (eg, Medicut, Angiocath).

Procedure (Figure III–11):

1. The most common site for a cutdown is the greater saphenous vein. The best location for a cutdown is approximately one fingerbreadth anterior and superior to the medial malleolus. Other sites on the foot, hand, or arm can be used.

2. Apply a tourniquet proximal to the site. Children may need to be restrained. Prep the skin with antiseptic solution, drape the patient, and put on sterile gloves.

3. Infiltrate the skin over the vein with 1% lidocaine. Incise the skin transversely.

4. Spread the incision in the direction of the vein with a hemostat until the excess tissue is cleaned off. Lift the vein off the posterior tissues.

5. Pass two chromic or silk ties (3-0 or 4-0) behind the vein. Tie off the distal vein. The upper tie is used for traction.

6. Make a transverse nick in the vein. You may need a catheter introducer ("banana") to hold open the lumen of the vein.

7. Insert the plastic catheter or IV cannula into the vein and tie the proximal suture to secure it in place. The catheter may also be inserted through a separate stab wound and then passed into the vein.

8. Attach the fluid, release the tourniquet, and close the skin with silk or nylon. Apply a sterile dressing.

TABLE III–8. MOST PROCEDURES CAN BE ACCOMPLISHED WITH COMMERCIALLY AVAILABLE KITS. IN THE EVENT THESE KITS ARE NOT AVAILABLE, THE FOLLOWING GUIDELINES ARE PROVIDED AND REFERRED TO IN EACH PROCEDURE SECTION WHERE APPROPRIATE. A USEFUL NEEDLE GAUGE AND FRENCH CATHETER GUIDE CAN BE FOUND IN FIGURE III–12, PAGE 336.

Minor procedure tray

- Sterile gloves
- Sterile towels/drapes
- 4 × 4 gauze sponges
- Povidone-iodine (Betadine) prep solution
- Syringes 5, 10, 20 mL
- Needles 18, 20, 22, 25 gauge
- 1% lidocaine (with or without epinephrine)
- Adhesive tape

Instrument tray

- Scissors
- Needle holder
- Hemostat
- Scalpel and blade (No. 10 for adult, No. 15 for children or delicate work)
- Suture of choice

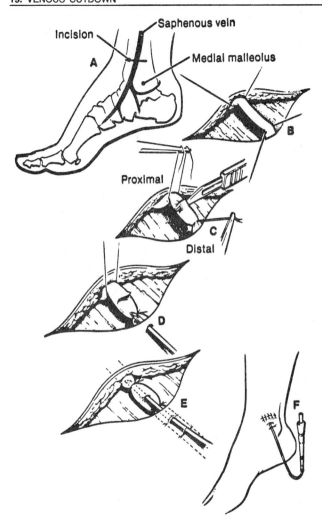

Figure III–11. Venous cutdown using the saphenous vein. Here the catheter is inserted through a separate stab wound. *(Reproduced, with permission, from Gomella LG (editor): Clinician's Pocket Reference, 5/e. Appleton-Century-Crofts, 1986.)*

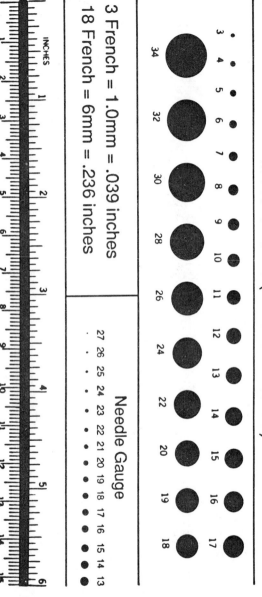

Figure III–12. French catheter guide and needle gauge reference.

IV. Fluids & Electrolytes

ORDERING IV FLUIDS

The following are general guidelines to ordering maintenance and replacement fluids in patients. Clinical judgment is needed to modify these appropriately.

A. Maintenance Fluids

    1. 70 kg male. D5 ¼ NS with 20 mEq KCl/L at 125 mL/hr.

    2. Other patients. Also use D5 ¼ NS with 20 mEq KCl/L. Determine their 24-hour water requirement by the following formula, called the "Kg Method":

- For the first 10 kg body weight: 100 mL/kg/d plus
- For the second 10 kg body weight: 50 mL/kg/d plus
- For weight above 20 kg: 20 ml/kg/d

and divide by 24 hours to determine the hourly rate.

    3. Pediatric patients. Use the same solution, but determine the daily fluid requirements by either of the following:

        a. Kg Method: As previously outlined.

        b. Meter Squared Method: Maintenance fluids are 1500 mL/m²/d. Divide by 24 to get the flow rate per hour. To calculate the surface area, use the body surface area charts in the Appendix.

B. Specific Replacement Fluids. Table IV–1 gives general guidelines to the daily production of various body fluids.

    1. Gastric (NG tube, emesis). D5 ½ NS with 20 mEq/L KCl.

TABLE IV–1. COMPOSITION AND DAILY PRODUCTION OF BODY FLUIDS.

Fluid	Na	Cl	K	HCO₃	Average Daily Production[1] (mL)
		(mEq/L)			
Sweat	50	40	5	0	Varies
Saliva	10	15	26	50	1500
Gastric juice	60–100	100	10	0	1500–2000
Duodenum	130	90	5	0–10	300–2000
Bile	145	100	5	15–35	100–800
Pancreatic juice	140	75	5	70–115	100–800
Ileum	140	100	5	15–30	2000–3000
Diarrhea	50	40	35	45	—

[1]In adults.

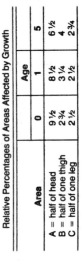

Relative Percentages of Areas Affected by Growth

Area	0	Age 1	5
A = half of head	9½	8½	6½
B = half of one thigh	2¾	3¼	4
C = half of one leg	2½	2½	2¾

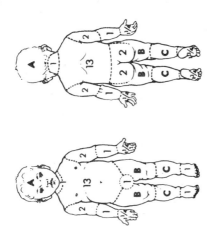

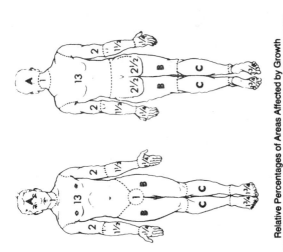

Relative Percentages of Areas Affected by Growth

Area	10	Age 15	Adult
A = half of head	5½	4½	3½
B = half of one thigh	4¼	4¼	4¾
C = half of one leg	3	3¼	3½

TABLE IV–2. COMPOSITION OF COMMONLY USED CRYSTALLOIDS.

Fluid	Glucose (gm/L)	Na	Cl (mEq/L)	K	Ca	HCO₃[1]	Mg	HPO₄	kcal/L
D5W (Dextrose 5% in water)	50	—	—	—	—	—	—	—	170
D10W (Dextrose 10% in water)	100	—	—	—	—	—	—	—	340
D20W (Dextrose 20% in water)	200	—	—	—	—	—	—	—	680
D50W (Dextrose 50% in water)	500	—	—	—	—	—	—	—	1700
1/2 NS[2] (0.45% NaCl)	—	77	77	—	—	—	—	—	0
3% NS[2]	513	513	—	—	—	—	—	—	0
NS[2] (0.9% NaCl)	—	154	154	—	—	—	—	—	0
D 5% 1/4 NS[2]	50	38	38	—	—	—	—	—	17
D 5% 1/2 NS[2] (0.45% NaCl)	50	77	77	—	—	—	—	—	17
D 5% NS[2] (0.9% NaCl)	50	154	154	—	—	—	—	—	17
D 5% Lactated Ringer's (D5LR)	50	130	110	4	3	27	—	—	18
Lactated Ringer's	—	130	110	4	3	27	—	—	<1
Ionosol MB	50	25	22	20	—	23	3	3	17
Normosol M	50	40	40	13	—	16	3	—	17

[1]HCO_3 is administered in these solutions as lactate that is converted to bicarbonate.
[2]NS = normal saline.

2. **Diarrhea.** D5LR with 15 mEq/L KCl. Use body weight as a re-placement guide (about 1 L for each 1 kg or 2.2 lb lost).
3. **Bile.** D5LR with 25 mEq/L (½ amp) of HCO_3.
4. **Pancreatic.** D5LR with 50 mEq/L (1 amp) HCO_3.
5. **Burn patients.** See Figure IV–1. Use the "Parkland Formula":

Total fluid required during the first 24 hours = (percentage of body burn) × (body weight in kg) × 4 mL.

Figure IV–1. Tables for estimating the extent of burns in adults and children. In adults, a reasonable system for calculating the percentage of body burned is the "Rule of nines": Each arm equals 9%; the head equals 9%; the anterior and posterior trunk each equal 18%; each leg equals 18%; and the perineum equals 1%. *(Reproduced, with permission, from Demling RH, Way LW: Burns & Other Thermal Injuries. In: Current Surgical Treatment & Diagnosis, 10/e. Way LW (editor). Appleton & Lange, 1994.)*

Replace with lactated Ringer's solution over 24 hours:

- ½ total over first 8 hours (from time of burn)
- ¼ total over second 8 hours
- ¼ total over third 8 hours.

COMPOSITION OF PARENTERAL FLUIDS

Parenteral fluids are generally classified based on molecular weight and oncotic pressure. Colloids are generally > 8000 dalton molecular weight and have high oncotic pressure (albumin, blood, dextran, hetastarch, plasma protein fraction). Crystalloids are < 8000 dalton molecular weight and have low oncotic pressure (most IV fluids, see Table IV–2 on page 339).

V. Nutritional Management of the Surgical Patient

Although the occurrence of malnutrition is well-described, suboptimal responses to therapeutic modalities occur in the malnourished patient and complications such as poor wound healing, impaired organ function and compromised immunity are observed. Therefore when the nutritional status of the patient is not addressed, clinical management of the patient is often more complex, and patient outcome may be compromised. Specialized nutritional support, whether enteral or parenteral, when used appropriately can help to prevent the nutrition related morbidities in the surgical patient population. However, the approach to specialized nutritional support may not always be clear. There is no data to support the use of routine nutritional support in the preoperative period except in the severely malnourished patient.

Assessment (Table V–1)

Differentiation of acute and chronic malnutrition is helpful in the decision of when to initiate specialized nutritional support. Acute malnutrition, also called kwashiorkor or acute hypoalbuminemia, is defined as starvation occurring during a catabolic stress such as surgery, infection, burn, or trauma and is a more aggressive nutritional insult than simple starvation for a brief period. Chronic malnutrition, also called **marasmus,** is characterized by growth retardation and wasting of muscle and subcutaneous fat while maintaining an appetite. Frequently in the surgical patient population, the two nutritional insults may be superimposed. The most recent guidelines from the American Society for Parenteral and Enteral Nutrition state, "patients should be considered malnourished or at risk of developing malnutrition if they have inadequate nutrient intake for 7 days or more or if they have a weight loss of 10% or more of their pre-illness body weight." The formula for determination of percentage weight loss is:

$$\% \text{ weight loss} = \frac{\text{usual weight} - \text{present weight}}{\text{usual weight}} \times 100$$

Formal evaluation is important to identify patients at nutritional risk and to provide a baseline to assess the achievement of therapeutic goals with the specialized nutritional support. The patient's history is useful to evaluate weight loss and dietary intolerance (eg, glucose or lactose and disease states that may influence nutritional tolerance). Anthropometric evaluations such as midarm muscle circumference (MAMC) and triceps skin fold (TSF) have much interobserver variability and are generally not useful unless performed by an experienced evaluator. Absolute lymphocyte count and response to skin test antigens provide insight to the patient's immune function.

TABLE V–1. PARAMETERS OF NUTRITIONAL ASSESSMENT.

Parameter	Type of Malnutrition	Comment
Weight loss	Chronic	Affected by volume status
Anthropometric measurements (MAMC, TSF[1])	Chronic	Interobserver variability
Lymphocyte count	Acute or chronic	Reflects immune function
Anergy testing	Acute or chronic	Reflects immune function
Albumin	Acute	Affected by hydration status
Prealbumin	Acute	More sensitive visceral protein marker of nutritional status than albumin
Retinol binding protein	Acute	Limited availability
Transferrin	Acute	Affected by iron status
Urinary urea nitrogen	Acute or chronic	Indicates nitrogen balance and efficacy of nutritional regimen. Potential for collection problems

[1]MAMC = midarm muscle circumference; TSF = triceps skin fold.

Visceral protein markers such as prealbumin and transferrin may be helpful in evaluating nutritional insult as well as catabolic stress. Although the most commonly quoted laboratory parameter of nutritional status is serum albumin, its concentration often reflects hydration status and metabolic response to injury (ie, the acute phase response) more than the nutritional state of the patient, especially in the patient with intravascular volume deficits. Because of its long half-life, albumin may be normal in the malnourished patient. Prealbumin is superior as an indicator of malnutrition only because of its shorter half-life. However, these serum proteins as an indicator of malnutrition are subject to the same limitations because they are affected by catabolic stress.

Urinary urea nitrogen collected over a 24 hour period is an important tool to evaluate nitrogen balance and the adequacy of the patient's nutritional regimen if the specimen is collected accurately.

- Nitrogen balance = Nitrogen input − nitrogen output
  1 g of nitrogen = 6.25 g of protein.
- Nitrogen input = Protein in grams/6.25 g nitrogen.
- Nitrogen output = 24-hour urinary urea nitrogen (UUN) + 4 g/d (nonurine loss).

Certain disease states, including high output fistulas or massive diarrhea, will increase the amount of nonurine losses for nitrogen. Fecal nitrogen measurements are difficult to obtain, but are most useful in the patient's assessment.

Example of Nitrogen Balance

A patient receives 2 L TPN per 24 hours with 27.5 g synthetic amino acid (protein) solution per liter.

1. 27.5 g protein/L $\times$ 2 L = 55 g protein/24 hours.
2. Recall that 1 g of nitrogen = 6.25 g of protein.
3. Nitrogen input = 55 g protein/6.25 g protein/gram N 8.8 gN
4. Patient voided 22.5 dL urine/24 hours with UUN 66 mg/dL
5. Nitrogen lost in urine = 22.5 dL $\times$ 66 mg/dL = 1485 mg or about 1.5 g
6. Add 4.0 g for nonurine nitrogen loss
7. Nitrogen output = 1.5 g + 4.0 = 5.5 g
8. Nitrogen balance = input − output = 8.8 − 5.5 = positive (+) 3.3 g nitrogen.

A positive nitrogen balance assures that the amount of protein being administered is sufficient to cover the losses of endogenous protein, which occur secondary to catabolism. This is the best therapeutic goal for TPN patients because statements as to whether the prescribed protein prevents muscle breakdown cannot be made. Once positive balance has been achieved, protein replacement has been optimized. This may not be possible in the acute phase of injury, in severe trauma or burn patients. Thus a minimization of loss (between −2 and −4 g/d) may be the goal during this period.

A negative nitrogen balance indicates insufficient protein replacement for the degree of skeletal muscle loss. Under most circumstances, an attempt to achieve positive balance should be made. Patients with renal dysfunction or severe stress may not be able to achieve a positive balance owing to safety concerns.

There are a number of considerations including preexisting illnesses and coexisting metabolic abnormalities commonly present in the critically ill patient. Preexisting conditions such as hepatic insufficiency, congestive heart failure, and renal impairment must be taken into consideration when instituting nutritional support. For example, a high carbohydrate load in patients with respiratory failure can lead to a significant increase in P_{CO_2}. In general, it is important to correct coexisting metabolic abnormalities, such as hypophosphatemia or hyperglycemia before instituting nutritional support, particularly parenteral nutrition. In general, other metabolic abnormalities are not critical to correct before instituting TPN.

The decision to begin nutritional support is not an "On-Call Problem" in the literal sense. It is never a decision that must be made late at night by the house officer. Rather, it should be a considered decision made by the team responsible for the care of the patient. Clear indications for nutritional support include:

- Weight loss >12% or more of body weight (or weight <85% of ideal body weight).
- Expected >5–7 days of no oral intake.
- Inadequate nutrient intake for 7 or more days.
- Albumin <3.5 g/dL, transferrin <200 mg/dL.

Hospital Diets

There are a number of standard dietary formulations available in the hospital. Most hospitals have a manual available for reference that provides details of the available diets. In addition, registered dieticians are available for consultation. This service should be used when questions arise about the use of specialized diets in the care of individual patients.

Regular. Used for adult patients without dietary restrictions. The composition is based on Recommended Dietary Allowances.

Soft. Calorically and nutritionally similar to a regular diet, but tender foods are used (this is not a ground/pureed diet). Useful in patients with oral problems preventing the chewing of food.

Mechanical Soft. Uses ground foods, also useful for those with chewing difficulties (eg, edentulous patients).

Pureed. Foods are ground finely, also useful in patients with difficulty chewing.

Clear Liquids. Usually used in the immediate preoperative or postoperative period, particularly in the transition from NPO to starting oral feedings. This diet leaves little residue and requires minimal digestive activity for absorption. In general, this diet should not be used for more than 3 days without supplementation.

Full Liquids. Includes foods that are liquid at room temperature, such as, milk or milk-products (eg, puddings, ice cream, etc). In the past, this diet was used widely as a transition diet from clear liquids to regular, but it is used less often now. This diet can be difficult for many patients because it contains high-fat, lactose-containing ingredients.

Low Fiber (Residue). Indicated for patients with colitis, ileitis, or diarrhea. Decreases fecal volume.

High Fiber. Useful for atonic constipation, diverticular disease, irritable bowel syndrome, and diabetes.

Diabetic (ADA). Used for patients with IDDM or NIDDM. These diets are prescribed at a specified number of calories per day (eg, 2000 calories ADA, 2400 calories ADA, etc). Assessment by a clinical dietician helps to determine the appropriate calorie level, as well as help the patient maintain the correct diet after leaving the hospital.

Reduction. Used to assist in weight loss to achieve ideal body weight. Assessment by a clinical dietician is helpful in determining the appropriate calorie level.

Pediatric. Usually ordered as "Diet for age."

Hyperlipidemia. Used for patients with lipid abnormalities. Diet is written as type I, IIa, IIb, III, IV, or V depending on the diagnosis.

Low Fat. Designed to limit fat intake to approximately 50 g/d. Indicated for some diseases of the gallbladder, liver, or pancreas.

Protein Restricted. Useful in patients with renal failure or hepatic disorders. Specify number of grams of protein to be given.

Sodium Restricted. Used for the management of patients with congestive heart failure (CHF), hypertension, or other diseases resulting in fluid retention. Specify amount of sodium in milligrams or grams. Sodium restriction at levels <1000 mg/d is not recommended because of the poor palatability of such diets.

5–6 g sodium	Includes table salt, average person in the United States consumes 12.5–15 g salt.
4 g sodium	Regular diet without added salt, approx 180 mEq = 10 g salt.
2 g sodium	Restricted sodium diet, no sodium in food preparation, avoids processed meats. Practical for home use with a cooperative patient, approx 87 mEq sodium or 5 g salt.
1 g sodium	Limitations of most foods including breads. Practical for home use only with an exceptionally cooperative patient, approx 2.5 g salt.

Potassium Restricted. Used mostly for patients with renal failure. Specify in grams or milliequivalents. A typical renal diet is limited to 40 mEq of potassium daily.

Nutritional Requirements

Overall, nutritional requirements are the same whether feeding the patient enterally or parenterally. Appropriate calculations of calories and protein are important to achieve optimal anabolism while avoiding the metabolic complications associated with overfeeding.

Caloric Requirements. Caloric requirements are dictated by the patient's needs for energy to support metabolic processes and activity. Catabolic patients with stresses from infections, burns, surgery, or trauma require additional energy to allow for the increased basal metabolic rate and increased metabolic demands associated with these conditions. Using the appropriate weight to predict energy needs is important for the patient who is not at ideal body weight. For an underweight patient, it is important to use the actual weight to avoid the complications associated with overfeeding. Similarly, for the overweight patient, it is important to estimate the amount of mass that is metabolically active to avoid unnecessary metabolic stress. This weight is 25% of the difference between the ideal weight and the actual weight added to the ideal weight.

Ideal body weight:

Males: 50 kg + 2.3 kg/in >5 feet.
Females: 45.5 kg + 2.3 kg/in >5 feet.

Metabolically active weight for obese patients:

(Actual weight − ideal body weight) × 0.25 + ideal body weight.

The amount of energy to support metabolic process can be estimated from a number of equations or a nomogram. The Harris-Benedict equation is frequently used to provide an estimation of basal energy expenditure (see below). The predicted basal energy expenditure should be approximately 22 kcal/kg when calculated correctly. To estimate a patient's caloric requirement, the basal energy expenditure is multiplied by a factor for activity and injury.

Factors used to adjust the basal energy expenditure are less than originally published as the risks of overfeeding became apparent. Modified factors can be seen in Table V–2. Overall, total caloric provision (protein + nonprotein calories) should not exceed 25–30 kcal/kg for the nonstressed patient and 30–35 kcal/kg for the catabolically stressed patient. The burn victim will have higher requirements based on the amount of body surface area involved. In general, target nutritional support can be estimated to be:

Nonstressed: 25–30 kcals/kg/d.
Stressed: 30–35 kcals/kg/d.

Protein Requirements. Protein is required to minimize endogenous net catabolism by supporting anabolic processes. Daily maintenance protein requirements are 0.8–1 g/kg. Patients with mild to moderate physiologic stress require 1.2–1.5 g/kg/d. Those with severe injuries may require as much as 2.5 g/kg/d. Protein administration may be limited by relative hepatic or renal insufficiency. In patients with a history of hepatic encephalopathy, protein doses >0.8 g/kg are rarely tolerated. Such patients may benefit from amino acid formulations with higher concentrations of branched chain amino acids.

Carbohydrates & Fat. Generally, the caloric goal is achieved using carbohydrate and fat when feeding a patient parenterally. The protein is not counted as calories in the acutely stressed patient. Conceptually, this is to provide adequate calories for nitrogen incorporation and to allow adequate protein for tissue anabolism, although this practice differs in various medical centers. Optimal calorie to nitrogen ratios to achieve nutritional anabolism are estimated to 150:1 for the nonstressed patient and 100:1 in the catabolic patient. On the average, protein is comprised of 16% nitrogen.

TABLE V–2. CALCULATION OF CALORIC REQUIREMENTS. THE CALCULATION RELIES ON THE HARRIS-BENEDICT EQUATION FOR MEN AND WOMEN AND IS ADJUSTED FOR ACTIVITY LEVEL OR INJURY FACTORS.

Caloric requirement (men) = 66.47 + (13.75 × wgt[kg]) + (5.0 × hgt [cm])
    − (6.76 × age [yrs]) × (activity factor) × (injury factor)

Caloric requirement (women) = 655.10 + (9.56 × wgt[kg]) + (1.85 × hgt [cm])
    − (4.68 × age [yrs]) × (activity factor) × (injury factor)

Activity	Factor
Paralyzed	1.1
Confined to bed	1.2
Out of bed	1.3
Normal activity	1.5
Injury (choose highest factors)	
Surgery	
Minor	1.1
Major	1.1–1.3
Infection	
Minor	1.1
Severe	1.1–1.3
Trauma	
Skeletal	1.2–1.3
Head injury with steroids	1.6
Burns	
Up to 20% BSA[1]	1–1.5
20–40% BSA	1.5–1.85
>40% BSA	1.85–1.95

[1]BSA = % body surface area.

The majority of calories are provided as carbohydrate. This is consistent with the typical diet. Carbohydrate administration, either enterally or parenterally may be limited owing to hyperglycemia, increased CO_2 production, or fatty liver infiltration. Generally, the maximal glucose administration tolerated is 4–5 mg/kg/min or 20–25 kcal/kg/d.

A minimum amount of fat needs to be given to the parenterally fed patient to prevent the development of essential fatty acid deficiency (EFAD). This minimum is 4% of the total calories in the form of linoleic acid. However, additional fat calories are used to provide energy and to decrease the metabolic stress of glucose in the intolerant patient. Maximal intravenous fat administration is between 1 and 2.5 g/kg/d. Fat emulsions should not be infused in patients with triglyceride values >300–400 mg/dL. Although at one time, practitioners considered intravenous fat emulsion contraindicated in pancreatitis, IV fat may be a better tolerated fuel source in patients with pancreatitis without hypertriglyceridemia.

Intravenous fat emulsion has been associated with impaired immune function in animal studies. For this reason, IV fat emulsion should not be administered to acutely septic patients or during the immediate perioperative period.

Determining the Route of Nutritional Support

Having determined that nutritional support is indicated, select the route to be utilized. Clinical and laboratory studies demonstrate that the intestinal tract plays a critical role in the progress of numerous disease states. Enteral nutrition helps to preserve gut morphology, is better tolerated metabolically, and is less expensive. In addition, in animal studies, enteral nutrition has been shown to prevent translocation of bacteria across the gut mucosa; therefore, enteral nutrition may have a role in preventing septicemia although this has not been demonstrated in humans yet. Furthermore, there is no advantage to parenteral nutrition in the patient with a functioning gastrointestinal tract. Parenteral nutrition does not achieve greater anabolism nor provide greater control over a patient's nutritional regimen. Thus, parenteral nutrition is indicated only when the enteral route is not usable. In other words: **"If the gut works, use it."**

The factors involved in choosing the route for enteral nutrition include the duration, gastrointestinal tract pathophysiology, and the risk for aspiration. Nasally placed tubes are the most frequently used. Patient comfort is maximized when a small bore flexible tube is used. However, such tubes do not allow aspiration for residual volumes that may be significant if gastric emptying is questionable. Patients at risk for aspiration require longer tubes into the jejunum or duodenum. When long-term feeding is anticipated, a tube enterostomy is required. Percutaneous endoscopic gastrostomy tubes (PEG) are usually placed without general anesthesia. However, patients with tumors, gastrointestinal obstruction, adhesions, or abnormal anatomy may require open surgical placement. A jejunal feeding tube may be threaded through a PEG for small bowel feeding. The placement of a needle catheter or Witzel jejunostomy during surgery generally allows earlier postoperative feeding with an elemental formulation than if one needed to wait for the return of gastric emptying and colonic function (see page 311 for enteral tube placement procedures).

Some patients, because of their disease states, are unable to be fed enterally and require parenteral feedings. Enteral nutrition is avoided in patients with active, massive gastrointestinal bleeding, obstruction, high-output fistulas, or short-gut syndrome. Other contraindications for enteric feeding include severe diarrhea of small bowel origin, peritonitis, severe acute pancreatitis, shock, or intestinal hypomotility.

1. ENTERAL NUTRITION: Enteral nutrition is best tolerated when instilled into the stomach because there are less problems with osmolarity or feeding volumes. Remember that the stomach serves as a barrier to hyperosmolarity, thus the use of isotonic feedings is mandated only when instilling nutrients directly into the small intestine. The use of gastric feedings is thus preferable and should be used whenever appropriate. Patients at risk for aspiration or with impaired gastric emptying may need to be fed past the pylorus into the jejunum or the duodenum. Feedings via a jejunostomy placed at the time of surgery can often be initiated on the first postoperative day obviating the need for parenteral nutrition.

Although enteral nutrition is generally safer than parenteral nutrition, aspiration can be a significant morbid event in the care of the patient. Appropriate monitoring for residual volumes in addition to keeping the head of the bed elevated can help prevent this complication. A significant residual may be defined as 1½ times the instillation rate. This can be treated in a number of ways. There may be a transient postoperative ileus treated best by waiting. Metoclopramide, erythromycin, or cisapride may be useful pharmacologic therapy. Patients who have been tolerating feedings and develop a new high residual should be carefully assessed for the cause, concentrating on intra-abdominal infections.

The question of when to start enteral feedings in the postoperative patient needs to be clarified. Often, the presence of bowel sounds is used as the single criterion. It is important to realize that the presence of bowel sounds may not be a reliable indicator of gastrointestinal motility. The passage of flatus indicates colonic motility, and because the colon is the last part of the gastrointestinal tract to regain motility after laparotomy in most cases, this may be a more useful indicator.

However, a more global approach to assessment of the gastrointestinal tract is warranted. If feeding into the stomach, gastric emptying should be evaluated. Generally, if an adult patient "puts out" <600 mL per 24 hour shift on nasogastric suction, the pylorus is functioning appropriately. Minimal gastrointestinal output should be collected on straight drain. Clamping of the nasogastric tube to evaluate gastric emptying is contraindicated as it exposes the patient to the risk of aspiration unnecessarily. Tolerance to enteral feeding can be assessed with the instillation of an isotonic diet given for 24 hours at 30 mL/hr as a trial. Feeding intolerance is characterized by vomiting, abdominal distention, diarrhea, or high gastric residual volumes.

The nutritional components and osmolality of the enteral product help classify the formulations to simplify selection. The protein component can be supplied as intact proteins, partially digested hydrolyzed proteins, or crystalline amino acids. Each gram of protein provides 4 calories when oxidized. The carbohydrate source may be intact complex starches, glucose polymers, or simpler disaccharides such as sucrose. Carbohydrates provide 4 calories/g. Fat in enteral products usually is supplied as long-chain fatty acids. However, some enteral products contain medium-chain triglycerides (MCT), which are transported directly in the portal circulation rather than via chyle production. Because MCT oil does not contain essential fatty acids, it cannot be used as the sole fat source. Long-chain fatty acids provide 9 calories/g and MCT oil provides 8 calories/g.

The osmolality of an enteral product is determined primarily by the concentration of carbohydrates, electrolytes, amino acids, or small peptides.

The clinical importance of osmolality is often debated. Hyperosmolal formulations with osmolalities exceeding 450 mosm/L may contribute to diarrhea by acting in a manner similar to osmotic cathartics. Hyperosmolal feedings are well tolerated when delivered into the stomach (as opposed to the small bowel) because gastric secretions dilute the feeding before it leaves the pylorus to traverse the small bowel. Thus, feedings administered directly to the small bowel (eg, via feeding jejunostomy) should not exceed 450 mosm/L.

Based on osmolality and macronutrient content, the clinician can classify enteral products into several categories. Low osmolality formulas are isotonic and contain intact macronutrients. They usually provide 1 calorie/mL and require approximately 2 L to provide the RDA for vitamins. These products are appropriate for the general patient population. Two examples are Ensure and Isocal.

High-density formulas may provide up to 2 calories/mL. These concentrated solutions are hyperosmolar and also contain intact nutrients. The RDA for vitamins can be met with volumes of 1500 mL or less. These products are used for volume restricted patients. Examples are Nutren 2.0 and Ensure Plus HN Liquid.

Chemically defined or elemental formulas provide the macronutrients in the predigested state. These formulations are usually hyperosmolar and have poor palatability. Patients with compromised nutrient absorptive abilities or gastrointestinal function may benefit from elemental type feedings. Vivonex TEN and Peptamen are two such products.

Several enteral formulas have been developed that have been altered for various disease states. Products for pulmonary patients, such as Pulmocare, contain a higher percent of calories from fat to decrease the carbon dioxide load from the metabolism of excess glucose. A low carbohydrate, high-fat product for persons with diabetes, is available that also contains fiber that may help regulate glucose control. Other fiber containing enteral feedings are available to help regulate bowel function, eg, Enrich. Patients with hepatic insufficiency may benefit from formulations containing a higher concentration of the branched chain amino acids and less aromatic amino acids in an attempt to correct their altered serum amino acid profile, eg, Hepatic-Aid II. Formulas containing only essential amino acids have been marketed for the renal failure patient. The clinical usefulness of many specialty products remains controversial.

Oral supplements differ from other enteral feedings by design so that they are more palatable to improve compliance. Furthermore, oral supplements contain lactose, which is inappropriate for patients with lactase deficiency; whereas, most enteral products do not contain lactose.

Guidelines for ordering enteral feedings are outlined in Table V–3. In summary, when using enteral feedings–

- Determine nutritional needs.
- Assess gastrointestinal tract function and appropriateness of enteral feedings.
- Determine fluid requirements and volume tolerance based on overall status and concurrent disease states.

TABLE V-3. ROUTINE ORDERS FOR ENTERAL NUTRITION.

1. Confirm tube placement.
2. Elevate head of bed to 45 degrees.
3. Check gastric residuals in patients receiving gastric feedings. Hold feedings if >1.5–2× infusion rate. Significant residuals should be reinstilled and rechecked in 1 hour. If continues to be elevated, hold tubefeeding and begin NG suction.
4. Check patient's weight 3 times per week.
5. Record strict input and output (I&O).
6. Routine laboratory studies.

- Select an appropriate enteral feeding product.
- Verify that the regimen selected satisfies micronutrient requirements.
- Monitor and assess nutritional status to evaluate the need for changes in the selected regimen.

Complications of Enteral Nutrition

A. Diarrhea: A common complication of enteral feeding is diarrhea. It occurs in about 10–60% of patients receiving enteral feedings. The clinician must be certain to evaluate the patient for other causes of diarrhea (see Section I, Problem 22, page 84). Formula-related causes include contamination, excessive cold temperature, lactose intolerance, osmolality, and the method and/or route of delivery. Eliminate potential causes before using antidiarrheal medications:

- Check medication profile for possible drug-induced cause.
- Rule out *C difficile* colitis in patients receiving antibiotics.
- Attempt to decrease rate.
- Change formulation: Limit lactose, reduce osmolality.
- Pharmacologic therapy used only after eliminating treatable causes.

B. Constipation: Although less common than diarrhea, constipation can occur in the enterally fed patient. Check to be sure that adequate fluid volume is being given. Patients with additional requirements may benefit from water boluses or dilution of the enteral formulation. Fiber can be added to help regulate bowel function.

C. Aspiration: Aspiration is a serious complication of enteral feedings and is more likely to occur in the patient with diminished mental status. The best approach here is prevention by elevating the patient's head and carefully monitoring residual fluid volume. Any patient suspected of possible aspiration or assessed to be at increased risk of aspiration before instituting enteral feedings should be further evaluated and may not be a candidate for gastric feedings, necessitating small bowel feedings (see Section I, Problem 8, page 28).

D. Drug Interactions: The vitamin K content of various enteral products varies from 22 µg to 156 µg per 1000 calories. This can significantly affect the anticoagulation profile of a patient receiving warfarin. Tetracycline products should not be administered 1 hour before or 2 hours after enteral feedings to avoid the inhibition of absorption. Similarly, enteral feedings should be stopped 2 hours before and after the administration of phenytoin.

2. PARENTERAL NUTRITION:

Peripheral Versus Central Parenteral Nutrition. The use of total parenteral nutrition (TPN) necessitates a central venous catheter with its concomitant risks.

Although some patients require parenteral nutrition, they have additional nutritional needs that can be met better with the use of peripherally administered parenteral nutrition (PPN).

The limiting factor in the use of PPN is the osmolality of the solution. Because centrally administered fluids are rapidly diluted at the catheter tip, osmolality is not a concern, whereas peripherally administered fluids of high osmolality rapidly result in venous sclerosis owing to the relatively low flow and slow dilution of these fluids. Thus, only patients with modest nutritional requirements will be able to meet these criteria for the necessarily low-calorie-containing solutions that can be administered peripherally.

PPN can be up to 900 mosm/kg and can be prepared from amino acid mixtures (5%), dextrose solutions (10%), and fat emulsions (20%). They have a low caloric density (0.3–0.6 kcal/mL) compared to TPN solutions and can thus only provide 1200–2300 kcal/d in 2000–3500 mL of solution. Thus, with PPN, the ability to provide caloric needs in relatively small volumes is lost; this may be clinically significant in patients requiring fluid restriction.

In general, the largest bore intravenous catheter should be used. The site should be changed frequently, usually every 72 hours. Fat emulsion can be given through a Y-connector or using a three-in-one bag as is commonly used for centrally administered parenteral nutrition. Septic complications are uncommon, but thrombophlebitis can occur at the infusion site.

While peripherally administered parenteral nutrition alleviates some of the complications associated with central TPN, its use is limited by the inability to provide the level of nutritional support frequently needed in the surgical patient. Patients with large nutritional requirements owing to stress or chronic malnutrition, high electrolyte needs, fluid restrictions, or prolonged intravenous feeding are inappropriate candidates for PPN.

Prescribing Total Parenteral Nutrition (Central TPN). Central vein infusions allow greater concentrations of both macronutrients and electrolytes. Therefore, central TPN is much more flexible in meeting a patient's requirements. With the use of permanent types of catheters (eg, the tunneled subclavian catheter, the implantable port, or a peripherally inserted central line), TPN can be administered in the hospital or home setting depending on the patient's overall clinical condition.

When calculating caloric provision of parenteral nutrition, intravenous fat emulsion 10% provides 1.1 kcal/mL, and 20% provides 2 kcal/mL.

Intravenous dextrose provides 3.4 kcal/g rather than 4 kcal/g because it is a monohydrate and therefore less calorically dense.

Centrally administered TPN is given through a central venous catheter (placed percutaneously or an operatively placed tunneled catheter) (see Section III, page 295). The solutions are usually >1900 mosm/kg and contain at least 1 kcal/mL. Thus the usual infusion of 2000–2500 L/d provides at least 2000–2500 kcal/d. This is sufficient to meet the needs of most surgical patients.

The solutions are formulated in the hospital pharmacy and are typically ordered using a standard "check-list" available in most hospitals. A commonly used method uses a single infusion bag containing all components to be infused over a 24-hour period. A typical 24-hour single bag will contain:

Amino acids (10%)	1000 mL
Dextrose (50%)	500 mL
Fat emulsion (20%)	500 mL
Total	2000 mL

Electrolytes and vitamins to create a solution containing all nutrient requirements:

Sodium	30	mEq/L
Potassium	30	mEq/L
Phosphate	15	mmol/L
Magnesium	8	mEq/L
Calcium gluconate	4.7	mEq/L
Chloride	50	mEq/L
Acetate	70	mEq/L

The values given here represent commonly used amounts, but must be adapted to the nutritional and electrolyte needs of individual patients, as well as taking into account concurrent disease states, such as renal or hepatic failure.

Electrolyte administration must be changed to reflect losses as well. Salts are usually administered as chloride or acetate, usually in similar amounts. However, patients losing fluid by nasogastric suction require increased amounts of chloride. Similarly, patients with high output pancreatic or small bowel fistulae will require more acetate.

Trace elements are added daily. Commercially available mixtures are usually adequate to provide needed amounts. Similarly, vitamins are usually added as pre-made mixtures. In addition to these mixtures (eg, MVI-12 Table V–4), the clinician must administer vitamin K, 5–10 mg IM weekly. Increased amounts of zinc are necessary with small bowel losses.

Trace element	Parenteral daily dose
Zinc	2.5–6 mg
Copper	0.3–0.5 mg
Selenium	20–50 μg
Chromium	10–15 μg
Manganese	0.4–8 mg

TABLE V-4. VITAMINS PROVIDED BY TWO VIALS
OF MVI-12.

Ascorbic acid	100 mg
Vitamin A	1 mg
Vitamin D	5 µg
Biotin	60 µg
Folic acid	40 µg
Vitamin B_{12}	5 µg
Pyridoxine (B_6)	4 mg
Dexpanthenol	15 mg
Vitamin E	10 mg
Thiamine (B_1)	3 mg
Riboflavin (B_2)	3.6 mg

Starting TPN (Table V–5). TPN is usually begun at 25–50 mL/hr, with increases of 25 mL/h until the precalculated final rate is achieved. Glucose is carefully monitored, especially in the early phase of TPN administration because glucose intolerance is very common. Be sure to check serum electrolytes (especially PO_4-) and glucose before starting TPN. Remember that glucose intolerance in a patient who had normal glucose levels while on TPN may be an early sign of sepsis. If a patient is undergoing surgery, the TPN usually is tapered to help prevent stress related hyperglycemia (usually ⅓–½) and assist in fluid administration.

TABLE V–5. SAMPLE ORDERS FOR PATIENTS ON CENTRAL TOTAL PARENTERAL
NUTRITION (TPN).

Routine orders on starting TPN
   Specify infusion (typically start 25–50 mL/hr for 24 hours; if tolerating well, especially
      sugars, can increase up to 2 L/d)
   Daily electrolytes
   Liver function tests twice weekly
   CBC daily
   Vital signs qshift
   Fingerstick blood sugar qshift
   Strict intake and output
   Prealbumin

Routine orders once stabilized on TPN
   Electrolytes and liver function tests twice weekly
   Weight weekly
   Prealbumin (weekly)
   Urinary nitrogen (weekly)

Stopping TPN. Although commonly practiced, weaning is generally not necessary. Most patients tolerate cessation of TPN, especially if they are taking oral nutrition at the time TPN is stopped. If there are concerns about hypoglycemia, the TPN rate can be halved for 1 hour and then stopped completely.

Complications. Complications associated with parenteral nutrition are generally divided into mechanical, infectious, and metabolic problems.

A. *Mechanical Complications:* Following placement of the central venous catheter, a chest x-ray is obtained to evaluate the tip position and the presence of a pneumothorax. The tip should be at the atrial-caval junction. A catheter tip well into the right ventricle can cause arrhythmias and may damage the tricuspid valve. Pneumo- and hydrothorax should be treated with appropriate chest tube drainage.

B. *Infectious Complications:* The use of central lines always has the potential for infectious problems. Always consider infection in a patient with new glucose intolerance on TPN. The line is usually the source of infection. Once suspected, the line should be removed. If TPN is still necessary, then a new site should be used. The catheter tip should be carefully removed and cultured. Secondary infection of the catheter, seeding from another septic site is also possible and also may necessitate catheter removal.

C. *Hyperglycemia:* The most frequently occurring metabolic complication is hyperglycemia. Hyperglycemia for the patient receiving TPN is defined as a glucose >200 mg/dL. The approach to hyperglycemia should be dictated by first determining its cause. The initial step in this process is to assess the appropriateness of overall caloric provisions and to clarify the fuel sources. Carbohydrate calories in excess of 30–35 kcal/kg should be decreased. In patients who are diabetic, on steroids, or otherwise glucose intolerant, glucose in excess of 150–200 g/d may be tolerated poorly. Fat calories should be increased to approximately 30% of the nonprotein calories in the nonseptic patient. If after adjustments hyperglycemia persists, a review of the patients clinical condition and medications is warranted.

Patients with new onset hyperglycemia should always be evaluated for an infection. Corticosteroids are the leading culprit in hyperglycemia. In patients with infections or changing steroid doses management of hyperglycemia can be achieved with sliding scale insulin or insulin infusions if the patient is in ICU. Insulin should not be incorporated in the TPN of patients with new onset hyperglycemia because their hyperglycemia is due to increased hepatic gluconeogenesis as well as a relative insulin resistance, not to a lack of endogenously released insulin. Hyperglycemia associated with parenteral nutrition generally requires aggressive sliding scale coverage (Table V–6.) Only regular insulin should be used to manage hyperglycemia in TPN patients. Patients who are stable on a given amount of insulin may have the insulin placed in the TPN bag.

Insulin infusions are typically compounded by adding 150 units of regular insulin to 150 mL of 0.9% sodium chloride. The infusion is started at

TABLE V–6. SLIDING SCALE DOSAGE FOR SUBCUTANEOUS INSULIN ADMINISTRATION.

	Dose of Regular Insulin (in units)	
Blood Sugar (mg/dl)	Adequate Renal Function	Renal Failure
200–250	5	2
251–300	10	4
301–350	15	6
351–400	20	8

1–2 U/hr and titrated upward to control the glucose at 200 mg/dL. When insulin infusions exceed 8–10 U/hr, insulin resistance is occurring. At this point, it is often best to discontinue the TPN and to correct the hyperglycemia.

D. *Refeeding Syndrome:* Often when malnutrition is recognized, the inclination is to rapidly and aggressively initiate specialized nutritional support. Unfortunately, this approach is associated with more hazards than the underlying malnutrition. The refeeding syndrome and morbidity associated with overfeeding are real clinical hazards associated with both parenteral and enteral nutrition. The refeeding syndrome is a constellation of severe fluid and electrolyte shifts associated with initiating nutrition in the chronically malnourished individual.

Typically, hypophosphatemia, hypomagnesemia, and hypokalemia are the electrolyte abnormalities that can result in cardiac and respiratory dysfunction and failure. Thiamine deficiency, hyperglycemia, and volume overload have also occurred. The best approach to the refeeding syndrome is prevention. TPN should be started at no more than 1000 kcals or 20 kcal/kg on the first day and titrated based on patient tolerance as defined by glucose monitoring and electrolyte values. Empiric replacement of vitamins, phosphorous, magnesium, and potassium is appropriate in the patient at risk.

E. *Electrolyte Abnormalities:* In general, when electrolyte deficiencies are present in the patient before initiating TPN, it is best to correct the problems and delay intravenous feeding. Electrolyte deficiencies that occur once the patient is receiving parenteral nutrition should be corrected with runs outside of the parenteral nutrition. If the patient has increased maintenance requirements because of chronic gastrointestinal losses or other reasons, the maintenance requirements should be incorporated into the parenteral nutrition mixture. The use of inadequate or excessive amounts of any additive results in the corresponding electrolyte abnormality. The amount of the corresponding electrolyte must be adjusted to correct the abnormality.

F. *Acid-Base Disturbances:* Hyperchloremic metabolic acidosis is fairly common in patients receiving TPN and may result from bicarbonate loss, which can be caused by severe diarrhea, pancreatic fistulas, or small bowel losses. The treatment is to administer more Na and K as acetate salts (instead of the Cl salt) because the acetate covers the amino acids in the TPN.

G. *Impaired Liver Function Tests:* Hepatic and biliary complications associated with parenteral nutrition are generally characterized by the duration of parenteral nutrition. Abnormal liver function tests are common in both short-term and long-term patient populations. The most common hepatic complication associated with short-term TPN administration is hepatic steatosis. This fatty liver infiltration is thought to be a result of overfeeding, especially of carbohydrate calories. The incidence of hepatic steatosis has decreased with the introduction of IV fat emulsion and the growing consideration of conservative caloric feeding. Biliary sludge formation and cholelithiasis with its associated complications have been noted in patients receiving TPN for 3 weeks or longer. Biliary stasis owing to the lack of stimulation resulting from bowel rest or short-gut is thought to be the primary mechanism. Long-term TPN administration is associated with hepatic steatonecrosis. Its pathogenesis is unclear at this time.

The diagnosis of TPN-associated hepatotoxicity is a diagnosis of exclusion. Once other causes have been ruled out, management of hepatotoxicity includes reformulation of the caloric regimen, cyclic administration of TPN, and metronidazole.

H. *Prerenal Azotemia:* Excessive amino acid infusion with inadequate calorie administration can result in prerenal azotemia. A rising BUN should be monitored, but probably not treated until it is >100 mg/dL. This is treated by reducing the amino acid intake and increasing calories administered as glucose. Prerenal azotemia resulting from intravascular volume depletion should be ruled out.

I. *Bleeding Abnormalities:* These can be caused by inadequate amounts of vitamin K, iron deficiency, folate deficiency, or vitamin B_{12} deficiency. Adjust the nutrient administration to the required amount.

J. *Overfeeding:* It is imperative to nutritionally support a patient on a rational and quantitative basis. In order to do this, the clinician must know the requirements for each nutritional component. Energy requirements are dependent on gender, weight, height, age, energy expenditure, and seriousness of the injury. Overfeeding places patients at risk for hepatic complications, increased carbon dioxide production, and hyperglycemia.

3. TPN IN SPECIFIC DISEASE STATES:

Cardiac Failure. Fluid administration is limited in these patients. Instead of the usual 1 mL water per calorie (as in tube feedings), water is given at 0.5 mL/calorie. Alternatively, water can be given at a rate equal to 500 mL (insensible losses) plus measured losses. Protein can be limited to 0.8–1 g/kg, and sodium limited to 0.5–1.5 g/d.

Diabetes. Use increased calories from fat in these patients to limit the carbohydrate calories while providing sufficient calories for protein anabolism. Insulin can be added to the bag in a patient with stable insulin requirements. In general, fat should provide no more than 50% of total caloric intake and no more than 2.5 g/kg/d.

Hepatic Dysfunction. Patients with hepatic dysfunction usually benefit from increased amounts of branched chain amino acids (eg, leucine, valine and isoleucine) and reduced amounts of aromatic amino acids, which are precursors to centrally active amines and thus contribute to hepatic encephalopathy. Specialized mixtures of amino acids are available and should be used only in patients with hepatic encephalopathy. Lipid emulsions should be limited in those with severe hepatic dysfunction.

Renal Disease. These patients have a number of specific restrictions that must be carefully accounted for in the administration of TPN including fluid, protein, potassium, magnesium, and sodium. Protein must be restricted to 0.6–0.8 g/kg/d in patients not undergoing dialysis. Patients receiving hemodialysis generally require 1.2 g/kg of protein per day, and patients undergoing peritoneal dialysis need 1.5 g/kg. The latter patient also absorbs approximately 500 kcals/d of dextrose from the dialysate, which needs to be taken into account when designing their nutritional regimen. Patients on hemodialysis may receive the usual protein load of 1–1.5 g/kg/d. Specially formulated amino acid mixtures are used in these patients containing higher amounts of essential amino acids. In general, TPN should not contain potassium or magnesium in renal failure patients. Reduced sodium may also be necessary.

Pulmonary Dysfunction. Carbohydrate metabolism (including overfeeding) results in production of CO_2. Thus, patients with impaired ventilation, who already may retain CO_2, are further stressed if high carbohydrate loads are administered. This may be treated by increasing the percentage of calories provided by fat (up to 50%). Overall, calories should not exceed 30–35 kcal/kg. These patients also may be sensitive to phosphate depletion and should be monitored carefully for the development of hypophosphatemia. Once identified, this is treated with phosphate supplementation.

REFERENCES

ASPEN Board of Directors. Guidelines for the use of parenteral and enteral nutrition in adult and pediatric patients. J Parent and Ent Nutr 1993;17:6SA.

Gomella LG (editor): Total parenteral nutrition. In: *Clinician's Pocket Reference,* 7/e. Appleton & Lange, 1993.

McCarthy MC: Nutritional support in the critically ill surgical patient. Surg Clin NA 1991;71:831.

Rombeau JL, Rolandelli RH, Wilmore DW: Nutritional support. In: *Care of the Surgical Patient,* Wilmore DW et al (editors). Scientific American, 1989.

Rosen GH: An overview of enteral nutrition. *Pharmacy Times.* Sept 1991:33.

VI. Blood Component Therapy

BLOOD BANKING PROCEDURES

Type & Screen (T & S): The blood bank will type the patient's blood and screen it for antibodies. If a rare antibody is found, the physician will usually be notified, and if it is likely that blood will be needed, the type and screen order may be changed to a type and cross.

Type & Cross (T & C): The blood bank will type and screen the patient's blood and match the patient with specific donor units. If the request is made "stat," the bank will set up blood immediately and usually hold it for 12 hours. For routine requests, the blood is set up at a date and time that the physician specifies, and the blood is usually held for 36 hours.

PREOPERATIVE BLOOD SET UP

Many institutions have established parameters for setting up blood before procedures. General guidelines are given here for the number of units of packed red cells or if only a type and screen (T & S) is requested (Table VI–1).

BLOOD BANK PRODUCTS & BLOOD COMPONENT THERAPY

Table VI–2 and Table VI–3 describe products used in blood component therapy and give some common indications for their use.

TRANSFUSION PROCEDURE

1. Draw a clot tube (red top) and sign the lab slips to verify it is the sample from the correct patient. The patient should be identified by the identification (ID) bracelet. If the patient is able to speak, ask the patient their name. The patient's name, hospital number, date, and physician's signature should be placed on the test tube label. **Prestamped labels are not accepted by most blood banks.**
2. When the blood products become available, make sure that the patient has good venous access for the transfusion (18 gauge or larger is preferred in an adult).
3. Remember to verify the information with another person, such as a nurse, on the request slip, blood bag, and with the patient's identification (ID) bracelet. **Note:** Many hospitals have defined protocols for this procedure; check guidelines for specific institution.
4. Blood products to be transfused may be mixed with only isotonic normal saline. Using hypotonic products, such as D5W, may result in hemolysis of the blood in the tubing. Lactated Ringer's should not be used because the calcium could chelate the anticoagulant citrate.

TABLE VI–1. TYPICAL PARAMETERS FOR SETTING UP BLOOD BEFORE PROCEDURES.

Procedure	Guidelines
Amputation (lower extremity)	2 units
Cardiac procedure (CABG, valve)	4 units
Cholecystectomy (open and laparoscopic)	T & S
Colostomy	T & S
Colon resection	2 units
Cystectomy (radical with diversion)	4 units
Esophageal resection	2 units
Exploratory laparotomy	2 units
Gastrectomy	2 units
Gastrostomy	T & S
Hemorrhoidectomy	T & S
Hernia	T & S
Hysterectomy	2 units
Liver resection	6 units
Liver transplant	6 units
Mastectomy	T & S
Nephrectomy	2 units
Pancreatectomy	4 units
Parathyroidectomy	T & S
Pulmonary resection	2 units
Radical neck dissection	2 units
Radical prostatectomy	3–4 units
Renal transplant	2 units
Small bowel resection	2 units
Splenectomy	2 units
Thyroidectomy	T & S
Tracheostomy	2 units
Total hip	2 units
Transurethral resection of prostate (TURP)	2 units
Vascular procedures	
Abdominal aortic aneurysm	6 units
Carotid endarterectomy	T & S
Aortofemoral bypass	4 units
Aortoiliac bypass	4 units
Femoral popliteal bypass	4 units
Iliofemoral bypass	4 units
Portacaval shunt	6 units
Splenorenal shunt	6 units
Vein stripping	T & S

TABLE VI–2. BLOOD BANK PRODUCTS THAT USUALLY REQUIRE A "CLOT TUBE" TO BE SENT FOR TYPING.

Product	Description	Common Indications
Whole blood	No elements removed; 1 unit = 450 mL +/− 45 mL; contains red cells, white cells, plasma and platelets (platelets may be nonfunctional)	Not for routine use; acute, massive bleeding; open heart surgery; neonatal total exchange
Packed red blood cells (PRBC) (also see page 363)	Most plasma removed; unit = 250–300 mL; 1 unit should raise Hct 3%	Replacement in chronic and acute (PRBC) blood loss, GI bleeding, trauma
Universal pedi-packs	250–300 mL divided into 3 bags; contains red cells, some white cells, some plasma and platelets	Transfusion for infants
Platelets (also see page 363)	1 "pack" should raise count by 5–8000; "6-pack" means a pool of platelets from 6 units of blood; 1 pack = about 50 mL	Decreased production or destruction (ie, aplastic anemia, acute leukemia, postchemo, etc); counts <5000 (risk of spontaneous hemorrhage); counts 5–30,000 if risk of bleeding (headache, GI losses, contiguous petechiae) or active bleeding; counts <50,000 if life-threatening bleed or preop; counts <100,000 in some cases of post-CABG bleeding or with neuro- or ophthalmic surgery; usually not indicated in idiopathic thrombocytopenic purpura [ITP] or thrombotic thrombocytopenic purpura [TTP] unless life-threatening bleed or preoperatively
Leukocyte poor red cells	Most WBC removed to make it less antigenic; 1 unit = 200–250 mL	Potential renal transplant patients; previous febrile transfusion reactions; patients requiring multiple transfusions (eg, leukemia)
Washed RBCs	Like leukocyte poor red cells, but WBC almost completely removed; 1 unit = 300 mL	As for leukocyte poor red cells, but very expensive and much more purified

(*continued*)

TABLE VI–2. BLOOD BANK PRODUCTS THAT USUALLY REQUIRE A "CLOT TUBE" TO BE SENT FOR TYPING (continued).

Product	Description	Common Indications
Cryoprecipitated antihemophilic factor ("cryo")	Contains factor VIII, factor XIII, von Willebrand's factor, and fibrinogen; 1 unit = 10 mL	Hemophilia A (factor VII deficiency), when safer factor VIII concentrate not available; von Willebrand's disease; fibrinogen deficiency, fibrin surgical glue
Fresh frozen plasma (FFP)	Contains factors II, VII, IX, X, XI, XII, XIII and heat labile V and VII; about 1 hr to thaw; 150–250 mL (400–600 mL if single donor pheresis)	Emergency reversal of Coumadin; massive transfusion (>5 L in adults); hypoglobunemia (IV immune globulin preferred); suspected or documented coagulopathy (congenital or acquired) with active bleeding or before surgery; clotting factor replacement when concentrate unavailable; no longer recommended for volume replacement
Single donor plasma	Like FFP, but lacks factors V and VIII; about 1 hr to thaw; 150–200 mL	No longer routinely used for plasma replacement; stable clotting factor replacement; Coumadin reversal, Hemophilia B (Christmas disease)
RhoGam (Rho D immune globulin)	Antibody against Rh factor	Rh⁻ mother with Rh⁺ baby, within 72-hr of delivery

5. When transfusing large volumes of packed red cells (>6–8 units), it is necessary to also transfuse platelets and fresh frozen plasma (FFP) periodically. Also, a calcium replacement is sometimes needed because the preservative used in the blood is a calcium binder and hypocalcemia can result after large amounts of blood are transfused. Also, the blood should be warmed in massive transfusions (usually >50 mL/min) to prevent hypothermia and cardiac arrhythmias.

BLOOD GROUPS

Table VI–4 gives information on the major blood groups and their relative occurrences. O⁻ is the **universal donor** and AB⁺ is the **universal recipient**.

TABLE VI–3. BLOOD BANK PRODUCTS THAT ARE DISPENSED BY MOST HOSPITAL PHARMACIES AND ARE ORDERED AS MEDICATION.

Product	Description	Common Indications
Factor VIII (purified antihemophilic factor)	From pooled plasma, pure factor VIII	Routine for hemophilia A (factor VII deficiency); increased hepatitis risk
Factor IX concentrate (prothrombin complex)	Increased hepatitis risk; factors II, VII, IX, and X; equivalent to 2 units of plasma	Active bleeding in Christmas disease (Hemophilia B or factor IX deficiency)
Immune serum globulin	Precipitate from plasma; gamma globulin	Immune globulin deficiency; disease prophylaxis (eg, hepatitis A, measles)
5% albumin or 5% plasma protein fraction	Precipitate from plasma (see Section IX)	Plasma volume expanders in acute blood loss
25% albumin	Precipitate from plasma	Hypoalbuminemia, volume expander, burns; draws extravascular fluid into circulation

TRANSFUSION FORMULA

Red Blood Cells

As a rule of thumb, 1 unit of packed red cells raises the hematocrit by 3% (hemoglobin 1 g/dL) in the average adult. To roughly determine the volume of whole blood or packed red cells needed to raise a hematocrit to a specific amount, use the following formula:

$$\text{Volume of cells} = \frac{\text{Total blood volume of patient} \times (\text{desired Hct} - \text{actual HCT})}{\text{Hct of transfusion product}}$$

where total blood volume = 70 mL/kg in adults, 80 mL/kg in children; Hematocrit (Hct), packed cells = approximately 70%; Hematocrit (Hct), whole blood = approximately 40%.

Platelets

Platelets are often transfused at a dose of 1 unit/10 kg body weight. After administration of 1 unit of multiple donor platelets, the count should rise 5–8,000/μL within 1 hour of transfusion and 4,500 μL within 24 hours. Normally, stored platelets that are transfused should survive in-vivo 6–8 days after infusion. Clinical factors (DIC, alloimmunization) can significantly shorten these intervals. To standardize the corrected platelet count to an individual patient use the corrected count increment (CCI). Measure

TABLE VI–4. BLOOD GROUPS.

Type (ABO/Rh)	Occurrences	Can Usually Receive Blood From
O$^+$	1 in 3	O($^{+/-}$)
O$^-$	1 in 15	O($^-$)
A$^+$	1 in 3	A($^{+/-}$) or O($^{+/-}$)
A$^-$	1 in 16	A($^-$) or O($^-$)
B$^+$	1 in 12	B($^{+/-}$) or O($^{+/-}$)
B$^-$	1 in 67	B($^-$) or O($^-$)
AB$^+$	1 in 29	AB, A, B or O (all^{+or-})
AB$^-$	1 in 167	AB, A, B or O (all$^-$)

the platelet count immediately before and 1 hour after the platelet infusion. If the correction is less than expected, workup of platelet refractoriness (antibodies, splenomegaly, etc) should be performed.

$$CCI = \frac{\text{posttransfusion count} - \text{pretransfusion count} \times \text{body surface area (m}^2)}{\text{platelets given} \times 10^{11}}$$

EMERGENCY TRANSFUSIONS

The transfusion of non-crossmatched blood is rarely indicated because most blood banks can do a complete crossmatch within 1 hour. In cases of massive, exsanguinating hemorrhage, type-specific blood (ABO and Rh matched only), usually available in 10 minutes, can be used. If this is too long, type O, Rh negative, packed red cell blood can be used as a last resort. It is generally preferable to support blood pressure with colloid and/or crystalloid until properly crossmatched blood is available.

TRANSFUSION REACTIONS

See Section I, Problem 68, page 217. Over 85% of adverse hemolytic transfusion reactions relate to clerical error.

AUTOLOGOUS BLOOD TRANSFUSIONS

Because of concerns over the transmission of disease by blood transfusion therapy, prehospital autologous blood banking (predeposit phlebotomy) has become popular in the elective surgery patient. General guidelines for autologous banking include good overall health status, a hematocrit >34% and arm veins that can accommodate a 16-gauge needle. Patients can usually donate up to 1 unit every 3–7 days, until 3–7 days before surgery (individual blood banks have their own specifications) depending on the needs of the planned surgery. Iron supplements (such as ferrous gluconate 325 mg PO tid) are usually given before and several months after the donation. Units of whole blood can be held for up to 35 days.

DIRECTED DONOR BLOOD PRODUCTS

Because of concerns over disease transmission, this form of donation is becoming more widely used, although this varies by region. This involves a person, often a relative, donating blood for a specific patient. This cannot be used in the emergency setting because it takes up to 48 hours to process the blood for transfusion.

There are some drawbacks to this system—relatives may be unduly pressured to give blood, risk factors that would normally exclude the use of the blood (eg, hepatitis or HIV positivity) become problematic, and ultimately the routine donation of blood for emergency transfusion may be adversely affected. These units are usually stored as packed red cells and released into the general transfusion pool 8 hours after surgery unless otherwise requested.

APHERESIS

Apheresis procedures are used to collect single donor platelets (**platelet-pheresis**) or white blood cells (**leukapheresis**); the remaining components are returned to the donor. **Therapeutic apheresis** is the separation and removal of a particular component to achieve a therapeutic effect (eg, **erythrocytapheresis** to treat polycythemia).

HEPATITIS & AIDS RISKS

Incidence of posttransfusion hepatitis is 0.3–0.9 cases/1000 units transfused. Anicteric hepatitis is much more common than hepatitis with jaundice. Screening of donors for HBsAg has almost eliminated this form of hepatitis, but most posttransfusion hepatitis is now hepatitis C (formerly non-A, non-B) variety. The greatest risk is with pooled factor products, such as concentrates of factor VIII. Use of albumin and globulins involves no risk of hepatitis.

HIV antibody testing is routinely performed on the donor's blood. A positive antibody test means that the donor may have been infected by the HIV virus; a Western blot to confirm the diagnosis is necessary. This allows blood centers to detect blood that should not be transfused and hopefully decrease the chance of AIDS transmission by transfusion. **A Western blot is not an absolute test for HIV and does not imply that the individual will develop AIDS. Follow-up testing of the donor who is HIV positive should be done because false-positives can occur.**

VII. Ventilator Management

INDICATIONS & SET-UP

I. Indications

A. Ventilatory Failure. Rigid criteria for defining ventilatory failure are found in Table VII–1. In general, ventilatory failure is based on the degree of hypercarbia. A $Paco_2$ >50 mm Hg indicates ventilatory failure; however, many patients will have chronic ventilatory failure with renal compensation (retaining HCO_3^-) to adjust the pH toward normal. Thus, absolute pH is often a better guide than $Paco_2$ to determine the need for ventilatory assistance. A respiratory acidosis with a rapidly falling pH or an absolute pH <7.24 is an indication for ventilatory support. The typical example of pure ventilatory failure is the drug overdose patient in whom there is a sudden loss of central respiratory drive with uncontrolled hypercarbia. Patients with sepsis, neuromuscular disease, and chronic obstructive pulmonary disease (COPD) may also have hypercarbic ventilatory failure.

B. Hypoxemic Respiratory Failure. Inability to oxygenate is an important indication for ventilatory support. A Pao_2 <60 mm Hg on ≥50% inspired fraction of oxygen (Fio_2) constitutes hypoxemic respiratory failure. Although these patients can sometimes be managed with higher Fio_2 delivery systems (eg, partial or nonrebreather masks or continuous positive airway pressure (CPAP) delivered by mask), they are at high risk for respiratory arrest and should be closely monitored in an intensive care unit (ICU). Worsening of the respiratory status necessitates prompt intubation and ventilatory support. The most common cause for hypoxemic respiratory failure is adult respiratory distress syndrome (ARDS) in which the high shunt fraction leads to refractory hypoxemia.

C. Mixed Respiratory Failure. Most patients have failure of both ventilation and oxygenation (eg, COPD with acute bronchitis). The indications for ventilatory support remain the same as listed earlier. The threshold for initiating ventilatory support will be even lower for patients with ventilation and oxygenation failure because oxygen management may further compound hypercarbia. Bronchospasm alters the ventilation-perfusion ratio (V/Q) relationships leading to worsening hypoxemia. Bronchospasm and accumulated secretions lead to a high work of breathing and consequent hypercarbia.

D. Neuromuscular Failure. This is a category of ventilatory failure but deserves special mention because the management is different. Hypercarbia occurs just before arrest and thus criteria other than arterial blood gases (ABGs) are needed.

TABLE VII–1. CRITERIA FOR DIAGNOSIS OF ACUTE RESPIRATORY FAILURE.[1]

Parameter	Normal	Respiratory Failure
Respiratory rate	12–20	>35
Vital capacity (mL/kg body wt)[2]	65–75	<15
FEV_1 (mL/kg body wt)[2]	50–60	≤10
Inspiratory force (cm H_2O)	⁻(75–100)	≥25
Compliance (mL/cm H_2O)	100	<20
P_aO_2 (mm/cm H_2O)	80–95 room air	<70
A-aDO_2 (mm Hg) (FIO_2 = 1.0)	25–65	>450
Qs/Qt (%)	5–8	>20
$PaCO_2$	35–45	>55[3]
VD/VT	0.2–0.3	>0.60

[1](Reproduced, with permission, from Demling RH, Goodwin CW: Pulmonary Dysfunction. In: Care of the Surgical Patient. Wilmore DW (editor). Scientific American, 1989.)
[2]Ideal body weight should be used.
[3]Chronic lung disease constitutes the exception.
FEV_1–Forced expiratory volume in 1 second; P_aO_2–Partial pressure of oxygen in arterial blood; A-aDO_2–Aveolar-arterial oxygen gradient; FIO_2–Fraction of inspired oxygen Qs/Qt–shunt fraction; P_aCO_2–Partial pressure of carbon dioxide in arterial blood; VD/VT–Ratio of dead space to tidal volume.

1. In progressive tachypnea, breathing rates >24/min are an early sign of respiratory failure. A progressive rise in the breath rate or sustained breathing rates >35/min are an indication for ventilatory support.
2. Abdominal paradox indicates dyssynergy of chest wall muscles and hemidiaphragms with impending respiratory failure. It is manifested by inward movement of the abdominal wall during inspiration rather than the normal outward motion.
3. A vital capacity <15 mL/kg (1000 mL for a normal body-sized person) is associated with acute respiratory arrest as well as an inability to clear secretions. Similarly, a negative inspiratory force less negative than −25 cm H_2O implies impending respiratory arrest. Guillain-Barré syndrome is the typical example of a neuromuscular disease in which the preceding criteria need strict attention. A patient with Guillain-Barré syndrome should be observed closely and followed with frequent vital capacity (VC). A rapidly falling VC or VC <1000 mL requires initiation of respirator support.

II. Endotracheal Intubation (see Section III, page 295). Endotracheal intubation is often the most difficult and potentially hazardous part of

ventilator initiation. Skill and experience are required for correct placement. Aspiration, esophageal intubation, and right mainstem bronchus
intubation are common complications. Bilateral breath sounds always
need to be confirmed by chest auscultation in each axilla. An immediate postintubation portable chest x-ray should be obtained. Intubation
can be accomplished by three routes.

A. Nasotracheal Intubation. This can be accomplished blindly and
in an awake patient. It requires experience and adequate local
anesthesia. Complications include esophageal intubation, nose-
bleeds, kinking of the endotracheal tube (ETT), and postobstructive sinusitis. A smaller ETT is usually required for nasotracheal
versus orotracheal intubation; this leads to a higher work of
breathing because of increased resistance, difficulties with adequate suctioning, and higher ventilation pressures. Nasotracheal
ETTs are more comfortable than orotracheal ETTs and are less
damaging to the larynx because of better stabilization in the
airway.

B. Orotracheal Intubation. Placement of orotracheal tubes requires
normal neck mobility to allow hyperextension of the neck for direct
visualization of the vocal cords. Larger ETTs can be placed by this
route. Adequate local anesthesia or sedation is necessary for safe
placement without aspiration.

C. Tracheostomy. Tracheostomy is a surgical procedure most often
done in acute cases for upper airway obstruction; however, in patients who require more than 14–21 days of ventilatory support, a
formal surgical tracheostomy is recommended to prevent tracheal
stenosis and vocal cord damage. Tracheostomy tubes facilitate
the weaning process by decreasing tube resistance as the tube is
shorter and of greater radius. Patients are able to eat and find the
tubes more comfortable

III. Ventilator Set-up

A. The Ventilator. Almost all modern adult ventilators are time- and
volume-cycled and can be used in adults and in children older
than two years. Children younger than two years and infants are
usually managed on pressure limited continuous flow. High frequency or "jet" ventilators are not used commonly. Elaborate
alarm systems are present to alert personnel to inadequate ventilation, high pressure, disconnection of the ETT, and so forth.
Effective ventilation is measured by changes in $Paco_2$. Minute
ventilation (V_e) is tidal volume × respiratory rate. Thus, ventilation
may be adjusted by changing the respiratory rate, the tidal volume, or both. Tidal volumes above 12 mL/kg may cause overdis-
tention of alveoli and increase the risk of pneumothorax. Most initial tidal volumes are therefore set at 10–12 mL/kg. Oxygenation

is adjusted by changing Fio_2. Prolonged Fio_2 >60% may cause pulmonary fibrosis. Thus, down-adjustment to "safe levels" sufficient to maintain O_2 saturation >90% should be attempted if indicated by ABGs. If an O_2 saturation >90% cannot be maintained when decreasing the Fio_2 <60%, other means, eg, positive end-expiratory pressure (PEEP), can be used. The mode of ventilation should be specified.

1. Control mode delivers a set rate and tidal volume irrespective of patient efforts and used in patients who are paralyzed or unable to initiate a breath. (Rarely, if ever, used.)

2. Assist control (AC) mode allows patient triggering of machine breaths once a threshold of inspiratory flow or effort is made. It also supplies a back-up rate in case of apnea or paralysis.

3. Intermittent mandatory ventilation (IMV) provides a set number of machine breaths per minute and allows the patient to make spontaneous breaths as well. Synchronized intermittent mandatory ventilation (SIMV) allows synchronization of the IMV breaths with patient efforts and is the generally preferred method. As the rate is decreased, the patient assumes more and more of the work of breathing.

4. Continuous positive airway pressure (CPAP) allows completely spontaneous respirations while the patient is still connected to the ventilator. A set amount of continuous pressure is applied during inspiration and expiration (from 0 to 30 cm H_2O).

5. Pressure support ventilation is used to help decrease the inspiratory work of breathing. Pressure support supplies a positive pressure when the patient initiates a breath. The patient sets the flow, respiratory rate, and tidal volume. Used in association with the AMV (augmented minute ventilation), this is becoming a popular technique to wean patients from ventilatory support because both the inspiratory pressure and the minute ventilation back-up can be weaned.

6. Currently, high frequency (jet) ventilation is not used widely except in specific situations. The process relies on low airway pressure, low tidal volumes (4 mL/kg), and very high rates (typically 100–400) cycles per minute.

B. **Ventilator Settings**

1. Initial ventilator settings should be dictated by the underlying condition as well as previous blood gas results. There are 5 parameters to order when writing initial ventilator orders. The patient's PO_2 is affected by the Fio_2 and the PEEP level. The patient's Pco_2 is affected by the rate and the tidal volume. Lastly, the mode of ventilation should be specified.

a. **Fraction of inspired oxygen (Fio_2):** There are many approaches to the first orders for oxygen, but the most prudent is to start every patient on 90–100% oxygen. The problem with high oxygen concentrations is toxicity. While oxygen at every amount greater than room air (21%) is toxic, the phenomenon is time-related. Many clinicians recommend 100% until the first blood gas result is available. This should not exceed 1 hour, minimizing any toxic effect of 100% oxygen. In general, try to keep F_{IO_2} <50% to maintain acceptable oxygenation (generally >90% saturated on ABG).

b. Positive-end expiratory pressure (PEEP): People are subject to about 5 cm H_2O of PEEP in a normal nonintubated condition. Because the normal closing of the glottis at the end of respiration is lost with an intubated patient, PEEP maintains the functional residual capacity above the critical closing volume. Usually start with 3–5 cm H_2O of PEEP. Adjust PEEP higher later to enable adequate oxygenation with lower F_{IO_2} as needed. High levels of PEEP (>10–15 cm H_2O) are associated with increased risk of barotrauma and decreased cardiac output; hemodynamic monitoring is usually needed for high levels of PEEP.

c. Rate: Normal respiratory rate is 12–20 per minute. Initially the ventilator should be set at 12 breaths per minute.

d. Tidal volume: Normal tidal volume is 8–10 mL/kg body weight.

e. Mode: There are several modes of operation of most volume cycled ventilators including IMV, SIMV, etc as previously noted. A basic understanding of these modes is important to order the optimum support for a given patient.

The following list is an example of settings for a patient who is status post respiratory arrest:

- F_{IO_2} 100%
- Assist control mode
- Rate 14
- Tidal volume 800 mL
- PEEP 5 cm H_2O.

An attempt should be made to supply the patient with at least as much minute ventilation as was required before intubation. Thus, patients with pulmonary edema, ARDS, or neuromuscular disease may require minute ventilation rates of 14–22 L/min. The AC mode will generally be more comfortable and will alleviate the work of breathing to a large extent. The following list shows sample settings for these patients:

- F_{IO_2} 100%
- Assist control mode
- Rate 18
- Tidal volume 750 mL
- PEEP 5 cm H_2O.

The patient with COPD, on the other hand, should not be overventilated initially. Such patients may have a chronically high bicarbonate because of renal compensation, and over-ventilation could cause a severe alkalosis. The following is a list of sample settings:

- Fio_2 50%
- SIMV mode
- Pressure support 15 cm
- Rate 12
- Tidal volume 800 mL
- PEEP 5 cm H_2O.

2. Secondary ventilator controls. Most major ventilator controls (inspired oxygen, tidal volume, PEEP, rate, and mode) are or-dered by the physician and accomplish the major control of the ventilators functions. However, there are a series of secondary ventilator controls that can be used to "optimize" or fine-tune the ventilator. Often, secondary controls are determined by lo-cal protocol. However, secondary ventilator control settings can be specified including:

a. Sigh: During normal breathing, the lungs are inflated to their maximum capacity up to 6 times an hour. The sigh mode de-livers a large tidal volume several times an hour to duplicate this normal physiologic breathing pattern. At very high peak inspiratory pressures, the sigh is not needed. To order sigh, specify the rate, volume delivered, and maximum pressure.

b. Peak inspiratory pressure (PIP): This represents the max-imum pressure generated and is typically set at 20–30 cm H_2O. Pressures above 45 cm are associated with significant barotrauma.

c. Inspiratory/expiratory ratio (I:E): Normal is approximately 1 : 3. Higher ratios favor oxygenation, lower ratios enhance CO_2 removal. Most ventilator alarms sound if the parame-ters chosen result in an I : E ratio of <1 : 1.

C. Additional Set-up Requirements

1. It may be necessary to restrain the patient's hands because the natural reaction to the ETT upon awakening is to pull it out.

2. Place a nasogastric tube to decompress the stomach and/or to continue essential oral medications and monitor gastric pH.

3. Obtain an immediate portable chest x-ray to confirm ETT placement and to reassess any underlying pulmonary disease.

4. Treat any underlying pulmonary disease (maximize bron-chodilators in status asthmaticus or vasodilators and diuretics in pulmonary edema).

5. Consider prophylactic measures. Heparin 5000 U subcuta-neously every 12 hours may reduce the incidence of pulmonary embolism while the patient is on bed rest. Stress ulceration bleeding can be prevented by the use of agents such as antacids, ranitidine (Zantac), or sucralfate (Carafate).

6. Order other medications (eg, morphine for pain, lorazepam (Ativan) for restlessness, and haloperidol (Haldol) for agitation) as needed.

ROUTINE MODIFICATION OF SETTINGS

Arterial blood gases should be monitored and adjusted to a normal pH (7.37–7.44) and a Pao_2 >60 mm Hg on <60% O_2. Tachypnea should be investigated for adequacy of ventilation or for any new cause, such as a fever, before sedating the patient.

I. Adjusting Pao_2

A. To Decrease. Fio_2 should be decreased in increments of 10–20% with either ABGs or oximetry checked in between. The "rule of 7s" states that there will be a 7 mm Hg fall in Pao_2 for each 1% decrease in Fio_2.

B. To Increase

1. Ventilation has some effect on Pao_2 (as shown by the alveolar air equation); therefore, correction of the respiratory acidosis will improve oxygenation.

2. Positive-end expiratory pressure (PEEP) can be added in increments from 2 to 4 cm H_2O. PEEP recruits previously collapsed alveoli, holds them open, and restores functional residual capacity (FRC) to a more physiologic level. It counteracts pulmonary shunts and raises Pao_2. PEEP increases intrathoracic pressure and thus may impede venous return and decrease cardiac output. This is particularly true in the presence of volume depletion and shock. If PEEP levels >10–12 cm H_2O are needed, the placement of a Swan-Ganz catheter is recommended to monitor mixed venous oxygen levels and cardiac output.

3. Increase I:E ratio.

II. Adjusting $Paco_2$

A. To Decrease

1. Increase the rate/decrease I : E ratio.
2. Check for leaks in the system.

B. To Increase

1. Decrease the rate/increase I : E ratio.
2. May have to switch from AC mode to SIMV mode to eliminate patient-driven central hyperventilation (not recommended).

3. An old but reliable method is to place increased exhalation tubing to increase deadspace and have the patient rebreathe CO_2.

4. The cause of the hyperventilation should be determined (ie, anxiety, sepsis) and treated appropriately.

TROUBLESHOOTING

Common problems with intubated patients are discussed in Section I, page 000. Typical ventilator management problems discussed include

- Agitation, Problem 71, page 225.
- High Inspired Oxygen (FiO_2), Problem 72, page 227.
- High Peak Pressure Problem 73, page 230.
- Low Arterial Oxygen (PO_2)/High Arterial Carbon Dioxide (PCO_2), Problem 74, page 233.

WEANING

I. Requirements. Once the underlying cause of respiratory failure has been corrected, it is time for the most arduous task of all—weaning the patient from the respirator.

A. Stabilization. The underlying disease is under optimum control.

B. Initiation of Weaning. The process is typically begun in the early morning. Patients like to rest rather than work all night. The following is a list of parameters considered minimum by most clinicians:

- PaO_2 ≥60 mm Hg on no PEEP (or <5 cm PEEP) and FiO_2 ≤0.5.
- Minute ventilation <10 L/min.
- Negative inspiratory force more negative than −20 cm H_2O.
- Vital capacity >800 mL.
- Tidal volume >300 mL.

II. Techniques

A. T-Piece (or T-tube bypass). The patient is taken off the respirator for a limited period of time and the ETT is connected to a constant flow of O_2 (usually 40–50%). If the patient tolerates breathing independently, the length of time off the respirator is progressively increased. This is an extremely effective method. It is particularly easy to use in patients with no underlying lung disease (eg, in a patient recovering from a drug overdose). There are three significant drawbacks to this technique: (1) No alarms are available because the patient is totally disconnected from the ventilator, (2) it is time consuming for the respiratory therapists and nurses, and

(3) it is much more work than breathing spontaneously without an ETT. This is due to the relatively small diameter of the tube. Remember, resistance increases by the fourth power of the radius. Therefore, patients are usually placed on a T-piece for intervals of <2 hours at a time.

B. **Synchronized Intermittent Mandatory Ventilation.** In this method, fewer and fewer machine breaths are given as the patient begins taking spontaneous breaths in between. For example, a patient breathing at a rate of 14 in AC mode is switched to SIMV mode, rate 14. The rate is then decreased to 10, 6, 4, and then to 0. Most physicians either place the patient on continuous positive airway pressure mode at this juncture or observe the patient briefly on a T-piece. This method has several theoretical advantages over T-piece weaning: (1) Back-up alarms including automatic rates in case of apnea are in place, (2) a graded assumption of work is done allowing respiratory muscle "retraining", and (3) there is still a high work of breathing because of the ETT resistance as well as the inherent resistance of the SIMV circuit valves. However, this method has never been proven clearly superior to T-piece weaning.

One way to decrease the work of breathing with the SIMV weaning technique is to add pressure support (PS) to the system. Pressure support is a positive pressure boost that is initiated when a certain liter flow rate during inspiration is sensed by the respirator. It then supplies a set amount of positive pressure (and by Boyle's law, it also supplies some tidal volume). A PS level of 10–15 cm will overcome the increased work caused by the ETT resistance.

C. **Continuous Positive Airway Pressure and Pressure Support.** In this method, the patient is switched to the spontaneous breathing mode, which in modern ventilators is the CPAP mode. In current usage, CPAP is equivalent to PEEP except it is used exclusively in spontaneously breathing mode. Anywhere from 0–30 cm pressure may be used, but generally the lowest level possible (usually 0–5 cm) is preferred. Pressure support (PS) may be used concomitantly to augment patient spontaneous breaths. It can then be progressively decreased as the patient increases tidal volumes. For example, PS levels of 25, then 20, then 15, and finally 10 can be used while monitoring the patient's breath rate, tidal volumes, and ABGs. This method requires an alert, cooperative patient who is spontaneously breathing. Machine back-up functions remain in place in case of apnea or other inadequate parameters.

III. **Timing.** Deciding when to extubate the patient is part of the art of medicine. Still, fulfilling certain criteria ensures success. The following weaning parameters (as discussed earlier) are acceptable:

- Breath rate is <30/min.
- ABGs show a pH >7.35 and adequate oxygenation.
- The patient is awake and alert.
- A normal gag reflex is present.
- The stomach is not distended.

IV. Postextubation. After extubation, it is important that the patient be encouraged to cough frequently and forcefully. Respiratory therapy treatments should be continued. Incentive spirometry should be used several times an hour while awake to encourage deep breathing. The patient must be carefully observed for stridor, respiratory muscle fatigue, or other signs of failure. Oxygen should be given at the same level or at a level slightly higher than was given via the respirator before intubation, usually by face mask. The ABGs should be checked 2–4 hours after extubation to confirm adequate ventilation and oxygenation.

VIII. Management of Perioperative Complications

This section details specific surgical complications that can occur in the postoperative period and sometimes require action by the house officer while "on call." They are listed by complication, rather than by operation, because they can result from many different operations.

Certain complications occur acutely and initial diagnosis and management may be life-saving (eg, neck hematoma, bronchial stump leak). Each management section includes a discussion on **Immediate Action** detailing plans for life-threatening problems. (The **Immediate Action** appears in boldface; whereas, other management suggestions appear in regular typeface.)

Other complications discussed here are more subacute, but early recognition and management with an understanding of the differential diagnosis and pathophysiology of the problem lead to optimal outcomes. This section does not provide a comprehensive listing of the various specific complications that can occur following general surgical procedures because the majority of these problems are fixed or chronic (eg, recurrent laryngeal nerve injury, short gut syndrome) and have no acute management issues.

Acute Gastric Dilatation

A. Operations: Major thoracic procedures and some abdominal operations (eg, splenectomy) if a nasogastric tube is not functioning or was not placed intraoperatively.

B. Pathophysiology: Acute gastric dilatation is the thoracic equivalent of an ileus limited to the foregut.

C. Diagnosis: Tachypnea, tachycardia, diaphoresis, or hiccups. Often the patients do not highlight abdominal distress. Pay attention to the gastric shadow on a chest x-ray in this postthoracotomy patient population (see Problem 37, page 129).

D. Management:
Immediate Action: Place a nasogastric tube, or make the tube that is in place functional. The problem is rapidly resolved by decompression with a nasogastric tube.

E. Comments: In general, the patients with this problem look clinically ill and more serious diagnoses should be considered and ruled out. An awareness of this condition results in appropriate diagnosis and treatment. Acute gastric dilatation can cause further complications (eg, bleeding) following certain procedures, such as a splenectomy.

Anastomotic Leak

A. Operations: This complication occurs after abdominal operations in which one hollow viscus (bowel or pancreaticobiliary) is connected to another hollow viscus.

B. Pathophysiology: This complication may be caused by a technical problem with leakage of intestinal contents, bile, pancreatic juice, or urine through an anastomotic suture or staple line. It can be a result of late tissue necrosis or local infection at the site of anastomosis. If it is an esophageal anastomosis the leak may occur in the neck or the pleural cavity while other sites of leakage will be in the peritoneal cavity.

C. Diagnosis: Fever, leukocytosis, and pain are the hallmarks of this complication. There may be increased or change in drain output or even possible leakage of intestinal contents from the wound. The timing of this complication is typically 5–10 days after the procedure (see also Section I, Problem 77, page 241).

D. Management:
Immediate Action: Usually not necessary except in the patient who is septic because of the leak.
   The management must be individualized according to the patient's condition. A small disruption of a suture or staple line may be salvageable without reoperation and should be treated by decreasing passage of material through the lumen by making the patient NPO for bowel anastomoses and possibly inserting a nasogastric tube. Treatment with H_2-receptor blockers and possibly the somatostatin analogue octreotide will decrease bowel and pancreatic secretions and aid in healing. If there is a significant fluid collection of leaked contents adjacent to the anastomosis, this will need to be drained to facilitate healing. Percutaneous drainage of the leaking anastomosis immediately converts the situation to a bowel, pancreatic, or biliary fistula allowing assessment of ongoing leak and controlling internal infection. For major disruptions of anastomoses operative reconstruction will almost always be indicated. Depending on the situation and the clinical condition of the patient, operative reconstruction may be attempted initially or as a temporizing measure (eg, a diverting colostomy for a rectal anastomosis or defunctionalizing the esophagus for a leak in the chest) may be indicated.

E. Comments: Of the bowel anastomoses usually performed in general surgical procedures, leaks are a more frequent complication from esophageal and rectal procedures. These areas of the gastrointestinal tract do not have a serosal covering and have somewhat impaired healing compared to small bowel or gastric anastomoses. Another problematic area involves anastomoses of the pancreas to the small intestine such as that performed in the Whipple procedure (pancreaticoduodenectomy).

Bronchial Stump Leak

A. Operations: Pneumonectomy.

B. Pathophysiology: Disruption of staple or suture line on the mainstem bronchus after lung resection is the usual problem.

C. Diagnosis: This condition is usually heralded by sudden onset of severe shortness of breath or expectoration of large amounts of serosanguinous fluid. It may present more insidiously with cough, fever, sepsis or contralateral pneumonia. On chest x-ray there are often new air/fluid levels in the affected hemithorax.

D. Management:
Immediate Action: Position the patient on their side with the resected side down and the intact lung up. Intubation of the bronchus with a cuffed tube can prevent ongoing aspiration of pleural space fluid.
After undertaking the immediate action, the chest usually is drained with a chest tube. Intravenous fluids and antibiotics are usually indicated. While small leaks may seal with tube thoracostomy alone, repeat thoracotomy usually is required, often with flap coverage of the defect.

E. Comments: The incidence of bronchial stump disruption is much lower in the era of mechanical staplers to close the bronchus as opposed to handsewn closures. Nevertheless, the initial management of this complication, in which a patient with one lung essentially drowns due to aspiration of fluid, can be lifesaving.

Early Postoperative Bowel Obstruction

A. Operations: Any major intraperitoneal procedure.

B. Pathophysiology: Mechanical obstruction of the small intestine generally results from twists or kinks (the precursors for later adhesions). The possibility of an internal hernia must be considered based on the initial abdominal procedure the patient underwent.

C. Diagnosis: Abdominal distention, crampy pain, obstipation. Abdominal x-rays will show distended loops of small bowel with air-fluid levels. The main differential diagnosis is between a prolonged postoperative ileus, which is a functional problem, and a true mechanical bowel obstruction, which occurs early in the postoperative course. X-ray features of an adynamic ileus show a dilated colon primarily indicating no physical obstruction at the level of the small bowel (see Section I, Problem 1, page 1).

D. Management:
Immediate Action: Usually not necessary.

Mechanical bowel obstruction in the early postoperative period (5–20 days postop) is typically treated in a much more conservative (ie, nonoperative) manner than late mechanical obstruction. Decompression with a nasogastric tube and observation usually are indicated. The early adhesions at this time are filmy and unlikely to cause strangulation. Also, operative repair at this point is difficult because the bowel is friable and susceptible to injury. Some surgeons advocate the use of a long suction tube often identified by the trade name (Cantor tube, Dennis tube, Baker tube, etc) in this situation. These tubes have a weighted tip that is advanced by peristalsis into the small bowel to the point of obstruction and decompression via the tube may allow the mechanical obstruction to be resolved. However, there is little literature to suggest that these tubes are more effective than the usual sump-type nasogastric tubes.

E. Comments: The primary differential diagnosis for early postoperative bowel obstruction is whether it is a true mechanical problem or a prolonged adynamic ileus, which is a functional problem. If a postoperative ileus resolves and the patient tolerates a diet and then develops signs and symptoms of obstruction it is more obvious but often the problems blend together. Gas patterns on abdominal x-rays help with this diagnosis because in functional ileus the colon is typically most affected, whereas in mechanical obstruction it is the small bowel. Another consideration in a postoperative patient who develops abdominal distention and difficulty tolerating a diet is a focal infectious problem.

Major Lymphatic Leak

A. Operations: Cervical procedures in the left neck, left subclavian line placement, esophagectomy, or retroperitoneal dissection can all lead to thoracic duct or major lymphatic duct injury with subsequent chylothorax or chylous ascites.

B. Pathophysiology: Operative injury to major lymphatic vessel with large amount of lymph leaking out of neck incision or accumulating in pleural or peritoneal space.

C. Diagnosis: High output drainage (> 500 mL/d) from cervical drain or chest tube with high concentration of lymphocytes and high triglyceride content. The fluid is usually grossly chylous after fatty meal ingestion. For chylous ascites, postoperative ascites with fluid characteristics as above.

D. Management:
Immediate Action: Usually not necessary.

Restrict fatty foods or make patient NPO with TPN to decrease lymph flow and seal leak. Maintain closed suction drainage system while measuring the volume of output daily. Follow serum albumin and serum total lymphocyte counts, which may be depleted in patients with high output leaks. If there is persistent drainage, then surgical exploration with suture ligature of leaking lymphatic may be indicated. Preoperative ingestion of a fatty meal may help to identify the source of leak intraoperatively.

E. Comments: These major lymphatic leaks should be detected as fluid in the surgical field during the initial procedure. Knowledge of the anatomy of the thoracic duct is important to avoid this complication.

Neck Hematoma

A. Operations: Thyroidectomy, parathyroidectomy, carotid artery endarterectomy, cervical esophageal procedures (eg, repair of a Zenker's diverticulum).

B. Pathophysiology: Postoperative bleeding into the closed space under the deep cervical fascia where the trachea lies.

C. Diagnosis: Postoperative swelling in neck with difficulty breathing and stridor. Distortion or deviation of tracheal air column may be seen on x-ray.

D. Management:
Immediate Action: Open the skin and deep cervical fascial closure to release the hematoma.
    Patients who are stable should be brought to the operating room for this procedure. In patients where the airway is compromised, it may be necessary to perform this procedure at the bedside.
    Cover the open wound with sterile (possibly dilute povidone-iodine [Betadine] soaked gauze) before reclosing incision in operating room. Avoid attempts at endotracheal intubation because placement of the tube will be difficult as a result of tracheal compression. It should be noted however, that endotracheal intubation may be required.

E. Comments: Any cervical procedure that closes the deep cervical fascia can lead to a trapped hematoma, which can cause tracheal compression and stridor. Opening the wound quickly solves the problem and can be life-saving.

Pancreatic Fistula or Fluid Collection

A. Operations: Pancreatic resections or splenectomy where the tail of the pancreas may be injured.

B. Pathophysiology: Any violation of the pancreatic parenchyma transects small pancreatic ducts. The digestive enzymes in exocrine pancreatic juice may prevent normal healing or sealing of minor duct injuries with accumulation of a pancreatic fluid collection high in enzyme content. For this reason it is appropriate to drain any pancreatic resection procedure and high output of fluid from these drains rich in pancreatic juice defines a pancreatic fistula. Percutaneous drainage of a pancreatic fluid collection postoperatively often leads to continued drainage defining a pancreatic fistula.

C. Diagnosis: High amylase content in fluid from peripancreatic drains placed at the time of pancreatic resection. Pancreatic fluid in a drain has a characteristic dirty dishwater brown/gray color. Drain output may increase or change in character with initiation of oral intake.

D. Management:
Immediate Actions: Usually not necessary.

Continued and complete drainage of a pancreatic fistula is an imperative component of treatment, and daily monitoring of drain output in terms of volume with intermittent amylase content checks help assess progress in treatment. Additional measures aimed at decreasing exocrine pancreas stimulation are used to help heal the fistula. Making the patient NPO and using TPN (see Section V, page 341) may be necessary in patients with high output fistulas. Patients continuing oral intake should be given a non-fat diet to decrease pancreatic stimulation. The somatostatin analogue, octreotide, can be given to decrease exocrine pancreas secretions. In fact, in patients undergoing pancreatic procedures there is evidence that beginning this agent preoperatively decreases postoperative pancreatic leak. When the drain (or fistula) output decreases to acceptable levels (< 50 mL/d) with a low amylase content (< 3 times the serum level) then octreotide should be stopped. If output remains low, then the drain can be removed.

E. Comments: Dependent on the caliber and location of the pancreatic duct injury the fistula can be low, mid, or high output. Injuries of the main duct or immediate branches of the main duct and injuries in the pancreatic head, as opposed to the distal pancreas, result in greater problems that are more difficult to heal.

Peripheral Lymphatic Leak

A. Operations: Lymph node dissection, vascular procedure with groin or axillary incision.

B. Pathophysiology: Operative injury to lymphatic vessels with leakage of fluid (usually clear) from the incision.

C. Diagnosis: Persistently high drain output via postoperative closed drains in operative field. Fluid leak from wound onto dressings.

D. Management:

Immediate Actions: Usually not necessary.

If drainage is controlled via closed system alternative management options include:

1. Observation with continued drainage including limiting activity, elevation of extremity, and wrapping extremity to decrease drain output.
2. Surgical exploration with suture ligation of leak sites. Preoperative injection of vital dye (methylene blue, etc) subcutaneously in distal extremity may help identify leak sites. Closed drain placed at this operation and components of treatment option No. 1 instituted.
3. Pull drain and observe wound. Sometimes suction drains may induce leakage and by removing the drain the problem is solved. This plan works best for low output (75–150 mL/d) lymphatic leaks.

Avoid injecting sclerosing agents (eg, bleomycin, tetracycline) into drains because this treatment causes discomfort, increases risk of infection, and is not effective in a controlled trial.

If lymph leak occurs as open drainage through the wound, surgical exploration as in treatment option No. 2 (above) is usually indicated. Open drainage tends to macerate skin and increase chance of wound infection.

E. Comments:

Postoperative lymph leaks are often difficult to resolve quickly even by surgical reexploration. Attention to detail by clipping or ligating lymphatics at the initial procedure to prevent this complication should be emphasized. Lymph leaks in vascular procedures can lead to more serious secondary complications of graft infection when artificial graft material is present.

Postoperative Adrenal Insufficiency

A. Operations:

Any major surgical procedure, but especially after adrenalectomy, radical nephrectomy.

B. Pathophysiology:

Acute postoperative adrenal insufficiency may occur for one of two general reasons. First, the adrenals may not respond appropriately to the stress of the surgical procedure because of unrecognized underlying adrenal pathology or because of iatrogenic adrenal suppression owing to steroid medication. A second cause of acute adrenal insufficiency is bilateral adrenal hemorrhage. Patients who are anticoagulated are more susceptible to this complication, but the majority of patients suffering that have this life-threatening problem are not anticoagulated.

C. Diagnosis:

Often very difficult to diagnose other than the fact that patients do very poorly for no obvious reason. This must be kept in mind as a possible explanation for poor progress. Symptoms include hypotension, confusion, vomiting with inability to eat; however, the electrolyte manifestations of Addison's disease may not occur. CT scans of the adrenals may show large bilateral hematomas. The diagnosis can be confirmed by failure to have a cortisol response to ACTH injection.

D. Management:
Immediate Action: Intravenous steroid administration. Hydrocortisone 100 mg IV STAT.

Once the diagnosis is made (and it often is not realized until a postmortem exam), treatment with stress doses of steroid medication can be life-saving.

E. Comments: Awareness of this very rare, but very serious, problem is the most important factor. In patients who are failing rapidly but have no obvious source of infection and are not bleeding and have no other explanations for a downward clinical spiral, acute adrenal insufficiency should be considered.

Postoperative Bleeding

A. Operations: Any surgical procedure.

B. Pathophysiology: Surgical bleeding is usually a technical error with a bleeding vessel that was not controlled satisfactorily intraoperatively. Occasionally, because of the primary disease, patients may have a coagulopathy with medical bleeding from dissection planes, which normally would be hemostatic, oozing blood as a result of the inability to form clot.

C. Diagnosis: Minor wound bleeding typically presents as bloody drainage from the wound or a subcutaneous hematoma. Major postoperative bleeding presents as signs and symptoms of hemorrhagic shock with hypotension, tachycardia, low urine output, and falling hematocrit. (See On Call Problems 23 and 24 relating to drain output and problem 42 "Hypotension")

D. Management:
Immediate Action: Volume resuscitation, obtain cross-matched blood products, identify source of bleeding.

For major postoperative surgical bleeding the principles of care of hemorrhagic shock of any etiology apply. Volume resuscitation making certain adequate venous access lines are available and ordering blood products to treat the bleeding are the cornerstones of therapy. Assessment of ongoing bleeding and response to volume resuscitation in terms of blood pressure, urine output, and serial hematocrits guides the decision whether or not the bleeding mandates reoperation. Some situations are clinically obvious with dramatic acute bleeding with large transfusion requirements in which reoperation is needed as soon as possible. Other clinical situations are more subacute and may not require reoperation. In all cases, measurement of coagulation parameters (including protime, prothrombin time, and platelet count) is indicated as some cases of bleeding are primarily a result of coagulopathy, which must be treated with the appropriate blood products.

Minor bleeding resulting in a wound hematoma in the subcutaneous location almost never results in hemodynamically significant blood loss. In most locations this can be treated with observation possibly with direct pressure to halt the blood loss. In certain locations even small hematomas can be symptomatic (see previous section, "Neck Hematoma"). If the subcutaneous bleeding is saturating the wound dressings instead of causing a hematoma, direct pressure often controls the bleeding site. Sometimes the offending vessel is a skin vessel that can be identified by inspecting the wound, and a simple nylon stitch under local anesthesia at the bedside can solve the problem.

E. Comments: An understanding of the volume of blood that can hide in the peritoneal or pleural cavities is needed to appreciate the potential problem that can happen with acute postoperative hemorrhage. Serial measurements of abdominal girth (as is often done) is a ridiculously insensitive barometer for this potentially life-threatening complication.

Postoperative Intra-Abdominal Fluid Collection/Abscess

A. Operations: Any abdominal operation can result in this problem, particularly infected, contaminated, or clean/contaminated procedures.

B. Pathophysiology: Postoperative intra-abdominal fluid serves as a site for infection to develop from organisms typically originating from the bowel, biliary, or genitourinary tract during the surgical procedure. As patients recover in a supine position, the fluid settles in the most dependent areas of the greater peritoneal cavity in the subphrenic spaces, infrahepatic space (Morrison's pouch), paracolic gutters, and pelvis.

C. Diagnosis: This complication may be evident as leukocytosis, fever, increased abdominal pain, referred pain to shoulders or back, abdominal distention. Often patients who are recovering from an abdominal procedure after making normal progress, begin to feel worse or lose their ability to eat.

D. Management:
Immediate Action: Usually not necessary.

Current management involves imaging fluid collections by CT scan or ultrasound with a radiologically guided aspiration and drainage if possible. Aspirated fluid should be sent to the laboratory for Gram's stain and culture. If the operative procedure involved the pancreas, assay of the fluid for amylase content will indicate a pancreatic source. Checking the creatinine in the fluid may demonstrate that it is urine. Broad spectrum antibiotics to treat enteric organisms should be initiated as soon as cultures are obtained. For clinically significant fluid collections that cannot be safely approached percutaneously (eg, interloop fluid collections between loops of small bowel), operative drainage may be indicated.

E. Comments: Advancements in radiologic imaging techniques and interventions have revolutionized the management of this postoperative complication.

Postoperative Intestinal Fistula

A. Operations: Abdominal operations where an intestinal anastomosis was created. Reoperative procedures where significant adhesions exist and there is the possibility of an unintentional enterotomy or a leak from a repaired inadvertent enterotomy. Rarely, sutures used for fascial closure may include a bowel segment with subsequent fistula formation.

B. Pathophysiology: Postoperative fistulas require violation of the bowel wall with leakage of intestinal contents, which eventually find a path out of the body to the skin. The most common cause for bowel wall disruption is an anastomotic leak as previously discussed. However, if the bowel wall was injured or made ischemic during the initial procedure, then it may develop into an intestinal leak, not related to an anastomosis, which can progress to a fistula.

C. Diagnosis: This complication is diagnosed by leakage of intestinal contents to the wound or drain sites.

D. Management:
Immediate Action: Usually not necessary.
  Similar to the situation with both anatomic leak and intra-abdominal abscess discussed above, the principles of management of an intestinal fistula are bowel rest (use TPN, see Section V, page 341), antibiotics, and control of the leak with drainage of intra-abdominal fluid collections to limit infection. Obtaining radiologic studies, such as a CT scan, to look for undrained fluid collections and possibly a fistulogram by injecting contrast retrograde into the site of the fistula to define the anatomy of the leak are helpful to define the anatomy of the fistula.
  Fistulas are usually categorized as low output ($<$ 500 mL/d) or high output ($>$ 500 mL/d). It is critically important to protect the skin at the site of the fistula. A stoma appliance is usually helpful in this matter as well as collecting the effluent. High-output fistulas should be treated as above, but persistently high-output fistulas usually require operative repair, while low-output fistulas usually close gradually with nonoperative management as previously outlined (see also Section I, Problem 77, page 241).

E. Comments: The postoperative complications of intra-abdominal fluid collection, anastomotic leak, and intestinal fistula are all interrelated problems that can occur together in patients undergoing major abdominal procedures.

Seroma

A. Operations: Lymph node dissection, mastectomy, any soft tissue resection.

B. Pathophysiology: Accumulation of lymph or serous fluid in deep wound space with normal healing of skin.

C. Diagnosis: This problem presents as a nontender swelling in the wound that is usually fluctuant. A needle aspirate (performed using sterile technique) shows serous fluid.

D. Management:
Immediate Actions: Usually not necessary.
   Observation for signs of infection or enlargement. Repeated complete aspiration of fluid using sterile technique. Avoid placing an indwelling drain.

E. Comments: Seromas are more of a nuisance than a symptomatic complication. Secondary problems, such as infection or open lymphatic leak, are more worrisome.

Skin Flap Necrosis

A. Operations: Mastectomy, lymph node dissection, soft tissue tumor resection, neck dissection.

B. Pathophysiology: Ischemic necrosis of skin and subcutaneous tissue resulting from inappropriate construction of flap or closure of incision under tension stretching tissues and restricting blood flow.

C. Diagnosis: This is a clinical diagnosis with a variable area of skin along an incision that demarcates and appears various shades of gray or purple, has little or no capillary refill, and eventually becomes black and necrotic.

D. Management:
Immediate Actions: Usually not necessary.
   When flap necrosis is initially suspected several maneuvers can be done to minimize skin and soft tissue loss. The patient should be well hydrated to assure adequate tissue perfusion and placed on oxygen to maximize oxygen tension in the area at risk. Nitropaste may be applied to the endangered area to cause vasodilatation and increased blood flow. When the flap becomes a black eschar the damage is irreversible and debridement of the dead tissue with subsequent skin graft or flap coverage is done as quickly as possible.

E. Comments: Flap necrosis is a vascular problem at the outset—not an infectious one. However, early recognition of this complication and prompt action to increase oxygen delivery to the tissue may salvage some of the ischemic skin flap.

Wound Infection

A. Operations: Any surgical procedure. More common in dirty, contaminated, or clean-contaminated cases.

B. Pathophysiology: The subcutaneous tissue between the skin and fascia is the most susceptible to infection because it is the least vascularized.

C. Diagnosis: Erythema, pain, and warmth at the wound characterize superficial infections. Purulent drainage from a wound in which there is a thick layer of subcutaneous tissue may be the only symptom. Systemic signs, such as fever or leukocytosis, may be present. Inspection of the wound including palpation to identify and express trapped purulent fluid confirms the diagnosis.

D. Management:
Immediate Actions: Usually not necessary.
   After diagnosing a wound infection, treatment of superficial cellulitis involves antibiotics. Parenteral antibiotics are indicated in patients with acute surgical wound infections. Antibiotic coverage for enteric organisms is recommended in dirty cases, ie, when the subcutaneous tissue comes into contact with intestinal contents. For most wound infections the causative organism is a gram-positive bacteria from the skin (staphylococcus or streptococcus), and treatment should be directed toward these organisms. If there is suspicion of an abscess or known drainage of pus from the wound, then wound needs to be opened widely to achieve drainage. The wound is then managed with dressing changes 2–3 times a day and allowed to heal by secondary intention (see also Section I, Problem 77, page 241).

E. Comments: The assessment of postoperative fever includes evaluation and inspection of the surgical incision. Even early postoperative fever mandates inspection of the wound because the source may be an early streptococci or clostridial infection that can progress rapidly and cause a high morbidity rate.

IX. Commonly Used Medications

This section is designed to serve as a quick reference to commonly used medications. You should be familiar with all of the indications, contraindications, side effects, and drug interactions of the medications that you prescribe. Such detailed information is beyond the scope of this manual and can be found in the package insert, Physicians' Desk Reference (PDR), or the American Hospital Formulary Service.

Drugs in this section are listed in alphabetical order by generic names. Some of the more common trade names are listed for each medication. Where no pediatric dosage is provided, the implication is that the use of the agent is not well established in this age group or is infrequently used.

Drugs under the control of the Drug Enforcement Agency (Schedule 2–5 controlled substances) are indicated by the symbol [C].

GENERIC DRUGS: GENERAL CLASSIFICATION

Analgesic/Anti-inflammatory/Antipyretic

Acetaminophen
Acetaminophen with butalbital
   and caffeine
Acetaminophen with codeine
Alfentanil
Aspirin
Aspirin with butalbital and
   caffeine
Aspirin with codeine
Buprenorphine
Butorphanol
Codeine
Dezocine
Diclofenac sodium
Diflunisal
Etodolac
Fenoprofen
Fentanyl
Fentanyl transdermal system
Flurbiprofen
Hydromorphone

Ibuprofen
Indomethacin
Ketoprofen
Ketorolac
Levorphanol
Meclofenamate
Mefenamic acid
Meperidine
Methadone
Morphine sulfate
Nabumetone
Nalbuphine
Naproxen
Oxaprozin
Oxycodone
Pentazocine
Piroxicam
Propoxyphene
Sufentanil
Sulindac
Tolmetin

Antacids/Antigas

Aluminum carbonate
Aluminum hydroxide

Aluminum hydroxide with
   magnesium hydroxide

Aluminum hydroxide with
    magnesium hydroxide and
    simethicone
Aluminum hydroxide with
    magnesium trisilicate and
    alginic acid

Calcium carbonate
Dihydroxyaluminum sodium
    carbonate
Magaldrate
Simethicone

Antianxiety Agents

Alprazolam
Buspirone
Chlordiazepoxide
Clorazepate
Diazepam
Doxepin

Halazepam
Hydroxyzine
Lorazepam
Meprobamate
Oxazepam
Prazepam

Antiarrhythmics

Adenosine
Amiodarone
Bretylium
Disopyramide
Flecainide
Lidocaine

Mexiletine
Moricizine
Procainamide
Propafenone
Quinidine
Tocainide

Antibiotics

Amikacin
Amoxicillin
Amoxicillin/potassium
    clavulanate
Ampicillin
Ampicillin/sulbactam
Azithromycin
Aztreonam
Cefaclor
Cefadroxil
Cefamandole
Cefazolin
Cefixime
Cefmetazole
Cefonicid
Cefoperazone
Cefotaxime
Cefotetan
Cefoxitin
Cefpodoxime
Cefprozil

Ceftazidime
Ceftizoxime
Ceftriaxone
Cefuroxime
Cephalexin
Cephalothin
Cephapirin
Cephradine
Ciprofloxacin
Clarithromycin
Clindamycin
Clofazimine
Cloxacillin
Cortisporin, otic
Dapsone
Demeclocycline
Dicloxacillin
Doxycycline
Enoxacin
Erythromycin
Ethambutol

Gentamicin
Imipenem/cilastatin
Isoniazid
Lomefloxacin
Methicillin
Metronidazole
Mezlocillin
Nafcillin
Neomycin sulfate
Norfloxacin
Ofloxacin
Oxacillin
Penicillin G aqueous
Penicillin G benzathine
Penicillin G procaine
Penicillin V

Pentamidine
Piperacillin
Piperacillin/tazobactam
Pyrazinamide
Rifabutin
Rifampin
Silver sulfadiazine
Sulfasalazine
Sulfisoxazole
Tetracycline
Ticarcillin
Ticarcillin/potassium clavulanate
Tobramycin
Trimethoprim
Trimethoprim/sulfamethoxazole
Vancomycin

Anticoagulant/Thrombolytic and Related Agents

Alteplase, recombinant (TPA)
Aminocaproic acid
Anistreplase
Antihemophilic Factor VIII
Aprotinin
Desmopressin (DDAVP)
Dextran 40
Dipyridamole

Enoxaparin
Heparin
Pentoxifylline
Protamine
Streptokinase
Ticlopidine
Urokinase
Warfarin

Anticonvulsants

Carbamazepine
Clonazepam
Diazepam
Ethosuximide
Felbamate
Gabapentin

Lorazepam
Pentobarbital
Phenobarbital
Phenytoin
Valproic acid

Antidepressants

Amitriptyline
Amoxapine
Bupropion
Desipramine
Doxepin
Fluoxetine
Imipramine

Maprotiline
Nortriptyline
Paroxetine
Sertraline
Trazodone
Trimipramine
Venlafaxine

Antidiabetic Agents

Acetohexamide
Chlorpropamide
Glipizide
Glyburide

Insulin
Tolazamide
Tolbutamide

Antidiarrheals

Bismuth subsalicylate
Diphenoxylate with atropine
Kaolin/Pectin

Lactobacillus
Loperamide
Octreotide

Antidotes

Acetylcysteine
Charcoal
Digoxin immune FAB
Flumazenil

Ipecac syrup
Mesna
Naloxone

Antiemetics

Benzquinamide
Buclizine
Chlorpromazine
Cyclizine
Dimenhydrinate
Dronabinol
Droperidol
Granisetron

Meclizine
Metoclopramide
Ondansetron
Prochlorperazine
Promethazine
Scopolamine
Thiethylperazine
Trimethobenzamide

Antifungal Agents

Amphotericin B
Clotrimazole
Econazole
Fluconazole

Itraconazole
Ketoconazole
Miconazole
Nystatin

Antigout Agents

Allopurinol
Colchicine

Probenecid
Sulfinpyrazone

Antihistamines

Astemizole
Brompheniramine
Chlorpheniramine
Clemastine fumarate
Cyproheptadine

Diphenhydramine
Hydroxyzine
Loratadine
Terfenadine

Antihyperlipidemics

Cholestyramine
Clofibrate
Colestipol
Fluvastatin
Gemfibrozil

Lovastatin
Niacin
Pravastatin
Probucol
Simvastatin

Antihypertensives

Acebutolol
Amlodipine
Atenolol
Benazepril
Betaxolol
Captopril
Carteolol
Clonidine
Diazoxide
Diltiazem
Doxazosin
Enalapril
Felodipine
Fosinopril
Guanabenz
Guanadrel
Guanethidine
Guanfacine
Hydralazine
Isradipine
Labetalol

Lisinopril
Methyldopa
Metoprolol
Minoxidil
Nadolol
Nicardipine
Nifedipine
Nitroglycerin
Nitroprusside
Penbutolol
Perindopril
Pindolol
Prazosin
Propranolol
Quinapril
Ramipril
Sotalol
Terazosin
Timolol
Trimethaphan
Verapamil

Antineoplastic Agents

Aldesleukin (IL-2)
Altretamine
BCG
Bleomycin
Carboplatin
Chlorambucil
Cisplatin
Cyclophosphamide
Cytarabine
Dacarbazine
Dactinomycin
Diethylstilbestrol
Doxorubicin
Etoposide

Fludarabine phosphate
Fluorouracil
Flutamide
Goserelin
Hydroxyurea
Idarubicin
Ifosfamide
Leuprolide
Megestrol acetate
Melphalan
Methotrexate
Mitomycin
Mitoxantrone
Paclitaxel

Plicamycin
Tamoxifen citrate
Teniposide

Thiotepa
Vinblastine
Vincristine

Antiparkinsonian Agents

Amantadine
Benztropine
Bromocriptine
Carbidopa/levodopa

Pergolide
Risperidone
Selegiline
Trihexyphenidyl

Antipsychotic Agents

Chlorpromazine
Clozapine
Fluphenazine
Haloperidol
Lithium carbonate
Mesoridazine

Molindone
Perphenazine
Prochlorperazine
Thioridazine
Thiothixene
Trifluoperazine

Antitussives, Decongestants, Expectorants, and Mucolytic Agents

Acetylcysteine
Benzonatate
Codeine

Dextromethorphan
Guaifenesin
Pseudoephedrine

Antiviral Agents

Acyclovir
Amantadine
Didanosine
Foscarnet
Ganciclovir

Ribavirin
Rimantadine
Zalcitabine
Zidovudine

Bronchodilators

Albuterol
Aminophylline
Bitolterol
Ephedrine
Epinephrine
Isoetharine

Isoproterenol
Metaproterenol
Pirbuterol
Terbutaline
Theophylline

Cardiovascular Agents

Acebutolol
Amrinone
Atenolol
Atropine

Bepridil
Digoxin
Diltiazem
Dobutamine

Dopamine
Edrophonium
Ephedrine
Epinephrine
Esmolol
Isoproterenol
Isosorbide dinitrate
Isosorbide mononitrate
Labetalol
Metaraminol
Methoxamine
Metoprolol
Milrinone

Nadolol
Nicardipine
Nifedipine
Nitroglycerin
Norepinephrine
Penbutolol
Phenylephrine
Pindolol
Propranolol
Sodium polystyrene sulfonate
Timolol
Verapamil

Cathartics/Laxatives

Bisacodyl
Docusate calcium
Docusate potassium
Docusate sodium
Glycerin suppositories
Lactulose
Magnesium citrate

Magnesium hydroxide
Mineral oil
Polyethylene glycol-electrolyte
  solution
Psyllium
Sorbitol

Diuretics

Acetazolamide
Amiloride
Bumetanide
Chlorothiazide
Chlorthalidone
Ethacrynic acid
Furosemide
Hydrochlorothiazide
Hydrochlorothiazide and
  amiloride

Hydrochlorothiazide and
  spironolactone
Hydrochlorothiazide and
  triamterene
Indapamide
Mannitol
Metolazone
Spironolactone
Torsemide
Triamterene

Estrogens

Esterified estrogens
Esterified estrogens with
  methyltestosterone
Estradiol topical
Estradiol transdermal
Estrogen, conjugated

Estrogen, conjugated with
  methylprogesterone
Estrogen, conjugated with
  methyltestosterone
Ethinyl estradiol

Gastrointestinal Agents

Cimetidine
Cisapride
Dicyclomine
Famotidine
Hyoscyamine sulfate
Mesalamine enema
Metoclopramide
Misoprostol
Nizatidine

Olsalazine
Omeprazole
Pancreatin
Pancrelipase
Propantheline
Ranitidine
Sucralfate
Vasopressin

Hormones/Synthetic Substitutes

Cortisone
Desmopressin
Desoxycorticosterone acetate
   (DOCA)
Dexamethasone
Epoetin alfa (Erythropoietin)
Filgrastim (G-CSF)
Fludrocortisone acetate
Glucagon
Gonadorelin
Hydrocortisone

Interferon alpha
Levonorgestrel Implants
Medroxyprogesterone
Methylergonovine
Methylprednisolone
Metyrapone
Oxytocin
Prednisolone
Prednisone
Sargramostim (GM-CSF)
Vasopressin

Immunosuppressive Agents

Antithymocyte globulin (ATG)
Azathioprine

Cyclosporine
Muromonab-CD3

Local Anesthetic Agents

Anusol
Bupivacaine
Lidocaine

Muscle Relaxants

Atracurium
Baclofen
Carisoprodol
Chlorzoxazone
Cyclobenzaprine
Dantrolene
Diazepam

Metaxalone
Methocarbamol
Mivacurium
Pancuronium
Pipecuronium
Succinylcholine
Vecuronium

Ophthalmic Antibiotics

Chloramphenicol
Ciprofloxacin
Cortisporin
Erythromycin

Gentamicin
Sulfacetamide
Tobramycin

Plasma Volume Expanders

Albumin
Dextran 40

Hetastarch
Plasma protein fraction

Respiratory Inhalants

Acetylcysteine
Beclomethasone
Cromolyn sodium

Flunisolide
Ipratropium
Triamcinolone

Sedatives/Hypnotics

Chloral hydrate
Diphenhydramine
Estazolam
Flurazepam
Hydroxyzine
Midazolam
Pentobarbital

Phenobarbital
Quazepam
Secobarbital
Temazepam
Triazolam
Zolpidem

Supplements

Calcium salts
Cholecalciferol
Cyanocobalamin
Ferrous sulfate
Folic acid
Iron dextran
Leucovorin

Magnesium oxide
Magnesium sulfate
Phytonadione (vitamin K)
Potassium supplements
Pyridoxine
Sodium bicarbonate
Thiamine

Thyroids/Antithyroids

Levothyroxine
Liothyronine

Methimazole
Propylthiouracil

Toxoids/Vaccines/Serums

Hemophilus B conjugate
Hepatitis B immune globulin
Hepatitis B vaccine
Immune globulin, intravenous

Pneumococcal vaccine, polyvalent
Tetanus immune globulin
Tetanus toxoid

Urinary Tract Agents

Belladonna and opium
  suppositories
Bethanechol
Finasteride
Flavoxate
Nalidixic acid

Neomycin-polymyxin bladder
  irrigant
Nitrofurantoin
Oxybutynin
Phenazopyridine
Trimethoprim

Vaginal Preparations

Amino-Cerv pH 5.5 cream
Estradiol topical
Miconazole

Nystatin
Terconazole
Tioconazole

Miscellaneous

Beractant
Colfosceril palmitate
Disulfiram
Gallium nitrate
Lindane (gamma benzene
  hexachloride)

Nimodipine
Permethrin
Physostigmine
Sumatriptan
Tacrine

GENERIC DRUGS: INDICATIONS & DOSAGE

ACEBUTOLOL (SECTRAL)

See Table IX–2, page 409.

ACETAMINOPHEN (TYLENOL, OTHERS)

Indications   Mild pain, headache, fever.
Dosage   Adult: 650–1000 mg PO or PR q4–6h.
                  Peds: 10 mg/kg/dose PO or PR q4–6h.
Notes   Overdose causes hepatotoxicity, which is treated with N-
                  acetylcysteine; charcoal is not usually recommended; has
                  no anti-inflammatory or platelet-inhibiting action.

ACETAMINOPHEN WITH BUTALBITAL AND CAFFEINE (FIORICET)

Indications   Mild pain, headache especially associated with stress.
Dosage   1–2 tablets or capsules PO q4–6h prn.

ACETAMINOPHEN WITH CODEINE (TYLENOL NO. 1, NO. 2, NO. 3, NO. 4) [C]

Indications   No. 1, No. 2, No. 3 for relief of mild to moderate pain; No.
                  4 for relief of moderate to severe pain.
Dosage   Adult: 1–2 tablets q3–4h prn.

TABLE IX–1. ANTISTAPHYLOCOCCAL PENICILLINS.

Drug (Brand Name)	Daily Dosage Range Adult (Peds)	Usual Dosing Interval	Supplied	Notes
Methicillin (Staphcillin)	4–18 g	4–6 hr	Injection	Interstitial nephritis can occur with high doses. Use high dose (12–18 g/d) for *Staphylococcus meningitis*. Reduce dose in renal failure.
Oxacillin (Prostaphlin)	4–12 g	4–6 hr	Injection Oral	Poorly absorbed orally; cloxacillin or dicloxacillin better for PO use. Interstitial nephritis can occur with high doses. Reduce dose in renal failure.
Nafcillin	4–18 g (50 mg/kg/d divided q4–6h)	4–6 hr	Injection Oral	Poorly absorbed orally; (Unipen) cloxacillin or dicloxacillin better for PO use. Injectable highest activity against *Staphylococcus aureus*. Can use for *Staphylococcus meningitis*
Cloxacillin (Tegopen, Cloxapen)	1–2 g	6 hr	Oral	Administer on an empty stomach at least 1 hr a.c. or 2 hrs p.c.
Dicloxacillin (Dynapen)	0.5–1 g (12–25 mg/kg/d divided QID)	6 hr	Oral	See above

Peds: Acetaminophen 10–15 mg/kg/dose; codeine 0.5–1.0 mg/kg dose q4–6h (useful dosing guide: 3–6 years, 5 mL per dose; 7–12 years, 10 mL per dose).

Notes Codeine in No. 1 = 7.5 mg, No. 2 = 15 mg, No. 3 = 30 mg, No. 4 = 60 mg.

ACETAZOLAMIDE (DIAMOX)

Indications Diuresis, glaucoma, alkalinization of urine, refractory epilepsy.
Dosage Adult: Diuretic: 250–375 mg IV or PO q24h in divided doses.
Glaucoma: 250–1,000 mg PO qd in divided doses.
Peds: Epilepsy: 8–30 mg/kg/24 hr PO in 4 divided doses.
Diuretic: 5 mg/kg/24 hr PO or IV.
Alkalinization of urine: 5 mg/kg/dose PO bid-tid.
Glaucoma: 20–40 mg/kg/24 hr PO in 4 divided doses.
Notes Contraindicated in renal failure, sulfa hypersensitivity; follow Na^+ and K^+; watch for metabolic acidosis.

ACETOHEXAMIDE (DYMELOR)

See Table IX–11 on page 497.

ACETYLCYSTEINE (MUCOMYST)

Indications Mucolytic agent as adjuvant therapy of chronic bronchopulmonary diseases and cystic fibrosis; as antidote to acetaminophen hepatotoxicity within 24 hours of ingestion.
Dosage Adults and Peds: Nebulizer: 3–5 mL of 20% solution diluted with equal volume of water or normal saline administered tid-qid.
Antidote: PO or NG; 140 mg/kg diluted 1:4 in carbonated beverage as loading dose, then 70 mg/kg q4h for 17 doses.
Notes Watch for bronchospasm when used by inhalation in asthmatics; activated charcoal adsorbs acetylcysteine when given PO for acute APAP ingestion.

ACYCLOVIR (ZOVIRAX)

Indications Treatment of Herpes simplex and Herpes zoster viral infections.
Dosage Adults: Topical: Apply 0.5-inch ribbon q3h.
Oral: Initial genital herpes: 200 mg PO q4h while awake, for a total of 5 capsules/day for 10 days.
Chronic suppression: 400 mg PO bid-tid.
Intermittent therapy: As for initial treatment, except treat for 5 days initiated at the earliest prodrome.

Herpes zoster: 800 mg PO 5 times/day.
Intravenous: 5–10 mg/kg/dose IV q8h.
Peds: 5–10 mg/kg/dose IV or PO q8h or 750 mg/m^2/24h divided q8h.

Notes   Adjust dose in renal insufficiency.

ADENOSINE (ADENOCARD)

Indications   Paroxysmal supraventricular tachycardia, including that associated with Wolff-Parkinson-White syndrome.

Dosage   Adults: 6 mg rapid IV bolus, may be repeated in 1–2 minutes at 12 mg IV if no response.
Peds: 0.03–0.25 mg/kg IV bolus; may repeat higher dose in 1–2 minutes if no response.

Notes   Doses > 12 mg are not recommended; caffeine and theophylline antagonize the effects of adenosine.

ALBUMIN (ALBUMINAR, BUMINATE, ALBUTEIN, OTHERS)

Indications   Plasma volume expansion for shock resulting from burns, surgery, hemorrhage, or other trauma.

Dosage   Adult: 25 g IV initially; subsequent infusions should depend on clinical situation and response.
Peds: 0.5–1.0 g/kg/dose; infuse at 0.05–0.1 g/min.

Notes   Contains 130–160 mEq Na$^+$/L.

ALBUTEROL (PROVENTIL, VENTOLIN)

Indications   Treatment of bronchospasm in reversible obstructive airway disease, prevention of exercise-induced bronchospasm.

Dosage   Adult: 2–4 inhalations q4–6h; 1 Rotocap inhaled q4–6h; 2–4 mg PO tid-qid.
Peds: 2 inhalations q4–6h; 0.1–0.2 mg/kg/dose PO, to maximum dose of 2–4 mg PO tid.

ALDESLEUKIN [IL-2] (PROLEUKIN)

Indications   Treatment of metastatic renal cell carcinoma, melanoma, and colorectal cancer.

Dosage   600,000 IU/kg (0.037 mg/kg) administered every 8 hours by a 15 minute infusion for 14 doses. Following 9 days of rest, repeat schedule for another 14 doses, for a maximum of 28 doses per cycle.

Notes   Only administer in a hospital with an intensive care unit and specialist available; may cause severe hypotension and capillary leaking, resulting in reduced organ perfusion.

ALFENTANIL (ALFENTA) [C]

Indications	Adjunct in the maintenance of anesthesia.
Dosage	Adults and Peds older than 12 years: 8–75 μg/kg IV infusion, total dose depends on the duration of the procedure.

ALLOPURINOL (ZYLOPRIM, LOPURIN)

Indications	Gout, treatment of hyperuricemia of malignancy, uric acid urolithiasis.
Dosage	Adult: Initial 100 mg PO qd; usual 300 mg PO qd. Peds: Use only for treating hyperuricemia of malignancy in children; 10 mg/kg/24 hours divided q6–8h (maximum 600 mg/24 hr).
Notes	Aggravates acute gouty attack, do **not** begin until acute attack resolves.

ALPRAZOLAM (XANAX) [C]

Indications	Management of anxiety and panic disorders, and anxiety associated with depression.
Dosage	0.25–2 mg PO tid.
Notes	Reduce dose in elderly and debilitated patients.

ALTEPLASE, RECOMBINANT [TPA] (ACTIVASE)

Indications	Treatment of acute MI and pulmonary embolism.
Dosage	100 mg IV over 3 hours.
Notes	May cause bleeding.

ALTRETAMINE (HEXALEN)

Indications	Palliative treatment of ovarian cancer.
Dosage	260 mg/m^2/d PO divided q6h, for 14–21 consecutive days of a 28-day cycle.
Notes	May cause neurologic and hematologic toxicity.

ALUMINUM CARBONATE (BASALJEL)

Indications	Hyperacidity (peptic ulcer, hiatal hernia, etc); supplement to management of hyperphosphatemia.
Dosage	Adult: 2 capsules or tablets or 10 mL (in water) q2h prn. Peds: 50–150 mg/kg/24h PO divided q4–6h.

ALUMINUM HYDROXIDE (AMPHOJEL, ALTERNAGEL)

Indications	Hyperacidity (peptic ulcer, hiatal hernia, etc); supplement to the management of hyperphosphatemia.

Dosage   Adult: 10–30 mL or 2 tablets PO q4–6h.
                  Peds: 5–15 mL PO q4–6h.
Notes   Can be used in renal failure; may cause constipation.

ALUMINUM HYDROXIDE WITH MAGNESIUM HYDROXIDE (MAALOX)

Indications   Hyperacidity (peptic ulcer, hiatal hernia, etc).
Dosage   Adult: 10–60 mL or 2–4 tablets PO qid or prn.
                  Peds: 5–15 mL PO qid or prn.
Notes   Doses qid are best given after meals and at bedtime; may
                  cause hypermagnesemia in renal insufficiency.

ALUMINUM HYDROXIDE WITH MAGNALIUM HYDROXIDE AND SIMETHICONE (MYLANTA, MYLANTA II, MAALOX PLUS)

Indications   Hyperacidity with bloating.
Dosage   Adults: 10–60 mL or 2–4 tablets PO qid or prn.
                  Peds: 5–15 mL PO qid or prn.
Notes   May cause hypermagnesemia in renal insufficiency; My-
                  lanta II contains twice the amount of aluminum and mag-
                  nesium hydroxide as Mylanta.

ALUMINUM HYDROXIDE, MAGNESIUM TRISILICATE, AND ALGINIC ACID (GAVISCON)

Indications   Symptomatic relief of heartburn; hiatal hernia.
Dosage   2–4 tablets or 15–30 mL PO qid followed by water.

AMANTADINE (SYMMETREL)

Indications   Treatment or prophylaxis of influenza A viral infections;
                  Parkinsonism.
Dosage   Adults: Influenza A: 200 mg PO qd or 100 mg PO bid.
                  Parkinsonism: 100 mg PO qd-bid.
                  Peds: 1–9 years old: 4.4–8.8 mg/kg/24h to a maximum of
                  150 mg/24h divided qd-bid; older than 9 years: same as
                  adults.
Notes   Reduce dose in renal insufficiency.

AMIKACIN (AMIKIN)

Indications   Treatment of serious infections caused by gram-negative
                  bacteria.
Dosage   Adults and Peds: 15 mg/kg/24h divided q8–12h or based
                  on renal function; refer to Aminoglycoside dosing on page
                  503.
Notes   May be effective against gram-negative bacteria resistant
                  to gentamicin and tobramycin; monitor renal function care-
                  fully for dosage adjustments; monitor serum levels (see
                  Table IX–12).

AMILORIDE (MIDAMOR)

Indications Hypertension and congestive heart failure.
Dosage 5–10 mg PO qd.
Notes Hyperkalemia may occur; monitor serum potassium levels.

AMINOCAPROIC ACID (AMICAR)

Indications Treatment of excessive bleeding resulting from systemic hyperfibrinolysis and urinary fibrinolysis.
Dosage Adults and Peds: 100 mg/kg IV, then 1 g/m^2/hr to maximum of 18 g/m^2/d or 100 mg/kg/dose q8h.
Notes Administer for 8 hours or until bleeding is controlled; contraindicated in disseminated intravascular coagulation; **not for upper urinary tract bleeding.**

AMINO-CERV PH 5.5 CREAM

Indications Mild cervicitis, postpartum cervicitis/cervical tears, postcauterization, postcryosurgery, and postconization.
Dosage 1 applicator intravaginally qhs for 2–4 weeks.
Notes Contains 8.34% urea, 0.5% sodium propionate, 0.83% methionine, 0.35% cystine, 0.83% inositol, benzalkonium chloride.

AMINOPHYLLINE

Indications Asthma and bronchospasm.
Dosage Adults: Acute asthma: Load 6 mg/kg IV, then 0.4–0.9 mg/kg/h IV continuous infusion.
Chronic asthma: 24 mg/kg/24h PO or PR divided q6h.
Peds: Load 6 mg/kg IV, then 1.0 mg/kg/h IV continuous infusion.
Notes Individualize dosage; signs of toxicity include nausea, vomiting, irritability, tachycardia, ventricular arrhythmias, and seizures; follow serum levels carefully (see Table IX–12, page 501); aminophylline is about 85% theophylline; erratic absorption with rectal doses.

AMIODARONE (CORDARONE)

Indications Treatment of recurrent ventricular fibrillation or hemodynamically unstable ventricular tachycardia.
Dosage Adults: Loading dose: 800–1600 mg/d PO for 1–3 weeks; maintenance: 600–800 mg/d PO for 1 month, then 200–400 mg/d.
Peds: 10 mg/kg/24h divided q12h PO for 7–10 days, then 5 mg/kg/24h divided q12h or qd (infants and neonates may require a higher loading dose).

Notes   Average half-life is 53 days; potentially toxic effects leading to pulmonary fibrosis, liver failure, ocular opacities, as
well as exacerbation of arrhythmias; Response requires 1
month as a rule.

AMITRIPTYLINE (ELAVIL)

Indications   Depression, peripheral neuropathy, chronic pain, cluster
and migraine headaches.
Dosage   Adults: Initially, 50–100 mg PO qhs; may increase to
300 mg qhs.
Peds: Not recommended for children younger than 12
years unless for chronic pain: 0.1 mg/kg qhs initially, then
advance over 2–3 weeks to 0.5–2 mg/kg qhs.
Notes   Strong anticholinergic side effects; may cause urinary retention and sedation.

AMLODIPINE (NORVASC)

Indications   Treatment of hypertension, chronic stable angina, and vasospastic angina.
Dosage   2.5–10 mg PO qd.

AMOXAPINE (ASENDIN)

Indications   Depression and anxiety.
Dosage   Initially, 150 mg PO qhs or 50 mg PO tid; increase to
300 mg daily.
Notes   Reduce dose in elderly; taper slowly when discontinuing
therapy.

AMOXICILLIN (AMOXIL, LAROTID, POLYMOX, OTHERS)

Indications   Treatment of susceptible gram-positive bacteria (streptococci), and gram-negative bacteria (*Haemophilus influen-
zae, Escherichia coli, Proteus mirabilis*).
Dosage   Adults: 250–500 mg PO tid.
Peds: 25–100 mg/kg/24h PO divided q8h.
Notes   Cross-hypersensitivity with penicillin; may cause diarrhea;
skin rash is common; many hospital strains of *Escherichia
coli* are resistant.

AMOXICILLIN/POTASSIUM CLAVULANATE (AUGMENTIN)

Indications   Treatment of infections caused by β-lactamase producing
strains of *Haemophilus influenzae, Staphylococcus au-
reus,* and *Escherichia coli.*
Dosage   Adult: 250–500 mg as amoxicillin PO q8h.
Peds: 25–50 mg/kg/d as amoxicillin PO divided q8h.

Notes   Do not substitute two 250 mg tablets for one 500 mg tablets or an overdose of clavulanic acid will occur; may cause diarrhea and gastrointestinal intolerance. Combination of a β-lactamase antibiotic and a β-lactamase inhibitor.

AMPHOTERICIN B (FUNGIZONE)

Indications Severe, systemic fungal infections.
Dosage   Adults and Peds: Test dose of 1 mg, then 0.25–1.5 mg/kg/24 hr IV over 4–6 hours. Doses often range from 25 to 50 mg qd or every other day. Total dose varies with indication.
Notes   Severe side effects with IV infusion; monitor renal function; hypokalemia and hypomagnesemia may be seen from renal wasting; pretreatment with acetaminophen and antihistamines (Benadryl) to help minimize adverse effects such as fever.

AMPICILLIN (AMCILL, OMNIPEN)

Indications Treatment of susceptible gram-negative (*Shigella, Salmonella, Escherichia coli, Haemophilus influenzae, Proteus mirabilis*) and gram-positive (*streptococci*) bacteria.
Dosage   Adults: Between 500 mg and 2 g PO, IM, or IV q6h.
               Peds: Neonates younger than 7 days: 50–100 mg/kg/24 hr IV divided q8h.
               Term infants: 75–150 mg/kg/24 hr divided q6–8h IV or PO.
               Older than 1 month and children: 100–200 mg/kg/24 hr divided q4–6h IM or IV; 50–100 mg/kg/24 hr divided q6h PO up to 250 mg/dose. Meningitis: 200–400 mg/kg/24 hr divided q4–6h IV.
Notes   Cross-hypersensitivity with penicillin; can cause diarrhea and skin rash; Many hospital strains of *Escherichia coli* are now resistant.

AMPICILLIN/SULBACTAM (UNASYN)

Indications Treatment of infections caused by β-lactamase producing organisms of *Staphylococcus aureus, Enterococcus, Haemophilus influenzae, Proteus mirabilis,* and *Bacteroides* species.
Dosage   Adult: 1.5–3.0 g IM or IV q6h.
               Peds: Dosed by ampicillin content (see "Ampicillin," above.
Notes   2:1 ratio of ampicillin: sulbactam; adjust dosage in renal failure; observe for hypersensitivity reactions.

AMRINONE (INOCOR)

Indications   Short-term management of congestive heart failure.
Dosage   Adults and Peds: Initially give IV bolus of 0.75 mg/kg
                    over 2–3 minutes followed by maintenance dose of 5–
                    10 µg/kg/min.
Notes   Not to exceed 10 mg/kg/d; incompatible with dextrose-
                    containing solutions; monitor for fluid and electrolyte
                    changes and renal function during therapy.

ANISTREPLASE (EMINASE)

Indications   Treatment of acute MI.
Dosage   30 units IV over 2–5 minutes.
Notes   May not be effective if readministered more than 5 days
                    after anistreplase, streptokinase, or streptococcal infec-
                    tion due to production of antistreptokinase antibody.

ANTIHEMOPHILIC FACTOR [FACTOR VIII] (MONOCLATE)

Indications   Treatment of classical hemophilia A.
Dosage   Adults and Peds: 1 AHF U/kg increases factor VIII con-
                    centration in the body by approximately 2%. Units re-
                    quired = (kg) (desired factor VIII increase as % normal) ×
                    (0.5).
                    Prophylaxis of spontaneous hemorrhage = 5% normal.
                    Hemostasis following trauma or surgery = 30% normal.
                    Head injuries, major surgery or bleeding = 80–100%
                    normal.
                    Patient's percentage of normal level of factor VIII concen-
                    tration must be ascertained before dosing for these calcu-
                    lations.
Notes   Not effective in controlling bleeding of patients with von
                    Willebrand's disease.

ANTITHYMOCYTE GLOBULIN [ATG] (ATGAM)

Indications   Management of allograft rejection in renal transplant pa-
                    tients.
Dosage   Adults: 10–30 mg/kg/d.
                    Peds: 5–25 mg/kg/d.
Notes   Do not administer to a patient with a history of severe sys-
                    temic reaction to any other equine gamma globulin prepa-
                    ration; discontinue treatment if severe unremitting throm-
                    bocytopenia or leukopenia occurs.

ANUSOL, ANUSOL-HC

Indications   Symptomatic relief of pain from external and internal hem-
                    orrhoids and anorectal surgery.

Dosage	1 suppository every morning and bedtime and following each bowel movement; apply cream or ointment freely to anal area q6–12h.
Notes	Anusol-HC also contains 1% hydrocortisone for anti-inflammatory effect.

APROTININ (TRASYLOL)

Indications	Reduction or prevention of blood loss in patients undergoing CABG.
Dosage	**High-dose:** 2 million KIU load, 2 million KIU for the pump prime dose, followed by 500,000 KIU/hr until surgery ends. **Low-dose:** 1 million KIU load, 1 million KIU for the pump prime dose, followed by 250,000 KIU/hr until surgery ends. Maximum total dose of 7 million KIU.
Notes	1 KIU = 0.14 mg of aprotinin.

ASPIRIN (BAYER, ST. JOSEPH)

Indications	Mild pain, headache, fever, inflammation, prevention of emboli, and prevention of myocardial infarction.
Dosage	Adults: Pain, fever: 325–650 mg q4–6h PO or PR. Rheumatoid arthritis: 3–6 g/d PO in divided doses. Platelet inhibitory action: 325 mg PO qd. Prevention of MI: 325 mg PO qd. Peds: **Caution:** Use linked to Reye's syndrome; avoid use with viral illness in children. Antipyretic: 10–15 mg/kg/dose PO or PR q4h up to 80 mg/kg/24 hr. Rheumatoid arthritis: 60–100 mg/kg/24 hr PO divided q4–6h (monitor serum levels to maintain between 15–30 mg/dL).
Notes	Gastrointestinal upset and erosion are common adverse reactions; discontinue use 1 week before surgery to avoid postop bleeding complications.

ASPIRIN WITH BUTALBITAL AND CAFFEINE (FIORINAL) [C]

Indications	Mild pain, headache especially when associated with stress.
Dosage	1–2 tablets (capsules) PO q4–6h prn.
Notes	Also available with codeine: No. 1 = 7.5 mg; No. 2 = 15 mg; No. 3 = 30 mg; significant drowsiness associated with use.

ASPIRIN WITH CODEINE (EMPIRIN NO. 1, NO. 2, NO. 3, NO. 4) [C]

Indications	Relief of mild to moderate pain.

Dosage	Adults: 1–2 tablets PO q3–4h prn.
	Peds: Aspirin 10 mg/kg/dose; codeine 0.5–1.0 mg/kg/dose q4h.
Notes	Codeine in No. 1 = 7.5 mg, No. 2 = 15 mg, No. 3 = 30 mg, No. 4 = 60 mg.

ASTEMIZOLE (HISMANAL)

Indications	Allergic rhinitis.
Dosage	Adults and Peds older than 12 years: 10 mg PO daily.
Notes	Nonsedating; take on an empty stomach; may affect allergy skin testing for weeks after one dose; may cause ventricular arrhythmias when used concurrently with the macrolide antibiotics, itraconazole or ketoconazole.

ATRACURIUM (TRACRIUM)

Indications	Adjunct to anesthesia to facilitate endotracheal intubation.
Dosage	Adults and Peds: 0.4–0.5 mg/kg IV bolus, then 0.08–0.1 mg/kg every 20–45 minutes prn.
Notes	Patient must be intubated and on controlled ventilation. Use adequate amounts of sedation and analgesia.

ATENOLOL (TENORMIN)

See Table IX–2 on page 409.

ATROPINE

Indications	Preanesthetic, symptomatic bradycardia, asystole.
Dosage	Adults: Emergency cardiac care, bradycardia: 0.5 mg IV q5min up to 2.0 mg total.
	Asystole 1.0 mg IV, repeat in 5 min.
	Preanesthetic: 0.3–0.6 mg IM.
	Peds: Emergency cardiac care: 0.01–0.03 mg/kg IV q2–5 min up to 1.0 mg total dose; minimum dose of 0.1 mg.
	Preanesthetic: 0.01 mg/kg/dose s.c./IV (maximum 0.4 mg).
Notes	Can cause blurred vision, urinary retention, dried mucous membranes.

AZATHIOPRINE (IMURAN)

Indications	Adjunct for the prevention of rejection following organ transplantation; rheumatoid arthritis; systemic lupus erythematosus.
Dosage	Adults and Peds: 1–3 mg/kg IV or PO daily.
Notes	May cause gastrointestinal intolerance; injection should be handled with cytotoxic precautions.

TABLE IX–2. BETA-ADRENERGIC BLOCKING AGENTS.

Drug (Brand Name)	Receptor Activity	Half-Life	Excretion	Dosing Range and Frequency[1]	
				Angina Pectoris	Hypertension
Acebutolol (Sectral)	β_1	3–4 hr	Hepatic, renal	N/A	200 mg PO bid; 400 mg PO qd
Atenolol (Tenormin)	β_1	6–9 hr	Renal	50–100 mg PO qd[2]	50–100 mg PO qd[2]
Betaxolol (Kerlone)	β_1	14–22 hr	Hepatic	N/A	10–20 mg PO qd
Bisoprolol (Zebeta)	β_1			N/A	5–10 mg PO qd
Carteolol (Cartrol)	β_1, β_2	6 hr	Renal	N/A	2.5–10 mg PO qd
Labetalol (Normodyne, Trandate)	β_1, β_2 alpha	6–8 hr	Hepatic	N/A	100–400 mg PO bid
Metoprolol (Lopressor)	β_1	3–7 hr	Hepatic, renal	50–100 mg PO bid	50–100 mg PO bid-tid
Nadolol (Corgard)	β_1, β_2	20–40 hr	Renal	40–240 mg PO qd[2]	40–320 mg PO qd[2]
Penbutolol (Levatol)	β_1, β_2	5 hr	Hepatic, renal	N/A	20–40 mg PO qd
Pindolol (Visken)	β_1, β_2	3–4 hr	Hepatic, renal	N/A	10–40 mg PO bid
Propranolol[3] (Inderal)	β_1, β_2	3–5 hr	Hepatic	80–240 mg PO bid-tid	80–480 mg PO bid-tid
Sotalol (Betapace)	β_1, β_2			80 mg PO bid	
Timolol (Blocadren)	β_1, β_2	4 hr	Hepatic, renal	10–40 mg PO bid	N/A

[1]Other uses of β-blockers include postmyocardial infarction to reduce mortality, pheochromocytoma, hypertrophic subaortic stenosis; ophthalmic preparations for glaucoma.
[2]Reduce dose in renal failure.
[3]For arrhythmias: Adult: 80–120 mg PO divided tid-qid; migraine 80–240 mg PO divided bid-tid.

AZITHROMYCIN (ZITHROMAX)

Indications   Treatment of mild to moderate upper and lower respiratory tract infections, and nongonococcal urethritis.

Dosage   Respiratory tract: 500 mg on first day followed by 250 mg PO qd for 4 more days. Non-gonococcal urethritis: 1 g as a single dose.

Notes   Should be taken on an empty stomach; avoid concurrent use with terfenadine, astemizole, and loratadine.

AZTREONAM (AZACTAM)

Indications   Treatment of infections caused by aerobic gram-negative bacteria including *Pseudomonas aeruginosa*.

Dosage   Adults: 1–2 g IV/IM q6–12h.
                  Peds: Premature infants: 30 mg/kg/dose IV q12h.
                  Term infants, children: 30–50 mg/kg/dose q6–8h.

Notes   Not effective against gram-positive or anaerobic bacteria; may be given to penicillin-allergic patients.

BACLOFEN (LIORESAL)

Indications   Management of spasticity secondary to severe chronic disorders such as multiple sclerosis or spinal cord lesions.

Dosage   5 mg PO tid initially, increase every 3 days to maximum effect; maximum 80 mg/d.

Notes   Caution in epileptics and neuropsychiatric disturbances.

BCG (THERACYS, TICE)

Indications   Treatment and prophylaxis of superficial bladder cancer.

Dosage   1 ampule in 30–50 mL normal saline instilled into bladder by catheter and held for 2 hours (standard treatment weekly for 6 weeks).

Notes   Do not give if catheterization traumatic.

BECLOMETHASONE (BECONASE, VANCENASE NASAL INHALERS)

Indications   Allergic rhinitis refractory to conventional therapy with antihistamines and decongestants.

Dosage   Adults: 1 spray intranasally bid-qid.
                  Peds: 6–11 years: 1 spray intranasally tid.

Notes   Nasal spray delivers 42 µg/dose.

BECLOMETHASONE (BECLOVENT INHALER, VANCERIL INHALER)

Indications   Chronic asthma.

Dosage   Adults: 2–4 inhalations tid-qid (maximum 20/day).
                  Peds: 1–2 inhalations tid-qid (maximum 10/day).

Notes   Not effective for acute asthmatic attacks; may cause oral candidiasis.

BELLADONNA AND OPIUM SUPPOSITORIES (B & O SUPPRETTES) [C]

Indications   Treatment of bladder spasms; moderate to severe pain.
Dosage   Insert 1 suppository rectally q4–6h prn. 15A = 30 mg powdered opium; 16.2 mg belladonna extract. 16A = 60 mg powdered opium; 16.2 mg belladonna extract.
Notes   Anticholinergic side effects; caution subjects about sedation, urinary retention, constipation.

BENAZEPRIL (LOTENSIN)

Indications   Hypertension.
Dosage   10–40 mg PO qd.
Notes   May cause symptomatic hypotension in patients taking diuretics; may cause a nonproductive cough.

BENZONATE (TESSALON PERLES)

Indications   Symptomatic relief of nonproductive cough.
Dosages   100 mg PO tid.
Notes   May cause sedation.

BENZQUINAMIDE (EMETE-CON)

Indications   Nausea and vomiting.
Dosage   50 mg IM q3–4h prn.
Notes   Alternative antiemetic when phenothiazine or antihistamine is contraindicated.

BENZTROPINE (COGENTIN)

Indications   Treatment of Parkinson's disease and drug-induced extrapyramidal disorders.
Dosage   1–6 mg PO, IM, or IV in divided doses.
Notes   Anticholinergic side effects.

BEPRIDIL (VASCOR)

Indications   Treatment of chronic stable angina.
Dosage   200–400 mg PO daily.
Notes   May cause serious ventricular arrhythmias, including torsade de pointes and agranulocytosis.

BERACTANT (SURVANTA)

Indications   Prevention and treatment of respiratory distress syndrome in premature infants.
Dosage   4 mL/kg administered via endotracheal tube.

BETAXOLOL (KERLONE)

See Table IX–2 on page 409.

BETHANECHOL (URECHOLINE, DUVOID, VARIOUS)

Indications   Neurogenic atony of the bladder with urinary retention, acute postoperative and postpartum functional (nonobstructive) urinary retention.

Dosage   Adults: 10–50 mg PO tid-qid or 5 mg s.c. tid-qid and prn. Peds: 0.3–0.6 mg/kg/24 hr PO divided tid-qid or ⅓ the oral dose s.c.

Notes   Contraindicated in bladder outlet obstruction, asthma, coronary artery disease; do not administer IM or IV.

BISACODYL (DULCOLAX)

Indications   Constipation, bowel prep.

Dosage   Adults: 5–10 mg PO or 10 mg rectally prn. Peds younger than 2 years: 5 mg rectally prn; older than 2 years: 5 mg PO or 10 mg rectally prn.

Notes   Do not use with an acute abdomen or bowel obstruction; do not chew tablets; do not give within 1 hour of antacids or milk.

BISMUTH SUBSALICYLATE (PEPTO-BISMOL)

Indications   Indigestion, nausea, and diarrhea.

Dosage   Adults: 2 tablets or 30 mL PO prn. Peds: 3–6 years old: ⅓ tablet or 5 mL PO prn; 6–9 years old: ⅔ tablet or 10 mL PO prn; 9–12 years old: 1 tablet or 15 mL PO prn.

BISOPROLOL (ZEBETA)

See Table IX–2 on page 409.

BITOLTEROL (TORNALATE)

Indications   Prophylaxis and treatment of asthma and reversible bronchospasm.

Dosage   Adults and children older than 12 years: 2 inhalations q8h.

BLEOMYCIN (BLENOXANE)

Indications   Treatment of cervical, ovarian, squamous cell, testicular cancer, and lymphoma.

Dosage   0.25–0.5 U/kg/dose IV, IM, or s.c. once or twice weekly.

Notes   Pulmonary toxicity is increased with total doses of > 400 units.

BRETYLIUM (BRETYLOL)

Indications Acute treatment of ventricular fibrillation or tachycardia unresponsive to conventional therapy.

Dosage 5 mg/kg IV rapid injection (1 minute); may repeat q15–30min with 10 mg/kg (maximum of 30 mg/kg); maintenance, 1–2 mg/min IV infusion.

Notes Nausea and vomiting are associated with rapid IV bolus; should gradually reduce dose and discontinue in 3–5 days; effects are seen within first 10–15 minutes; transient rise in BP seen initially; hypotension is the most frequent adverse effect and occurs within the first hour of treatment.

BROMOCRIPTINE (PARLODEL)

Indications Hyperprolactinemia, prevention of lactation, and parkinsonian syndrome.

Dosage Hyperprolactinemia: 5–7.5 mg daily. Lactation: 2.5 mg PO qd-tid. Parkinson's: 1.25 mg PO bid initially, titrated to effect.

Notes Nausea and vertigo are common side effects.

BROMPHENIRAMINE (DIMETANE)

Indications Allergic reactions.

Dosage Adults: 4–8 mg PO tid-qid or 8–12 mg PO q8–12h (sustained release) or 10 mg IM q6–12h.
Peds: Younger than 6 years: 0.5 mg/kg/24 hr PO divided q6–8h.
Older than 6 years: 4 mg PO q6–8h or one 8–12 mg sustained release tablet q8–12h.

BUCLIZINE (BUCLADIN-S SOFTABS)

Indications Control of nausea, vomiting, and dizziness of motion sickness.

Dosage 50 mg dissolved in mouth bid; 50 mg PO prophylactically 30 minutes before travel.

Notes Not safe in pregnancy; contains tartrazine, observe patient for allergic reactions.

BUMETANIDE (BUMEX)

Indications Edema from congestive heart failure, hepatic cirrhosis, and renal disease.

Dosage Adults: 0.5–2.0 mg PO daily; 0.5–1.0 mg IV q8–24h.
Peds: 0.015–0.1 mg/kg/dose PO, IV, IM q6–24h.

Notes Monitor fluid and electrolyte status during treatment.

BUPIVACAINE (MARCAINE)

Indications   Local infiltration, lumbar epidural.
Dosage   Dose is dependent on the procedure, vascularity of the tissues, depth of anesthesia, and degree of muscle relaxation required. Maximum dose in 70 kg adult is 70 mL of 0.25%.

BUPRENORPHINE (BUPRENEX)

Indications   Relief of moderate to severe pain.
Dosage   0.3 mg IM or slow IV push every 6 hours prn.
Notes   May induce withdrawal syndrome in opioid dependent subjects.

BUPROPION (WELLBUTRIN)

Indications   Treatment of depression.
Dosage   200–450 mg/d divided bid-tid.
Notes   Has been associated with seizures; avoid use of alcohol and other CNS depressants.

BUSPIRONE (BUSPAR)

Indications   Short-term relief of anxiety.
Dosage   5–10 mg PO tid.
Notes   No abuse potential. No physical or psychological dependence.

BUTORPHANOL (STADOL)

Indications   Analgesic for moderate to severe pain.
Dosage   2 mg IM or IV every 3–4 hours prn.
Notes   May induce withdrawal syndrome in opioid-dependent patients.

CALCIUM CARBONATE (TUMS, ALKA-MINTS)

Indications   Hyperacidity associated with peptic ulcer disease, hiatal hernia, etc.
Dosage   From 500 mg to 1.5 g PO prn.

CALCIUM SALTS

Indications   Calcium replacement, ventricular fibrillation, electromechanical dissociation.
Dosage   Adults: Replacement: 1–2 g PO qd.
                  Cardiac emergencies: Calcium chloride 0.5–1.0 g IV every 10 minutes or Calcium gluconate 1–2 g IV every 10 minutes.
                  Peds: Replacement: 200–500 mg/kg/24h PO or IV divided qid.

Cardiac emergency: 100 mg/kg/dose IV every 10 minutes
of gluconate salt.

Notes   Calcium chloride contains 270 mg (13.6 mEq) elemental
calcium per gram, and calcium gluconate contains 90 mg
(4.5 mEq) elemental calcium per gram.

CAPTOPRIL (CAPOTEN)

Indications   Treatment of hypertension, congestive heart failure, and
diabetic nephropathy.

Dosage   Adults: Hypertension: Initially, 25 mg. PO bid-tid; titrate to
a maintenance dose every 1–2 weeks by 25 mg incre-
ments per dose (maximum 450 mg/d) to desired effect.
Congestive heart failure: Initially, 6.25–12.5 mg PO tid;
titrate to desired effect.
Peds: Infants younger than 2 months–0.05–0.1 mg/kg/dose
PO tid-qid.
Children: Initially, 0.15 mg/kg/dose PO; double q2h until
blood pressure is controlled, to maximum of 6 mg/kg/d;
maintenance, 0.5–0.6 mg/kg/d PO divided bid-qid.

Notes   Use with caution in renal failure. Give 1 hour before meals;
can cause rash, proteinuria, and cough.

CARBAMAZEPINE (TEGRETOL)

Indications   Epilepsy; trigeminal neuralgia.

Dosage   Adults: 200 mg PO bid initially; increase by 200 mg/d;
usual 800–1200 mg/d.
Peds 6–12 years: 100 mg/dose PO bid or 10 mg/kg/24h
PO divided qd-bid initially; increase to a maintenance
dose of 20–30 mg/kg/24h divided tid-qid.

Notes   Can cause severe hematologic side effects; monitor CBC;
monitor serum levels, see Table IX–12 (page 501); generic
products are **not** interchangeable.

CARBIDOPA/LEVODOPA (SINEMET)

Indications   Parkinson's disease.

Dosage   Start at 10/100 PO bid-tid; titrate as needed.

Notes   May cause psychiatric disturbances, orthostatic hypotension, dyskinesias, and cardiac arrhythmias.

CARBOPLATIN (PARAPLATIN)

Indications   Treatment of cervical, ovarian, and lung cancer.

Dosage   300–360 mg/m^2 on day 1 every 4 weeks.

Notes   May cause bone marrow suppression, vomiting, and anaphylaxis.

CARISOPRODOL (SOMA)

Indications   Adjunct to sleep and physical therapy for the relief of painful musculoskeletal conditions.
Dosage   350 mg PO qid.
Notes   Avoid alcohol and other CNS depressants.

CARTEOLOL (CARTROL)

See Table IX–2 on page 409.

CEFACLOR (CECLOR)

See Table IX–3 on page 417.

CEFADROXIL (DURICEF, ULTRACEF)

See Table IX–3 on page 417.

CEFAMANDOLE (MANDOL)

See Table IX–4 on page 418.

CEFAZOLIN (ANCEF, KEFZOL)

See Table IX–3 on page 417.

CEFIXIME (SUPRAX)

See Table IX–5 on page 419.

CEFMETAZOLE (ZEFAZONE)

See Table IX–4 on page 418.

CEFONICID (MONICID)

See Table IX–4 on page 418.

CEFOPERAZONE (CEFOBID)

See Table IX–5 on page 419.

CEFOTAXIME (CLAFORAN)

See Table IX–5 on page 419.

CEFOTETAN (CEFOTAN)

See Table IX–5 on page 419.

CEFOXITIN (MEFOXIN)

See Table IX–4 on page 418.

TABLE IX-3. FIRST GENERATION CEPHALOSPORINS.

Drug (Brand Name)	Daily Dosing Adult	Usual Interval	Pediatric (mg/kg/24 h)	Half-life	Supplied	Notes
Cefadroxil (Duricef, Ultracef)	1–2 g PO	12 hr		1.5 hr	Capsules, tablets	May be dosed bid.
Cephalothin (Keflin)	2–12 g[1]	4–6 hr	75–125	30–45 min	Injection	IV use causes phlebitis; IM use is painful.
Cephapirin (Cefadyl)	2–12 g[1]	4–6 hr	40–80	30–45 min	Injection	Possibly milder phlebitis, and less pain than cephalothin.
Cefaclor (Ceclor)	1–4 g[1]	4–6 hr	20–40	45 min	Oral	High level of activity against *Haemophilus influenza.*
Cephalexin (Keflex, Keftabs)	1–4 g[1]	4–6 hr	25–50	45 min	Oral	Keftabs has better absorption than Keflex.
Cephradine (Velocef, Anspor)	1–4 g PO 2–8 g IV	4–6 hr	25–50 PO 75–125 IM/IV	45 min	Oral, injection	Less active than cephalothin against *Staphylococcus aureus.*
Cefazolin (Ancef, Kefzol)	1.5–12 g[1]	8 hr	50–100	2 hr	Injection	Best first generation for surgical prophylaxis. IM dose fairly well tolerated.

[1]Reduce dose in renal failure.

417

TABLE IX-4. SECOND GENERATION CEPHALOSPORINS.

Drug (Brand Name)	Daily dosage	Interval	Pediatric (mg/kg/24h)	Half-life	Supplied	Notes
Cefamandole (Mandol)	3–12 g[1]	4–6 hr	50–150	40 min	Injection	High level of activity against *Haemophilus influenza.* Disulfiram reaction with alcohol use. Monitor PT closely with long-term use.
Cefoxitin (Mefoxin)	2–12 g[1]	4–6 hr	80–160	45 min	Injection	Best cephalosporin against *B fragilis;* good for mixed aerobic/anaerobic infections in OB/GYN, surgery.
Cefuroxime (Zinacef, Ceftin)	2.25–9 g IV[1] 500 mg–1 g PO	8 hr	75–150 divided q12h (200–240 in meningitis)	1.5 hr	Injection	Crosses blood-brain barrier; can be used for some organisms in meningitis at higher doses.
Ceforanide (Precef)	1–4 g[1]	12 hr		2.2 hr	Injection	Less effective against *Staphylococcus aureus.*
Cefonicid (Monocid)	1–4 g[1]	24 hr		4 hr	Injection	Less effective against *Staphylococcus aureus.*
Cefmetazole (Zefazone)	2–8 g[1]	6–12 hr		1.2 hr	Injection	*B fragilis* coverage.
Cefpodoxime (Vantin)	200–800 mg		10 divided bid			
Cefprozil (Cefzil)	250–500 mg					
Loracarbef (Lorabid)	200–400 mg	12 hr	15–30 divided bid			

[1]Reduce dose in renal failure.

TABLE IX–5. THIRD GENERATION CEPHALOSPORINS.

Drug (Brand Name)	Daily Dosage	Interval	Pediatrics (mg/kg/24h)	Half-life	Supplied	Notes
Cefixime (Suprax)	400 mg	12–24 hr	8 divided qd-bid	3.5 hr	Oral	May cause GI irritation. No *Staphylococcus* or *Pseudomonas* activity.
Cefoperazone (Cefobid)	2–12 g	8–12 hr		2.5 hr	Injection	Hepatic/renal excretion allows normal dosing in renal failure. Disulfiram reactions and hypoprothrombinemia can occur. Do not use alone for *Pseudomonas.*
Cefotaxime (Claforan)	2–12 g[1]	4–8 hr	50–180 divided q4–6h	1 hr	Injection	Excellent gram (−) activity except *Pseudomonas.* Crosses blood-brain barrier. Give 1/2 dose if Cr clear <20.
Cefotetan (Cefotan)	2–4 g	12 hr		4 hr	Injection	Activity against *B fragilis.* May cause hypoprothrombinemia.
Ceftazidime (Fortraz, Ceptaz, Tazidime, Tazicef)	2–12 g[1]	8–12 hr		2.5 hr	Injection	Best third generation against *Pseudomonas* No activity against *B fragilis.*
Ceftizoxime (Cefizox)	2–12 g[1]	8–12 hr	50 mg/kg/dose	2.5 hr	Injection	Spectrum similar to cefotaxime. Less activity against *B fragilis.*
Ceftriaxone (Rocephin)	1–4 g	24 hr	50–75 (2 g max)	8 hr	Injection	Long half-life allows once a day dose. Home therapy possible. No change in renal failure to 2 g/d.

[1]Reduce dose in renal failure.

CEFPODOXIME (VANTIN)

See Table IX–4 on page 418.

CEFPROZIL (CEFZIL)

See Table IX–4 on page 418.

CEFTAZIDIME (FORTAZ, CEPTAZ, TAZIDIME, TAZICEF)

See Table IX–5 on page 419.

CEFTIZOXIME (CEFIZOX)

See Table IX–5 on page 419.

CEFTRIAXONE (ROCEPHIN)

See Table IX–5 on page 419.

CEFUROXIME (CEFTIN, ZINACEF)

See Table IX–4 on page 418.

CEPHALEXIN (KEFLEX, KEFTAB)

See Table IX–3 on page 417.

CEPHALOTHIN (KEFLIN)

See Table IX–3 on page 417.

CEPHAPIRIN (CEFADYL)

See Table IX–3 on page 417.

CEPHRADINE (VELOSEF, ANSPOR)

See Table IX–3 on page 417.

CHARCOAL, ACTIVATED (SUPERCHAR, ACTIDOSE, LIQUI-CHAR)

Indications	Emergency treatment for poisoning by most drugs and chemicals.
Dosage	Adults: Acute intoxication: 30–100 g/dose. Gastrointestinal dialysis: 25–50 g q4–6h. Peds: Acute intoxication: 1–2 g/kg/dose. Gastrointestinal dialysis: 5–10 g/dose q4–8h.
Notes	Administer with a cathartic; liquid dosage forms are in sorbitol base; protect airway in lethargic or comatose patient.

CHLORAL HYDRATE (NOCTEC) [C]

Indications   Nocturnal and preoperative sedation.
Dosage   Adults: Hypnotic: Between 500 mg and 1 g PO or PR 30 minutes before sleep or procedure.
Sedative: 250 mg PO or PR tid.
Peds: Hypnotic: 50 mg/kg/24h PO or PR 30 minutes before sleep or procedure.
Sedative: 25 mg/kg/24h PO or PR tid.
Notes   Mix syrup in a glass of water or fruit juice.

CHLORAMBUCIL (LEUKERAN)

Indications   Treatment of ovarian cancer, leukemia, and lymphoma.
Dosage   Initially 0.1–0.2 mg/kg/d for 3–6 weeks, then maintenance therapy with no more than 0.1 mg/kg/d.

CHLORAMPHENICOL, OPHTHALMIC (CHLOROMYCETIN OPHTHALMIC)

Indications   Conjunctival infections.
Dosage   1% ointment apply q3h for 48 hours, then decrease if response. 0.5% solution apply 4–6 times a day, then for 72 hours, then decrease.

CHLORDIAZEPOXIDE (LIBRIUM)

Indications   Anxiety, tension, alcohol withdrawal.
Dosage   Adults: Mild anxiety, tension: 5–10 mg PO tid-qid or prn.
Severe anxiety, tension: 25–50 mg IM or IV tid-qid or prn.
Alcohol withdrawal: 50–100 mg IM or IV; repeat in 2–4 hours if needed, up to 300 mg in 24 hours; gradually taper daily dosage.
Peds: 0.5 mg/kg/24h PO or IM divided q6–8h.
Notes   Reduce dose in the elderly; absorption of IM doses can be erratic.

CHLOROTHIAZIDE (DIURIL)

Indications   Hypertension, edema, congestive heart failure.
Dosage   Adults: Between 500 mg and 1.0 g PO or IV qd-bid.
Peds: 20–30 mg/kg/24h PO divided bid.
Notes   Contraindicated in anuria.

CHLORPHENIRAMINE (CHLOR-TRIMETON, OTHERS)

Indications   Allergic reactions.
Dosage   Adults: 4 mg PO or IV q4–6h or 8–12 mg PO bid of sustained release.
Peds: 0.35 mg/kg/24h PO divided q4–6h or 0.2 mg/kg/24h sustained release.
Notes   Anticholinergic side effects and sedation are common.

CHLORPROMAZINE (THORAZINE)

Indications   Psychotic disorders, apprehension, intractable hiccups, control of nausea and vomiting.

Dosage   Adults: Acute anxiety, agitation: 10–25 mg PO or PR bid-tid.
Severe symptoms: 25 mg IM, can repeat in 1 hour, then 25–50 mg PO or PR tid.
Hiccups: 25–50 mg PO bid-tid.
Peds: 2.5–6.0 mg/kg/24h PO, PR or IM divided q4–8h.

Notes   Beware of extrapyramidal side effects, sedation, has α-adrenergic blocking properties.

CHLORPROPAMIDE (DIABINESE)

See Table IX–11 on page 497.

CHLORTHALIDONE (HYGROTON)

Indications   Hypertension, edema associated with congestive heart failure, steroid and estrogen therapy.

Dosage   Adults: 50–100 mg PO qd.
Peds: 2 mg/kg/dose PO 3 times weekly or 1–2 mg/kg PO daily.

Notes   Contraindicated in anuric patients.

CHLORZOXAZONE (PARAFLEX, PARAFON FORTE DSC)

Indications   Adjunct to rest and physical therapy for the relief of discomfort associated with acute, painful musculoskeletal conditions.

Dosage   250–500 mg PO tid-qid.

CHOLECALCIFEROL [VITAMIN D3] (DELTA D)

Indications   Dietary supplement for treatment of vitamin D deficiency.
Dosage   400–1000 IU PO daily.
Notes   1 mg cholecalciferol = 40,000 IU of vitamin D activity.

CHOLESTYRAMINE (QUESTRAN)

Indications   Adjunctive therapy for the reduction of serum cholesterol in patients with primary hypercholesterolemia; relief of pruritus associated with partial biliary obstruction.

Dosage   Individualize dose to 4 g 1–6 times a day.
Notes   Mix 4 g cholestyramine in 2–6 oz of noncarbonated beverages.

CIMETIDINE (TAGAMET)

Indications   Duodenal ulcer, ulcer prophylaxis in hypersecretory states such as trauma, burns, surgery, Zollinger-Ellison syndrome.

Dosage   Adults: Active ulcer: 2400 mg/d IV continuous infusion or 300 mg IV q6–4h; 400 mg PO bid or 800 mg qhs.
Maintenance therapy: 400 mg PO qhs.
Peds: Neonates: 10–20 mg/kg/24h PO or IV divided q4–6h.
Children: 20–40 mg/kg/24h PO or IV divided q4–6h.
Notes   Extend dosing interval with renal insufficiency; decrease dose in the elderly; has many drug interactions.

CIPROFLOXACIN (CILOXAN)

Indications   Conjunctival infections.
Dosage   0.06 or 0.12% solution, apply from every 15 min to every 4 hours.

CIPROFLOXACIN (CIPRO)

Indications   Broad spectrum activity against a variety of gram-positive and gram-negative aerobic bacteria.
Dosage   Adults: 250–750 mg PO q12h or 200–400 mg IV q12h.
Peds: Not recommended for use in children younger than 18 years, due to cartilage effects.
Notes   Little activity against streptococci; drug interactions with theophylline, caffeine, sucralfate, and antacids. Nausea, vomiting, and abdominal discomfort are common side effects. Contraindicated in pregnancy.

CISAPRIDE (PROPULSID)

Indications   Gastroesophageal reflux.
Dosage   10–20 mg PO qid.
Notes   Should be administered 15 minutes before meals.

CISPLATIN (PLATINOL)

Indications   Treatment of cervical, ovarian, testicular, and other solid tumors.
Dosage   20–70 mg/m^2 IV. Dosage and duration of therapy is dependent on individual treatment protocols.
Notes   Agent is nephrotoxic; hydrate patients with 1–2 L of fluid before infusion.

CLARITHROMYCIN (BIAXIN)

Indications   Treatment of upper and lower respiratory tract infections, skin and skin structure infections, and infections caused by nontubercular *Mycobacterium*.
Dosage   250–500 mg PO bid. *Mycobacterium:* 500–1000 mg PO bid.
Notes   Increases theophylline and carbamazepine levels; avoid concurrent use with astemizole, loratadine, and terfenadine.

CLEMASTINE FUMARATE (TAVIST)

Indications   Allergic rhinitis.
Dosage   1.34 mg bid to 2.68 mg tid, maximum 8.04 mg/d.

CLINDAMYCIN (CLEOCIN)

Indications   Susceptible strains of streptococci, pneumococci, staphylococci, and gram-positive and gram-negative anaerobes, no activity against gram-negative aerobes.
Dosage   Adults: 150–450 mg PO qid; 300–600 mg IV q6h or 900 mg IV q8h.
                   Peds: Neonates: 15–20 mg/kg/24h divided q6–8h.
                   Children older than 1 month: 15–40 mg/kg/24h divided q6–8h, to a maximum of 4 g/d.
Notes   Beware of diarrhea that may represent pseudomembranous colitis caused by *Clostridium difficile.*

CLOFAZIMINE (LAMPRENE)

Indications   Treatment of leprosy, and as part of combination therapy for *Mycobacterium avium* complex in AIDS patients.
Dosage   Adults and Peds: 100–300 mg PO qd.
Notes   Take with meals; may change skin pigmentation pink to brownish black; may cause skin dryness and gastrointestinal intolerance.

CLOFIBRATE (ATROMID-S)

Indications   Treatment of type III hyperlipidemia.
Dosage   500 mg PO qid.
Notes   Gastrointestinal intolerance is common.

CLONAZEPAM (KLONOPIN) [C]

Indications   Lennox-Gastaut syndrome, akinetic and myoclonic seizures, absence seizures.
Dosage   Adults: 1.5 mg/d PO in 3 divided doses; increase by 0.5–1.0 mg/d every 3 days prn up to 20 mg/d.
                   Peds: 0.01–0.05 mg/kg/24h PO divided tid; increase to 0.1–0.2 mg/kg/24h divided tid.
Notes   CNS side effects including sedation.

CLONIDINE (CATAPRES)

Indications   Hypertension, opioid and tobacco withdrawal.
Dosage   Adults: 0.10 mg PO bid adjusted daily by 0.1–0.2 mg increments (maximum 2.4 mg/d).
                   Peds: 5–25 μg/kg/24h divided q6h.

Notes   Dry mouth, drowsiness, sedation occur frequently; more effective for hypertension when combined with diuretics, rebound hypertension can occur with abrupt cessation of doses above 0.2 mg bid.

CLONIDINE TRANSDERMAL (CATAPRES TTS)

Indications   Hypertension.
Dosage   Apply one patch every 7 days to a hairless area on the upper arm or torso; titrate according to individual therapeutic requirements.
Notes   TTS-1, TTS-2, TTS-3 (programmed to deliver 0.1, 0.2, 0.3 mg respectively of clonidine per day, for 1 week). Doses above two TTS-3 are usually not associated with increased efficacy.

CLORAZEPATE (TRANXENE)

Indications   Acute anxiety disorders, acute alcohol withdrawal symptoms, adjunctive therapy in partial seizures.
Dosage   Adults: 15–60 mg/d PO in single or divided doses.
                  Peds: 3.75–7.5 mg/dose bid, to a maximum of 60 mg/d divided bid-tid.
Notes   Monitor patients with renal and hepatic impairment since drug may accumulate; CNS depressant effects.

CLOTRIMAZOLE (LOTRIMIN, MYCELEX)

Indications   Treatment of candidiasis and tinea infections.
Dosage   Orally: One troche dissolved slowly in mouth 5 times a day for 14 days.
                  Vaginal: Cream: One applicator qhs for 7–14 days; Tablets: 100 mg vaginally qhs for 7 days or 200 mg (2 tablets) vaginally qhs for 3 days or 500 mg tablet vaginally hs × 1.
                  Topical: Apply 3–4 times daily for 10–14 days.
Notes   Oral prophylaxis commonly used in immunosuppressed patients.

CLOXACILLIN (CLOXAPEN, TEGOPEN)

See Table IX–1 on page 398.

CLOZAPINE (CLOZARIL)

Indications   Severe schizophrenia that does not respond to standard therapy.
Dosage   Initial 25 mg qd-bid, increase dose to 300–450 mg/d over 2 weeks. Maintain patient at lowest dose possible.

Notes   Has limited distribution. Contact local pharmacy for drug availability. Monitor blood counts frequently because of the risk of agranulocytosis. May also cause drowsiness and seizures.

CODEINE [C]

Indications   Mild to moderate pain; symptomatic relief of cough.
Dosage   Adults: Analgesic: 15–60 mg PO, s.c., or IM qid prn.
                   Antitussive: 5–15 mg PO or s.c. q4h prn.
                   Peds: Analgesic: 0.5–1.0 mg/kg/dose PO or s.c. q4–6h prn.
                   Antitussive: 1.0–1.5 mg/kg/24hr divided q4h, maximum 30 mg/24 hr.
Notes   Most often used in combination with acetaminophen for pain or with agents such as terpin hydrate as an antitussive; 120 mg IM equivalent to 10 mg morphine IM.

COLCHICINE

Indications   Acute gout.
Dosage   Initially, 0.5–1.2 mg PO or IV, then 0.5–1.2 mg every 1–2 hours until gastrointestinal side effects develop (maximum of 8 mg/d).
Notes   Caution in elderly and patients with renal impairment. Colchicine 1–2 mg IV within 24–48 hours of an acute attack can be diagnostic and therapeutic in a monoarticular arthritis.

COLESTIPOL (COLESTID)

Indications   Adjunctive therapy for the reduction of serum cholesterol in patients with primary hypercholesterolemia.
Dosage   15–30 g/d divided into 2–4 doses.
Notes   Do not use dry powder; mix with beverages, soups, cereals, etc.

COLFOSCERIL PALMITATE (EXOSURF NEONATAL)

Indications   Prophylaxis and treatment of respiratory distress syndrome in infants.
Dosage   5 mL/kg/dose administered through the endotracheal tube as soon after birth as possible and again at 12 and 14 hours.
Notes   Monitor pulmonary compliance and oxygenation carefully. May cause pulmonary hemorrhage in infants weighing < 700 grams at birth. May cause mucous plugging of the endotracheal tube.

CORTISONE

See Table IX-10, page 491.

CORTISPORIN OTIC

Indications   Treatment of superficial bacterial infections of the external
auditory canal by organisms sensitive to neomycin or
polymyxin; suspension may also be used in the treatment
of infections in mastoidectomy and fenestration cavities.

Dosage   4 drops instilled into external auditory canal 3–4 times
daily.

Notes   Use suspension in cases of ruptured ear drum.

CROMOLYN SODIUM (INTAL, NASALCROM, OPTICROM)

Indications   Adjunct to the treatment of asthma; prevention of exercise
induced asthma; allergic rhinitis; ophthalmic allergic manifestations.

Dosage   Adults: Inhalation: 20 mg (as powder in capsule) inhaled
qid or metered dose inhaler 2 puffs qid.
Nasal instillation: Spray once in each nostril 2–6 times
daily.
Ophthalmic: 1–2 drops in each eye 4–6 times daily.
Peds: Older than 5 years: 2 puffs qid of metered dose inhaler.

Notes   Inhalation of dry powder can cause cough and bronchospasm; may need to switch to metered dose inhaler;
may require 2–4 weeks for maximal effect in perennial allergic disorders.

CYANOCOBALAMIN/VITAMIN B$_{12}$

Indications   Pernicious anemia and other vitamin B$_{12}$ deficiency
states.

Dosage   Adults: 100 μg, IM or s.c. qd for 5–10 days then 100 μg
IM twice a week for 1 month, then 100 μg IM monthly.
Peds: 100 μg qd IM or s.c. for 5–10 days, then 30–50 μg
IM every 4 weeks.

Notes   Oral absorption highly erratic, altered by many drugs and
not recommended; for use with hyperalimentation see
Section V.

CYCLIZINE (MAREZINE)

Indications   Prevention and treatment of nausea, vomiting, and dizziness of motion sickness.

Dosage   Adults: 50 mg PO 30 minutes before travel; may repeat
q4–6h to maximum dose of 200 mg/d; 50 mg IM q4–6h.
Peds: 6–10 years: 3 mg/kg/24h divided tid.

Notes   Anticholinergic and sedative side effects are common.

CYCLOBENZAPRINE (FLEXERIL)

Indications   Adjunct to rest and physical therapy for the relief of muscle spasm associated with acute painful musculoskeletal conditions.
Dosage   10 mg PO tid.
Notes   Do not use for longer than 2–3 weeks; has sedative and anticholinergic properties.

CYCLOPHOSPHAMIDE (CYTOXAN)

Indications   Treatment of breast, ovarian, and soft tissue sarcoma, leukemia, and lymphoma.
Dosage   Adults and children: Initially, 40–50 mg/kg IV divided over 2–5 days or 10–15 mg/kg IV every 7–10 days or 3–5 mg/kg IV twice weekly; oral–1–5 mg/kg/d.
Notes   May cause bone marrow suppression; SIADH has occurred with doses > 50 mg/kg. May cause hemorrhagic cystitis.

CYCLOSPORINE (SANDIMMUNE)

Indications   Prophylaxis of organ rejection in kidney, liver, heart, and bone marrow transplants in conjunction with adrenal cortico.
Dosage   Adults and Peds: Oral: 15 mg/kg/d beginning 12 hours before transplant; after 2 weeks, taper dose by 5 mg/wk to 5–10 mg/kg/d.
                  Intravenous: If patient unable to take orally, give ⅓ oral dose IV.
Notes   May elevate BUN/Cr, which may be confused with renal transplant rejection; should be administered in glass containers; has many drug interactions.

CYPROHEPTADINE (PERIACTIN)

Indications   Allergic reactions; especially good for itching.
Dosage   Adults: 4 mg PO tid, maximum of 0.5 mg/kg/dy.
                  Peds: 2–6 years–0.25/kg/24 hr divided tid-qid (maximum 12 mg/24 hr); 7–14 years–0.25 mg/kg/24 hr divided tid-qid (maximum of 16 mg/24 hr).
Notes   Anticholinergic side effects and drowsiness common; may stimulate appetite in some patients.

DACARBAZINE (DTIC-DOME)

Indications   Treatment of soft tissue and uterine sarcoma, melanoma, and Hodgkin's disease.
Dosage   Dependent on individual protocol.
Notes   May cause myelosuppression.

DACTINOMYCIN (COSMEGEN)

Indications   Treatment of Wilm's tumor, rhabdomyosarcoma, chorio-carcinoma, testicular carcinoma, Ewing's sarcoma, and sarcoma botryoides.
Dosage   Adults: 0.5 mg/d IV for 5 days.
Peds: 0.015 mg/kg/d IV for 5 days.
Notes   Severe soft tissue damage may occur with extravasation.

DANTROLENE SODIUM (DANTRIUM)

Indications   Treatment of clinical spasticity resulting from upper motor neuron disorders such as spinal cord injuries, strokes, cerebral palsy, or multiple sclerosis; treatment of malignant hyperthermic crisis.
Dosage   Adults: Spasticity: Initially, 25 mg PO qd, titrate to effect by 25 mg up to max dose of 100 mg PO qid prn.
Peds: Initially, 0.5 mg/kg/dose bid, titrate by 0.5 mg/kg to effectiveness up to max dose of 3 mg/kg/dose qid prn.
Adults and Peds: Malignant hyperthermia treatment: Continuous rapid IV push beginning at 1 mg/kg until symptoms subside or 10 mg/kg reached. Postcrisis follow-up: 4–8 mg/kg/d in 3–4 divided doses for 1–3 days to prevent recurrence.
Notes   Monitor ALT and AST closely.

DAPSONE

Indications   Leprosy, *Pneumocystis carinii* pneumonia.
Dosage   Adults: 50–100 mg PO qd.
Peds: 1–2 mg/kg/24h PO qd.

DAUNORUBICIN (CERUBIDINE)

Indications   Leukemia.
Dosage   Varies with individual protocol.
Notes   Severe tissue necrosis if extravasation occurs.

DEMECLOCYCLINE (DECLOMYCIN)

Indications   Treatment of SIADH.
Dosage   SIADH: 300–600 mg PO q12h; antimicrobial: 150–300 mg PO q12h.
Notes   Reduce dose in renal failure. May cause diabetes insipidus.

DESIPRAMINE (NORPRAMIN)

Indications   Endogenous depression.

Dosage   25–200 mg/d in single or divided doses; usually as a single bedtime dose.

Notes   Many anticholinergic side effects including blurred vision, urinary retention, and dry mouth.

DESMOPRESSIN (DDAVP, STIMATE)

Indications   Diabetes insipidus; bleeding due to hemophilia A and type I von Willebrand's disease (parenteral); Enuresis.

Dosage   Adults: Diabetes insipidus: 0.1–0.4 mL (10–40 μg) daily in 2–3 divided doses.

Parenteral: 0.5–1 mL (2–4 μg) daily in 2 divided doses. If converting from intranasal to parenteral dosing, use 1/10 of intranasal dose.

Peds: Between 3 months and 12 yr: 0.05–0.3 mL daily in single or 2 doses.

Hemophilia A and von Willebrand's disease (type I):

Adults and peds > 10 kg: 0.3 μg/kg diluted to 50 mL with NSS infused slowly over 15–30 minutes.

Peds < 10 kg: Same as above with dilution to 10 mL with NSS.

Notes   In very young and old patients, adjust fluid intake to avoid water intoxication and hyponatremia.

DESOXYCORTICOSTERONE ACETATE (DOCA, PERCORTEN)

Indications   Partial treatment for adrenocortical insufficiency.

Dosage   Injection: 2–5 mg/d IM into upper outer quadrant of gluteal region.

Pellets: by surgical implantation following 2–3 months of IM maintenance to determine dosage requirement.

Notes   Must be used in conjunction with a glucocorticoid.

DEXAMETHASONE (DECADRON)

See "Steroids," page 490.

DEXTRAN 40 (RHEOMACRODEX)

Indications   Plasma expander for adjunctive therapy in shock; prophylaxis of DVT and thromboembolism; adjunct in peripheral vascular surgery.

Dosage   Shock: 10 mL/kg infused rapidly with maximum dose of 20 mL/kg in the first 24 hours; total daily dosage beyond 24 hours should not exceed 10 mL/kg and should be discontinued after 5 days.

Prophylaxis of DVT and Thromboembolism: 10 mL/kg IV on day of surgery followed by 500 mL IV daily for 2–3 days; then 500 mL IV every 2–3 days based on patient's risk factors for up to 2 weeks.

Notes   Observe for hypersensitivity reactions; monitor renal function and electrolytes.

DEXTROMETHORPHAN (MEDIQUELL, BENYLIN DM, PEDIACARE 1)

Indications   To control nonproductive cough.

Dosage   Adults: 10–20 mg PO q4h prn.
Peds: 1–2 mg/kg/24hr divided tid-qid.

Notes   May be found in combination products with guaifenesin.

DEXTROTHYROXINE (CHOLOXIN)

Indications   Adjunct to diet for reduction of elevated serum cholesterol.

Dosage   Adults: 1–2 mg/d PO titrated a maximum of 4–8 mg/d.
Peds: Initial dose of 0.05 mg/kg/d PO titrated to a maximum of 0.4 mg/kg/d or 4 mg/d, then maintenance of 0.1 mg/kg/d.

Notes   If signs or symptoms of cardiac disease develop during treatment, discontinue use.

DEZOCINE (DALGAN)

Indications   Management of pain.

Dosage   5–20 mg IM or 2.5–10 mg IV q2–4h prn.

Notes   May cause withdrawal in patients dependent on narcotics.

DIAZEPAM (VALIUM) [C]

Indications   Anxiety, alcohol withdrawal, muscle spasm, status epilepticus, and preoperative sedation.

Dosage   Adults: Status epilepticus: 0.2–0.5 mg/kg/dose IV q15–30 min to maximum dose of 30 mg.
Anxiety, muscle spasm: 2–10 mg PO or IM q3–4h prn.
Preoperative: 5–10 mg PO or IM 20–30 minutes before procedure; can be given IV just before procedure.
Alcohol withdrawal: Initially, 2–5 mg IV, may require up to 1000–2000 mg in 24-hour period for severe withdrawal symptoms.
Peds: Status epilepticus: Younger than 5 years: 0.2–0.5 mg/kg/dose IV q15–30min up to maximum of 5 mg; older than 5 years: may administer up to maximum of 10 mg.
Sedation, muscle relaxation: 0.04–0.2 mg/kg/dose q2–4h IM or IV up to maximum of 0.6 mg/kg in 8 hours, or 0.12–0.8 mg/kg/24 hr PO divided tid-qid.

Notes   Do not exceed 5 mg/min IV as respiratory arrest can occur; absorption of IM dose may be erratic.

DIAZOXIDE (HYPERSTAT, PROGLYCEM)

Indications   Hypertensive emergencies; management of hypoglycemia owing to hyperinsulinism.

Dosage   Adults and Peds: Hypertensive crisis: 1–3 mg/kg/dose IV
up to maximum of 150 mg IV; may repeat at 15 minute intervals until desired effect is achieved. Hypoglycemia: 3–
8 mg/kg/24hr PO divided q8–12 hr.
Neonates: Hypoglycemia: 10 mg/kg/24hr divided in 3
equal doses; maintenance: 3–8 mg/kg/24h PO in 2 or 3
equal doses.

Notes   Sodium retention and hyperglycemia frequently occur;
possible thiazide diuretic cross-hypersensitivity; cannot be
titrated.

DICLOFENAC (CATAFLAM, VOLTAREN)

See Table IX–7 on page 457.

DICLOXACILLIN (DYNAPEN, DYCILL)

See Table IX–1 on page 398.

DICYCLOMINE (BENTYL)

Indications   Treatment of functional irritable bowel syndromes.

Dosage   Adults: 20 mg PO qid titrated to a maximum dose of
160 mg/d or 20 mg IM q6h.
Peds: Infants older than 6 months: 5 mg/dose tid-qid; children: 10 mg/dose tid-qid.

Notes   Anticholinergic side effects may limit dose.

DIDANOSINE [DDI] (VIDEX)

Indications   Treatment of HIV infection in patients who are zidovudine
intolerant.

Dosage   Adults: > 60 kg: 200 mg PO bid; < 60 kg: 125 mg PO bid.
Peds:

BSA (m^2)	Tablets	Powder
1.1–1.4	100 mg bid	125 mg bid
0.8–1	75 mg bid	94 mg bid
0.5–0.7	50 mg bid	62 mg bid
< 0.4	25 mg bid	31 mg bid

Notes   Reconstitute powder with water; side effects include pancreatitis, peripheral neuropathy, diarrhea, and headache.

DIETHYLSTILBESTROL (DES)

Indications   Treatment of breast and prostate cancer.
Dosage   50 mg PO tid; may be increased to 200 mg PO tid depending on patient tolerance (prostate dose 3–5 mg/d).

DIFLUNISAL (DOLOBID)

See Table IX–7 on page 457.

DIGOXIN (LANOXIN, LANOXICAPS)

Indications   CHF, atrial fibrillation and flutter, paroxysmal atrial tachycardia.
Dosage   Adults: PO digitalization: 0.50–0.75 mg PO, then 0.25 mg PO q6–8h until a total dose between 1.0 and 1.5 mg.
Intravenous or intramuscular digitalization: 0.25–0.50 mg IM or IV, then 0.25 mg q4–6h to a total dose of about 1 mg; daily maintenance: 0.125–0.500 mg PO, IM, or IV qd (average daily dose 0.125–0.250 mg).
Peds: Preterm infants: Digitalization: 30 μg/kg PO or 25 μg/kg IV, give ½ of dose initially then ¼ of dose at 8–12 hr intervals for 2 doses; maintenance: 10 μg/kg/24hr PO or 6–8 μg/kg/24hr IV divided q12 hours.
Term Infants: 2 years old: Digitalization: 65–75 μg/kg PO or 50 μg/kg IV give ½ dose initially then ¼ of dose at 8–12 hr intervals for 2 doses; maintenance: 15–20 μg/kg/24hr PO or 12–15 μg/kg/24hr IV divided q12h.
2–10 years old: Digitalization: 30–40 μg/kg PO or 25 μg/kg IV, give ½ dose initially, then ¼ dose at 8–12 hr intervals for 2 doses; maintenance: 8–10 μg/kg/24 hr PO or 6–8 μg/kg/24 hr IV divided q12h.
Older than 10 years: Same as adults.
Notes   Can cause heart block; low potassium can potentiate toxicity; reduce dose in renal failure; symptoms of toxicity include nausea, vomiting, headache, fatigue, visual disturbances (yellow-green halos around lights), cardiac arrhythmias (see Table IX–12, page 501); IM injection can be painful and has erratic absorption.

DIGOXIN IMMUNE FAB (DIGIBIND)

Indications   Treatment of life-threatening digoxin intoxication.
Dosage   Adults and Peds: Based on serum level and patient's weight. See dosing charts provided with the drug.
Notes   Each vial will bind approximately 0.6 mg of digoxin; in renal failure may require redosing in several days due to break down of the immune complex.

DIHYDROXYALUMINUM SODIUM CARBONATE (ROLAIDS)

Indications   Heartburn, gastroesophageal reflux, and acid ingestion.
Dosage   1–2 tablets prn.

DILTIAZEM (CARDIZEM, DILACOR)

Indications   Treatment of angina pectoris, prevention of reinfarction, hypertension; atrial fibrillation or flutter, and paroxysmal SVT.
Dosage   Oral: 30 mg PO qid initially; titrate to 180–360 mg/d in divided doses as needed.
                  Sustained release: 60–120 mg PO bid, titrate to effect, maximum dose 360 mg/d.
                  Continuous dose: 180–300 mg PO qd.
                  Intravenous: 0.25 mg/kg IV bolus over 2 minutes; may repeat dose in 15 minutes at 0.35 mg/kg. May begin continuous infusion of 5–15 mg/hr.
Notes   Contraindicated in sick-sinus syndrome, AV block, and hypotension. Cardizem CD and Dilacor XR are **not** interchangeable.

DIMENHYDRINATE (DRAMAMINE)

Indications   Prevention and treatment of nausea, vomiting, dizziness or vertigo of motion sickness.
Dosage   Adults: 50–100 mg PO q4–6h, maximum of 400 mg/d; 50 mg IM/IV prn.
                  Peds: 5 mg/kg/24hr PO or IV divided qid.
Notes   Anticholinergic side effects.

DIPHENHYDRAMINE (BENADRYL, OTHERS)

Indications   Allergic reactions, motion sickness, potentiate narcotics, sedation, cough suppression, treatment of extrapyramidal reactions.
Dosage   Adults: 25–50 mg PO, IV or IM bid-tid.
                  Peds: 5 mg/kg/24hr PO or IM divided q6h (maximum of 300 mg/d).
Notes   Anticholinergic side effects including dry mouth, urinary retention; causes sedation; increase dosing interval in moderate to severe renal failure.

DIPHENOXYLATE WITH ATROPINE (LOMOTIL) [C]

Indications   Diarrhea.
Dosage   Adults: Initially 5 mg PO tid or qid until under control, then 2.5–5.0 mg PO bid.
                  Peds older than 2 years: 0.3–0.4 mg/kg/24hr divided bid-qid.
Notes   Atropine-type side effects.

DIPYRIDAMOLE (PERSANTIN)

Indications   Prevention of postoperative thromboembolic disorders.
Dosage   75–100 mg PO tid-qid.
Notes   Aspirin potentiates the antiplatelet effects; may cause nausea and vomiting.

DISOPYRAMIDE (NORPACE, NAPAMIDE)

Indications   Suppression and prevention of premature ventricular contractions.
Dosage   Adults: 400–800 mg/d divided q6h for regular release products and q12h for sustained release products.
                  Peds younger than 1 year: 10–30 mg/kg/24hr PO; 1–4 years old: 10–20 mg/kg/24hr PO; 4–12 years old: 10–15 mg/kg/24hr PO; 12–18 years old: 6–15 mg/kg/24hr PO.
Notes   Has anticholinergic side effects (urinary retention); negative inotropic properties may induce CHF; decrease dose in impaired hepatic function.

DISULFIRAM (ANTABUSE)

Indications   Alcohol consumption deterrent.
Dosage   500 mg PO qd for 1–2 weeks, then 250 mg PO qd.
Notes   Patients must avoid all hidden forms of alcohol (cough syrup, sauces etc); CBC and LFTs should be checked periodically.

DOBUTAMINE (DOBUTREX)

Indications   Short term use in patients with cardiac decompensation secondary to depressed contractility.
Dosage   Adults and Peds: Continuous IV infusion of 2.5–15 μg/kg/min; rarely 40 μg/kg/min may be required; titrate according to response.
Notes   Monitor ECG for increase in heart rate, blood pressure, and increased ectopic activity; monitor pulmonary wedge pressure and cardiac output if possible.

DOCUSATE CALCIUM (SURFAK, OTHERS)
DOCUSATE POTASSIUM (DIALOSE)
DOCUSATE SODIUM (DOSS, COLACE, OTHERS)

Indications   Constipation-prone patient; adjunct to painful anorectal conditions (hemorrhoids).
Dosage   Adults: 50–500 mg PO qd.
                  Peds: Infants to 3 years old: 10–40 mg/24hr divided qd-qid; 3–6 years old: 20–60 mg/24hr divided qd-qid; 6–12 years old: 40–120 mg/24hr divided qd-qid.
Notes   No significant side effects, no laxative action.

DOPAMINE (INTROPIN, DOPASTAT)

Indications   Short term use in patients with cardiac decompensation secondary to decreased contractility; increases organ perfusion.

Dosage   Adults and Peds: 5 μg/kg/min by continuous infusion titrated by increments of 5 μg/kg/min to maximum of 50 μg/kg/min based on effect.

Notes   Dosage > 10 μg/kg/min may decrease renal perfusion; monitor urinary output; monitor ECG for increase in heart rate, blood pressure, and increased ectopic activity; monitor PCWP and CO if possible.

DOXAZOSIN (CARDURA)

Indications   Treatment of hypertension and benign prostatic hypertrophy.

Dosage   Initially 1 mg PO qd, may be increased to 16 mg PO qd.

Notes   Doses > 4 mg increase the likelihood of excessive postural hypotension.

DOXEPIN (SINEQUAN, ADAPIN)

Indications   Depression or anxiety.

Dosage   50–150 mg PO qd usually qhs but can be in divided doses.

Notes   Anticholinergic, central nervous system, and cardiovascular side effects.

DOXORUBICIN (ADRIAMYCIN)

Indications   Treatment of breast, endometrial, and ovarian cancer, and leukemia.

Dosage   60–75 mg/m^2 IV as a single dose, at 21-day intervals.

Notes   May cause myelosuppression and cardiotoxicity.

DOXYCYCLINE (VIBRAMYCIN)

Indications   Broad spectrum antibiotic including activity against *Rickettsiae, Chlamydia,* and *Mycoplasma pneumoniae.*

Dosage   Adults: 100 mg PO q12h first day, then 100 mg PO qd or bid or 100 mg IV q12h.
Peds older than 8 years: 5 mg/kg/24h PO up to a maximum of 200 mg/d, divided qd or bid.

Notes   Useful for chronic bronchitis; tetracycline of choice for patients with renal impairment.

DRONABINOL (MARINOL) [C]

Indications   Nausea and vomiting associated with cancer chemotherapy; appetite stimulation.

Dosage   Adults and Peds: Antiemetic: 5–15 mg/m^2/dose q4–6h prn.
               Adults: Appetite: 2.5 mg PO before lunch and supper.
Notes   Principle psychoactive substance present in marijuana;
               many CNS side effects.

DROPERIDOL (INAPSINE)

Indications Nausea and vomiting, premedication for anesthesia.
Dosage   Adults: Nausea: 1.25–2.5 mg IV prn; premedication:
                 2.5–10 mg IV.
                 Peds: 0.1–0.15 mg/kg/dose.
Notes   May cause drowsiness, moderate hypotension and occa-
                 sionally tachycardia.

ECONAZOLE (SPECTAZOLE)

Indications Treatment of most tinea, cutaneous *Candida,* and tinea
                 versicolor infections.
Dosage   Apply to affected areas bid (qd for tinea versicolor) for 2–4
                 weeks.
Notes   Relief of symptoms and clinical improvement may be seen
                 early in treatment, but course of therapy should be carried
                 out to avoid recurrence.

EDROPHONIUM (TENSILON)

Indications Diagnosis of myasthenia gravis; acute myasthenic crisis;
                 curare antagonist; paroxysmal atrial tachycardia.
Dosage   Adults: Test for myasthenia gravis: 2 mg IV in 1 minute; if
                 tolerated, give 8 mg IV; a positive test is a brief increase
                 in strength. PAT: 10 mg IV to a maximum of 40 mg.
                 Peds: Test for myasthenia gravis: total dose of 0.2 mg/kg.
                 Give 0.04 mg/kg as a test dose. If no reaction occurs, give
                 the remainder of the dose in 1 mg increments to a maxi-
                 mum of 10 mg.
Notes   Can cause severe cholinergic effects; keep atropine avail-
                 able.

ENALAPRIL (VASOTEC)

Indications Hypertension, CHF.
Dosage   Adults: 2.5–5 mg/d PO titrated by effect to 10–40 mg/d as
                 1–2 divided doses, or 1.25 mg IV q6h.
                 Peds: 0.05–0.08 mg/kg/dose PO q12–24h.
Notes   Initial dose can produce symptomatic hypotension, espe-
                 cially with concomitant diuretics; discontinue diuretic for
                 2–3 days before initiation if possible; monitor closely for
                 increases in serum potassium; may cause a nonproduc-
                 tive cough.

ENOXACIN (PENETREX)

Indications   Treatment of UTI and gonorrhea.
Dosage   200–400 mg PO bid. Gonorrhea: 400 mg as a single dose.
Notes   Significant drug interaction with theophylline and caffeine.

ENOXAPARIN (LOVENOX)

Indications   Prevention of DVT.
Dosage   30 mg s.c. twice daily.
Notes   Does not significantly affect bleeding time, platelet function, PT or APTT.

EPHEDRINE

Indications   Acute bronchospasm, nasal congestion, hypotension, narcolepsy, enuresis, myasthenia gravis.
Dosage   Adults: 25–50 mg IM or IV every 10 minutes to maximum 150 mg/d or 25–50 mg PO q3–4h prn.
                  Peds: 0.2–0.3 mg/kg/dose IM or IV q4–6h prn.

EPINEPHRINE (ADRENALIN, SUS-PHRINE, OTHERS)

Indications   Cardiac arrest, anaphylactic reactions, acute asthma.
Dosage   Adults: Emergency cardiac care: 0.5–1.0 mg (5–10 mL of 1:10,000) IV every 5 minutes to response. Anaphylaxis: 0.3–0.5 mL of 1:1000 dilution s.c.; may repeat q10–15 min to maximum of 1 mg/dose and 5 mg/d.
                  Asthma: 0.3–0.5 mL of 1:1000 dilution s.c. repeated at 20 minute to 4 hour intervals or 1 inhalation (metered dose) repeated in 1–2 minutes or suspension 0.1–0.3 mL s.c. for extended effect.
                  Peds: Emergency cardiac care—0.1 mL/kg of 1:10,000 dilution IV q3–5 min to response.
Notes   Sus-Phrine offers sustained action; in acute cardiac settings can be given via endotracheal tube if a central line is not available.

EPOETIN ALFA (EPOGEN, PROCRIT)

Indications   Treatment of anemia associated with chronic renal failure, zidovudine treatment in HIV-infected patients, and patients receiving cancer chemotherapy.
Dosage   Adults and Peds: 50–150 U/kg 3 times weekly, adjust dose every 4–6 weeks as needed.
Notes   May cause hypertension, headache, tachycardia, nausea and vomiting.

ERYTHROMYCIN (E-MYCIN, ILOSONE, ERYTHROCIN, ERYC, OTHERS)

Indications   Infections caused by Group A streptococci (*Streptococcus pyogenes*), alpha-hemolytic streptococci and *Neisseria gonorrhoeae* infections in penicillin allergic patients, *Streptococcus pneumoniae, Mycoplasma pneumoniae,* and Legionella.

Dosage   Adults: 250–500 mg PO qid or between 500 mg and 1 g IV qid.
Peds: 30–50 mg/kg/24hr PO or IV divided q6h, to a maximum of 2 g/d.

Notes   Frequent mild gastrointestinal disturbances; estolate salt is associated with cholestatic jaundice; erythromycin base not well absorbed from the gastrointestinal tract; some forms such as ERYC are better tolerated with respect to gastrointestinal irritation; lactobionate salt contains benzyl alcohol therefore use with caution in neonates; base used as part of the "Condon Bowel Prep."

ERYTHROMYCIN, OPHTHALMIC (ILOTYCIN)

Indications   Conjunctival infections.
Dosage   0.5% ointment, apply q6h.

ESMOLOL (BREVIBLOC)

Indications   Supraventricular tachycardia, noncompensatory sinus tachycardia.

Dosage   Initiate treatment with 500 μg/kg load over 1 minute then 50 μg/kg/min for 4 minutes; if inadequate response, repeat loading dose and follow with maintenance infusion of 100 μg/kg/min for 4 minutes; continue titration process by repeating loading dose followed by incremental increases in the maintenance dose of 50 μg/kg/min for 4 minutes until desired heart rate is reached or a decrease in blood pressure occurs; average dose is 100 μg/kg/min.

Notes   Monitor closely for hypotension; decreasing or discontinuing infusion will reverse hypotension in approximately 30 minutes.

ESTAZOLAM (PROSOM) [C]

Indications   Insomnia.
Dosage   1–2 mg PO qhs prn.

ESTERIFIED ESTROGENS (ESTRATAB, MENEST)

Indications   Vasomotor symptoms, atrophic vaginitis, or kraurosis vulvae associated with menopause, female hypogonadism.

Dosage   Menopause: 0.3–1.25 mg daily; hypogonadism: 2.5 mg
                  PO qd-tid.

ESTERIFIED ESTROGENS WITH
METHYLTESTOSTERONE (ESTRATEST)

Indications   Moderate to severe vasomotor symptoms associated with
                  menopause, postpartum breast engorgement.
Dosage   1 tablet qd for 3 weeks, then 1 week off.

ESTRADIOL TOPICAL (ESTRACE)

Indications   Atrophic vaginitis and kraurosis vulvae associated with
                  menopause.
Dosage   2–4 g daily × 2 weeks, then 1 g 1–3 times a week.

ESTRADIOL TRANSDERMAL (ESTRADERM)

Indications   Severe vasomotor symptoms associated with meno-
                  pause; female hypogonadism.
Dosage   0.05 system twice weekly, adjust dose as necessary to
                  control symptoms. Transdermal patches 0.05 mg, 0.1 mg
                  (delivers 0.05 mg or 0.1 mg/24hr).

ESTROGEN, CONJUGATED (PREMARIN)

Indications   Moderate to severe vasomotor symptoms associated with
                  menopause; atrophic vaginitis; palliative therapy of ad-
                  vanced prostatic carcinoma; prevention of estrogen defi-
                  ciency induced osteoporosis.
Dosage   0.3–1.25 mg/d PO cyclically; prostatic carcinoma requires
                  1.25–2.5 mg PO tid.
Notes   Do not use in pregnancy; associated with an increased
                  risk of endometrial carcinoma, gallbladder disease, and
                  thromboembolism and possibly breast cancer; generic
                  products are **not** equivalent.

ESTROGEN, CONJUGATED WITH METHYLPROGESTERONE
(PREMARIN WITH METHYLPROGESTERONE)

Indications   Vasomotor symptoms associated with menopause.
Dosage   1 tablet every day.

ESTROGEN, CONJUGATED WITH METHYLTESTOSTERONE
(PREMARIN WITH METHYLTESTOSTERONE)

Indications   Moderate to severe vasomotor symptoms associated with
                  menopause, postpartum breast engorgement.
Dosage   1 tablet every day for 3 weeks, then 1 week off.

ETHACRYNIC ACID (EDECRIN)

Indications Edema, CHF, ascites, any time rapid diuresis is desired.
Dosage Adults: 50–200 mg PO qd or 50 mg IV prn.
Peds: 1 mg/kg/dose IV. Repeated doses are not recommended.
Notes Contraindicated in anuria; many severe side effects.

ETHAMBUTOL (MYAMBUTOL)

Indications Pulmonary tuberculosis and other mycobacterial infections.
Dosage Adults and Peds older than 12 years: 15–25 mg/kg PO daily as single dose.
Notes May cause vision changes and gastrointestinal upset.

ETHINYL ESTRADIOL (ESTINYL, FEMINONE)

Indications Vasomotor symptoms associated with menopause, female hypogonadism.
Dosage 0.02–1.5 mg/d divided qd-tid.

ETHOSUXIMIDE (ZARONTIN)

Indications Absence seizures.
Dosage Adults: 500 mg qd PO initially; increase by 250 mg/d every 4–7 days as needed.
Peds: 20–40 mg/kg/24h PO qd to a maximum of 1500 mg/d.
Notes Blood dyscrasias, CNS and gastrointestinal side effects may occur; caution in patients with renal or hepatic impairment.

ETODOLAC (LODINE)

See Table IX–7 on page 457.

ETOPOSIDE (VEPESID)

Indications Treatment of gestational trophoblastic disease, ovarian, testicular, and lung cancer.
Dosage 35–100 mg/m^2/d IV. Number of doses and duration of therapy is dependent on individual protocols.
Notes May cause severe bone marrow suppression; has low stability in concentrated solutions.

FAMOTIDINE (PEPCID)

Indications Short-term treatment of active duodenal ulcer and benign gastric ulcer, maintenance therapy for duodenal ulcer; hypersecretory conditions.

Dosage   Ulcer: 20–40 mg PO hs or 20 mg IV q12h; hypersecretory: 20–160 mg PO q6h.
Notes   Decrease dose in severe renal failure.

FELBAMATE (FELBATOL)

Indications Treatment of partial seizures and Lennox-Gastaut syndrome.
Dosage   Adults: Initiate at 1200 mg/d PO in divided dose tid-qid. Titrate patients to no more than 3600 mg/d.
                 Peds: 15 mg/kg/d PO in divided doses tid-qid; lower adjunctive therapy doses by 20%.
Notes   There is no need to monitor felbamate serum levels.

FELODIPINE (PLENDIL)

Indications Treatment of hypertension.
Dosage   5–20 mg PO qd.
Notes   Closely monitor blood pressure in elderly patients and patients with impaired hepatic function; doses of > 10 mg should not be used in these patients.

FENOPROFEN (NALFON)

See Table IX–7 on page 457.

FENTANYL (SUBLIMAZE) [C]

Indications Short acting analgesic used in conjunction with anesthesia.
Dosage   Adults and Peds: 0.025–0.15 mg/kg IV/IM titrated to effect.
Notes   Causes significant sedation.

FENTANYL TRANSDERMAL SYSTEM (DURAGESIC) [C]

Indications Management of chronic pain.
Dosage   Apply patch to upper torso every 72 hours. Dose is calculated from the narcotic requirements for the previous 24 hours. Transdermal patches deliver 25 μg/hr, 50 μg/hr, 75 μg/hr, 100 μg/hr.
Notes   0.1 mg of fentanyl is equivalent to 10 mg of morphine IM.

FERROUS SULFATE

Indications Iron deficiency anemia; iron supplementation.
Dosage   Adults: 100–200 mg/d of elemental iron divided tid-qid.
                 Peds: 1–2 mg/kg/24h divided qd-bid.
Notes   May turn stools and urine dark; can cause gastrointestinal upset, constipation; vitamin C taken with ferrous sulfate increases the absorption of iron especially in patients with atrophic gastritis.

FILGRASTIM [G-CSF] (NEUPOGEN)

Indications To decrease the incidence of infection in febrile neutropenic patients with nonmyeloid malignancies.
Dosage Adults and Peds: 5 μg/kg/d s.c. or IV as a single daily dose. Administer until the patient is no longer neutropenic.
Notes May cause bone pain.

FINASTERIDE (PROSCAR)

Indications Symptomatic benign prostatic hypertrophy.
Dosage 5 mg qd indefinitely.
Notes Lowers PSA levels, can cause impotence, prostate enlarges after therapy is stopped.

FLAVOXATE (URISPAS)

Indications Symptomatic relief of dysuria, urgency, nocturia, suprapubic pain, urinary frequency, and incontinence.
Dosage 100–200 mg PO tid-qid.
Notes May cause drowsiness, blurred vision, and dry mouth.

FLECAINIDE (TAMBOCOR)

Indications Life-threatening ventricular arrhythmias.
Dosage 100 mg PO q12h; increase in increments of 50 mg q12h every 4 days to maximum of 400 mg/d.
Notes May cause new or worsened arrhythmias; therapy should be initiated in the hospital; may dose q8h if patient intolerant or uncontrolled at q12h interval; drug interactions with propranolol, digoxin, verapamil, and disopyramide; may cause CHF.

FLUCONAZOLE (DIFLUCAN)

Indications Oropharyngeal and esophageal candidiasis, cryptococcal meningitis, Candida infections of the lungs, peritoneum, and urinary tract; prevention of candidiasis in bone marrow transplant patients on chemotherapy or radiation.
Dosage Adults: 100–400 mg PO or IV qd.
Peds: 3–6 mg/kg PO or IV qd.
Notes Adjust dose in renal insufficiency; oral dosing produces the same blood levels as IV, therefore the oral route should be used whenever possible.

FLUDARABINE PHOSPHATE (FLUDARA)

Indications Treatment of leukemia.
Dosage 25 mg/m² IV for 5 consecutive days. Give every 28 days.
Notes May cause severe bone marrow suppression and neurologic toxicity.

FLUDROCORTISONE ACETATE (FLORINEF)

Indications   Partial treatment for adrenocortical insufficiency.
Dosage   Adult and Peds older than 1 year: 0.05–0.1 mg PO qd.
                  Infants: 0.1–0.2 mg PO qd.
Notes   For adrenal insufficiency, must be used in conjunction with
                  a glucocorticoid supplement; dosage changes based on
                  plasma renin activity.

FLUMAZENIL (ROMAZICON)

Indications   For complete or partial reversal of the sedative effects of
                  benzodiazepines.
Dosage   0.2 mg IV over 15 seconds, dose may be repeated if the
                  desired level of consciousness is not obtained to a maxi-
                  mum dose of 1 mg.

FLUNISOLIDE (AEROBID)

Indications   Control of bronchial asthma in patients requiring chronic
                  corticosteroid therapy.
Dosage   Adults: 2–4 inhalations bid.
                  Peds: 2 inhalations bid.
Notes   May cause oral candidiasis; not for acute asthma attack.

FLUOROURACIL (ADRUCIL)

Indications   Management of carcinoma of the colon, rectum, breast,
                  stomach, and pancreas.
Dosage   Varies with individual protocol.

FLUOXETINE (PROZAC)

Indications   Treatment of depression and obsessive-compulsive disor-
                  ders.
Dosage   20 mg PO qd initially; titrate to maximum dose of 80 mg/
                  24 hr.
Notes   May cause nausea, nervousness, weight loss, and in-
                  somnia.

FLUPHENAZINE (PROLIXIN, PERMITIL)

Indications   Psychotic disorders.
Dosage   0.5–10 mg/d in divided doses PO q6–8h; average mainte-
                  nance 5.0 mg/d or 1.25 mg IM initially then 2.5–10 mg/d in
                  divided doses q6–8h prn.
Notes   Reduce dose in elderly; monitor liver functions; may
                  cause drowsiness; do not administer concentrate with caf-
                  feine, tannic acid, or pectin-containing products.

FLURAZEPAM (DALMANE) [C]

Indications   Insomnia.

Dosage   Adults and Peds older than 15 years: 15–30 mg PO qhs prn.
Notes   Reduce dose in the elderly.

FLURBIPROFEN (ANSAID)

See Table IX–7 on page 457.

FLUTAMIDE (EULEXIN)

Indications   Prostate cancer in combination with LHRH analogue.
Dosage   3 capsules PO q8h.

FLUVASTATIN (LESCOL)

Indications   Adjunct to diet in the treatment of elevated total cholesterol.
Dosage   20–40 mg PO qhs.

FOLIC ACID

Indications   Macrocytic anemia.
Dosage   Adult: Supplement: 0.4 mg PO qd; pregnancy: 0.8 mg PO qd; folate deficiency: 1.0 mg PO qd-tid.
                  Peds: Supplement: 0.04–0.4 mg/24 hr PO, IM, IV, or s.c.; folate deficiency: 0.5–1.0 mg/24 hr PO, IM, IV or s.c.

FOSCARNET (FOSCAVIR)

Indications   Treatment of cytomegalovirus retinitis in patients with AIDS.
Dosage   Induction: 60 mg/kg IV q8h; maintenance: 90–120 mg/kg IV qd (Mon–Fri).
Notes   Dosage **must** be adjusted for renal function; nephrotoxic; monitor ionized calcium closely (causes electrolyte abnormalities); administer through a central line.

FOSINOPRIL (MONOPRIL)

Indications   Hypertension.
Dosage   Initially, 10 mg PO qd; may be increased to a maximum of 80 mg/d PO divided qd-bid.
Notes   Decrease dose in the elderly, do not need to adjust dose for renal insufficiency, may cause a nonproductive cough and dizziness.

FUROSEMIDE (LASIX)

Indications   Edema, hypertension, congestive heart failure.
Dosage   Adults: 20–80 mg PO or IV qd or bid.
                  Peds: 1 mg/kg/dose IV q6–12h; 2 mg/kg/dose PO q12h–24h.

Notes   Monitor for hypokalemia; use with caution in hepatic disease; high doses of the IV form may cause ototoxicity.

GABAPENTIN (NEURONTIN)

Indications   Adjunctive therapy in the treatment of partial seizures.
Dosage   900–1800 mg/d PO in 3 divided doses.
Notes   It is not necessary to monitor serum gabapentin levels.

GALLIUM NITRATE (GANITE)

Indications   Treatment of hypercalcemia of malignancy.
Dosage   100–200 mg/m^2/d for 5 days.
Notes   Can cause renal insufficiency; < 1% of patients developed acute optic neuritis.

GANCICLOVIR (CYTOVENE)

Indications   CMV retinitis.
Dosage   Adults and Peds: 5 mg/kg IV q12h for 14–21 days, then maintenance of 5 mg/kg IV qd for 7 days/week or 6 mg/kg IV qd for 5 days/week.
Notes   Not a cure for CMV; granulocytopenia and thrombocytopenia are the major toxicities; should be handled with cytotoxic precautions.

GEMFIBROZIL (LOPID)

Indications   Hypertriglyceridemia (types IV and V hyperlipoproteinemia).
Dosage   1200 mg/d PO in 2 divided doses 30 minutes before the morning and evening meals.
Notes   Monitor AST, ALT, LDH, Alk Phos and serum lipids during therapy; cholelithiasis may occur secondary to treatment; may enhance the effect of warfarin.

GENTAMICIN (GARAMYCIN)

Indications   Serious infections caused by susceptible *Pseudomonas, Proteus, Escherichia coli, Klebsiella, Enterobacter, Serratia,* and for initial treatment of gram-negative sepsis.
Dosage   Adults: 3–5 mg/kg/24h IV divided q8–24h.
                   Peds: Infants older than 7 days: 2.5 mg/kg/dose IV q12–24h; children: 2.5 mg/kg/d IV q8h.
Notes   Nephrotoxic and ototoxic; decrease dose with renal insufficiency; monitor creatinine clearance and serum concentration for dosage adjustments; see Table IX–12, page 501.

GENTAMICIN, OPHTHALMIC (GARAMYCIN OPHTHALMIC)

Indications   Conjunctival infections.
Dosage   0.3% ointment apply bid or tid

GLIPIZIDE (GLUCOTROL)

See Table IX–11 on page 497.

GLUCAGON

Indications   Treatment of severe hypoglycemic reactions in diabetic patients with sufficient liver glycogen stores.

Dosage   Adults: 0.5–1.0 mg s.c., IM, or IV repeated after 20 min as needed.
Peds: Neonates—0.3 mg/kg/dose s.c., IM, or IV q4h prn; children—0.03–0.1 mg/kg/dose s.c., IM or IV repeated after 20 min prn.

Notes   Administration of glucose IV is necessary; ineffective in states of starvation, adrenal insufficiency, or chronic hypoglycemia.

GLYBURIDE (DIABETA, MICRONASE)

See Table IX–11 on page 497.

GLYCERIN SUPPOSITORY

Indications   Constipation.

Dosage   Adult: 1 adult suppository PR, prn.
Peds: 1 infant suppository PR, qd-bid prn.

GONADORELIN (LUTREPULSE)

Indications   Primary hypothalamic amenorrhea.

Dosage   5–20 µg IV q90 min for 21 days using a reservoir and pump.

Notes   Risk of multiple pregnancies.

GOSERELIN (ZOLADEX)

Indications   Treatment of prostate cancer and endometriosis.

Dosage   3.6 mg s.c. every 28 days into the abdominal wall.

GRANISETRON (KYTRIL)

Indications   Prevention of nausea and vomiting associated with emetogenic cancer therapy.

Dosage   Adults and Peds: 10 µg/kg IV 30 minutes before initiation of chemotherapy.

GUAIFENESIN (ROBITUSSIN, OTHERS)

Indications   Symptomatic relief of dry nonproductive cough.

Dosage   Adult: 200–400 mg (10–20 mL) PO q4h.
Peds: 2–5 years: 50–100 mg (2.5–5 mL) PO q4h; 6–11 years: 100–200 mg (5–10 mL) PO q4h.

GUANABENZ (WYTENSIN)

Indications   Hypertension.
Dosage   Adult: Initially, 4 mg PO bid, increase by 4 mg/d incre-
                  ments at 1–2 week intervals up to 32 mg bid.
                  Peds older than 12 years: 0.5–4 mg/d initially, increase
                  by increments of 0.5–2 mg/d at 1-week intervals up to
                  24 mg/d divided bid.
Notes   Sedation, dry mouth, dizziness, and headache common.

GUANADREL (HYLOREL)

Indications   Hypertension.
Dosage   5 mg PO bid initially, increase up to 10 mg/d increments at
                  1 week intervals up to 75 mg PO bid.
Notes   Interactions with tricyclic antidepressants; less orthostatic
                  changes and impotence than guanethidine.

GUANETHIDINE (ISMELIN)

Indications   Hypertension.
Dosage   Adult: Initially, 10–25 mg PO qd, increase dose based on
                  response.
                  Peds: 0.2 mg/kg/24 hr PO initially, increase by 0.2 mg/
                  kg/24 hr increments q7–10 days up to maximum dose of
                  3 mg/kg/24 hr.
Notes   May produce profound orthostatic hypotension especially
                  with diuretic use; may potentiate effects of vasopressor
                  agents; increased bowel movements and explosive diar-
                  rhea possible; interaction with tricyclic antidepressants re-
                  duces the effectiveness of guanethidine.

GUANFACINE (TENEX)

Indications   Hypertension.
Dosage   1 mg qhs initially, increase by 1 mg/24 hr increments to
                  maximum dose of 3 mg/24 hr; split dose bid if BP in-
                  creases at the end of the dosing interval.
Notes   Use with thiazide diuretic is recommended; sedation,
                  drowsiness common; rebound hypertension may occur
                  with abrupt cessation of therapy.

HALAZEPAM (PAXIPAM) [C]

Indications   Anxiety disorders.
Dosage   20–40 mg PO tid-qid.
Notes   Reduce dosage in elderly.

HALOPERIDOL (HALDOL)

Indications Management of psychotic disorders; schizophrenia; agitation; Tourette's disorders; hyperactivity in children.

Dosage Adults: Moderate symptoms: 0.5–2.0 mg PO bid-tid. Severe symptoms or agitation: 3–5 mg PO bid-tid or 1–5 mg IM q4h prn (maximum 100 mg/d).
Peds: 3–6 years: 0.01–0.03 mg/kg/24h PO qd; 6–12 years: initially, 0.5–1.5 mg/24 hr PO, increase by increments of 0.5 mg/24 hr to maintenance of 2–4 mg/24 hr (0.05–0.1 mg/kg/24h) or 1–3 mg/dose IM q4–8h to a maximum of 0.1 mg/kg/24h. Tourette's syndrome may require up to 15 mg/24 hr PO.

Notes Can cause extrapyramidal symptoms, hypotension; reduce dose in the elderly.

HEMOPHILUS B CONJUGATE VACCINE (PROHIBIT)

Indications Routine immunization of children between the ages of 18 months and 5 years against diseases caused by *Haemophilus influenzae* type B.

Dosage Peds: 0.5 mL (25 µg) IM in deltoid or vastus lateralis.

Notes Booster not required; observe for anaphylaxis.

HEPARIN SODIUM

Indications Treatment and prevention of venous thrombosis and pulmonary emboli, atrial fibrillation with emboli formation, acute arterial occlusion.

Dosage Adult: Prophylaxis: 3000–5000 units s.c. q8–12h. Treatment of thrombosis: Loading dose of 50–75 units/kg IV, then 10–20 units/kg IV qh (adjust based on PTT).
Peds: Infants: Load 50 U/kg IV bolus then 20 U/kg/hr IV by continuous infusion. Children: Load 50 U/kg IV then 15–25 U/kg continuous infusion or 100 U/kg/dose q4h IV intermittent bolus.

Notes Follow PTT, thrombin time, or activated clotting time to assess effectiveness; heparin has little effect on the prothrombin time; with proper dose PTT is about 1½–2 times the control; can cause thrombocytopenia, follow platelet counts.

HEPATITIS B IMMUNE GLOBULIN (HYPERHEP, H-BIG, HEP-B-GAMMAGEE)

Indications Exposure to HBsAg-positive materials such as blood, plasma, or serum (accidental needle-stick, mucous membrane contact, oral ingestion).

Dosage   Adults and Peds: 0.06 mL/kg IM to maximum of 5 mL;
                  within 24 hr of needle-stick or percutaneous exposure;
                  within 14 days of sexual contact; repeat at 1 and 6 months
                  after exposure.
Notes   Administered in gluteal or deltoid muscle; if exposure con-
                  tinues should receive hepatitis B vaccine.

HEPATITIS B VACCINE (ENGERIX-B, RECOMBIVAX HB)

Indications   Prevention of type B hepatitis.
Dosage   Adult: 3 IM doses of 1 mL each, the first 2 given 1 month
                  apart, the third 6 months after the first.
                  Peds: 0.5 mL IM dose given on the same schedule as
                  adults.
Notes   IM injections for adults and older peds to be administered
                  in the deltoid; other peds to be administered in anterolat-
                  eral thigh; may cause fever, injection site soreness; de-
                  rived from recombinant DNA technology.

HETASTARCH (HESPAN)

Indications   Plasma volume expansion as an adjunct in treatment of
                  shock due to hemorrhage, surgery, burns, and other
                  trauma.
Dosage   500–1000 mL (do not exceed 1500 mL/d) IV at a rate not
                  to exceed 20 mL/kg/hr.
Notes   Not a substitute for blood or plasma; contraindicated in
                  patients with severe bleeding disorders, severe CHF, or
                  renal failure with oliguria or anuria.

HYDRALAZINE (APRESOLINE)

Indications   Moderate to severe hypertension.
Dosage   Adults: Begin at 10 mg PO qid, then increase to 25 mg qid
                  to a maximum of 300 mg/d.
                  Peds: 0.75–3 mg/kg/24h PO divided q12–6h.
Notes   Caution with impaired hepatic function, coronary artery
                  disease; compensatory sinus tachycardia can be elimi-
                  nated with the addition of propranolol; chronically high
                  doses can cause SLE-like syndrome; SVT can occur fol-
                  lowing IM administration.

HYDROCHLOROTHIAZIDE (HYDRODIURIL, ESIDRIX, OTHERS)

Indications   Edema, hypertension, CHF.
Dosage   Adults: 25–100 mg PO qd in single or divided doses.
                  Peds: 2–3 mg/kg/24h PO divided bid.
Notes   Hypokalemia is frequent; hyperglycemia, hyperuricemia,
                  hyperlipidemia, and hyponatremia are common side ef-
                  fects.

HYDROCHLOROTHIAZIDE AND AMILORIDE (MODURETIC)

Indications   Hypertension, adjunctive therapy for congestive heart failure.

Dosage   1–2 tablets PO qd.

Notes   Should not be given to diabetics or patients with renal failure.

HYDROCHLOROTHIAZIDE AND SPIRONOLACTONE (ALDACTAZIDE)

Indications   Edema (CHF, cirrhosis), hypertension.

Dosage   25–200 mg each component per day in divided doses.

HYDROCHLOROTHIAZIDE AND TRIAMTERENE (DYAZIDE, MAXZIDE)

Indications   Edema, hypertension.

Dosage   Dyazide: 1–2 capsules PO qd-bid. Maxzide: 1 tablet PO qd.

Notes   Hydrochlorothiazide component in Maxzide is more bioavailable than Dyazide; can cause hyperkalemia as well as hypokalemia; follow serum potassium.

HYDROCORTISONE

See "Steroids," page 490.

HYDROMORPHONE (DILAUDID) [C]

Indications   Moderate to severe pain.

Dosage   1–4 mg PO, IM, IV, or PR q4–6h prn.

Notes   1.5 mg IM equivalent to 10 mg morphine IM.

HYDROXYUREA (HYDREA)

Indications   Treatment of cervical and ovarian cancer, melanoma, and leukemia adjunct in sickle cell anemia.

Dosage   Continuous therapy: 20–30 mg/kg PO qd; intermittent therapy: 80 mg/kg every 3 days.

HYDROXYZINE (ATARAX, VISTARIL)

Indications   Anxiety, tension, sedation, itching.

Dosage   Adults: Anxiety or sedation: 50–100 mg PO or IM qid or prn (maximum of 600 mg/d); itching: 25–50 mg PO or IM tid-qid.
Peds: 0.6–1.0 mg/kg/24h PO or IM q6h.

Notes   Useful in potentiating the effects of narcotics; **not** for IV use; drowsiness, anticholinergic effects are common.

HYOSCYAMINE SULFATE (ANASPAZ, LEVSIN, CYTOSPAZ)

Indications   Control of gastric secretions, visceral spasm, spastic bladder, pylorospasm.
Dosage   Oral: 0.125–0.25 mg PO tid-qid. Intravenous: 0.25–0.5 mg s.c. Intramuscular or intravenous: 2–4 times daily as needed.
Notes   May cause dizziness, blurred vision, dry mouth, difficulty in urination.

IBUPROFEN (MOTRIN, RUFEN, ADVIL, OTHERS)

See Table IX–7 on page 457.

IDARUBICIN (IDAMYCIN)

Indications   Treatment of leukemia.
Dosage   12 mg/m^2 daily for 3 days.
Notes   Do not administer if bilirubin is > 5 mg/dL.

IFOSFAMIDE (IFEX)

Indications   Treatment of testicular, breast, sarcoma, and ovarian cancer.
Dosage   1.2 g/m^2/d for 5 consecutive days. Repeat course every 3 weeks.
Notes   Causes hemorrhagic cystitis; hydrate patients well and administer with MESNA.

IMIPENEM/CILASTATIN (PRIMAXIN)

Indications   Treatment of serious infections caused by a wide variety of susceptible bacteria; inactive against *Staphylococcus aureus,* group A and B streptococci, and others.
Dosage   Adults: 250–500 mg (Imipenem) IV q6h.
                   Peds: Children younger than 3 years: 100 mg/kg/24h IV divided q6h; children older than 3 years: 60 mg/kg/24h IV divided q6h.
Notes   Seizures may occur if drug accumulates; adjust dosage for renal insufficiency to avoid drug accumulation if calculated creatinine clearance is < 70 mL/min.

IMIPRAMINE (TOFRANIL)

Indications   Depression, enuresis.
Dosage   Adults: Hospitalized: Start at 100 mg/24 hr PO or IV in divided doses, can increase over several weeks to 250–300 mg/24 hr.
                   Outpatient: maintenance of 50–150 mg PO qhs not to exceed 200 mg/24hr.

Peds: Antidepressant: 1.5–5.0 mg/kg/24h divided tid; enuresis: 10–25 mg PO qhs; increase by 10–25 mg at 1–2 week intervals, treat for 2–3 months, then taper.

Notes Do not use with MAO inhibitors; less sedation than amitriptyline.

IMMUNE GLOBULIN INTRAVENOUS (GAMIMUNE N, SANDOGLOBULIN, GAMMAR IV)

Indications IgG antibody deficiency diseases such as congenital agammaglobulinemia, common variable hypogammaglobulinemia; idiopathic thrombocytopenic purpura (ITP).

Dosage Adults and Peds: Immunodeficiency: 100–200 mg/kg IV monthly at rate of 0.01–0.04 mL/kg/minute up to maximum of 400 mg/kg/dose; ITP: 400 mg/kg/dose IV qd × 5 days.

Notes Adverse effects associated mostly with rate of infusion.

INDAPAMIDE (LOZOL)

Indications Hypertension, congestive heart failure.

Dosage 2.5–5.0 mg PO qd.

Notes Doses greater than 5 mg do not have additional effects on lowering blood pressure.

INDOMETHACIN (INDOCIN)

Also see Table IX–7 on page 457.

Indications Closure of patent ductus arteriosus.

Dosage Infants: 0.2–0.25 mg/kg/dose IV, may be repeated in 12–24h for up to 3 doses.

Notes Monitor renal function carefully.

INSULIN

Indications Diabetes mellitus that cannot be controlled by diet and/or oral hypoglycemic agents.

Dosage Based on serum glucose levels; usually given s.c. can also be given IV or IM (only regular insulin can be given IV). See Table IX–6 on page 454.

Notes The highly purified insulins provide an increase in free insulin; monitor patients closely for several weeks when changing doses.

INTERFERON ALPHA (ROFERON-A, INTRON A)

Indications Hairy cell leukemia.

Dosage Alpha-2A: 3 million IU daily for 16–24 weeks s.c. or IM; alpha-2B: 2 million IU/m^2 IM or s.c. 3 times a week for 2–6 months.

TABLE IX–6. COMPARISON OF INSULINS.

Type of Insulin	Onset (hr)	Peak (hr)	Duration (hr)
Rapid			
Regular Iletin II	0.25–0.5	2.0–4.0	5–7
Humulin R	0.5	2.0–4.0	6–8
Novolin R	0.5	2.5–5.0	5–8
Intermediate			
NPH Iletin II	1.0–2.0	6–12	18–24
Lente Iletin II	1.0–2.0	6–12	18–24
Humulin N	1.0–2.0	6–12	14–24
Novolin L	2.5–5.0	7–15	18–24
Novolin 70/30	0.5	7–12	24
Prolonged			
Ultralente	4.0–6.0	14–24	28–36
Humulin U	4.0–6.0	8–20	24–28

Notes   Is being used in many investigational protocols (including bladder cancer); flu-like symptoms are a common reaction with systemic use.

IPECAC SYRUP

Indications   Treatment of drug overdose and certain cases of poisoning.

Dosage   Adults: 15–30 mL PO followed by 200–300 mL water; if no emesis occurs in 20 minutes, may repeat × 1.
Peds: 6–12 months of age: 5–10 mL PO followed by water.
1–12 years old: 15 mL PO followed by water.

Notes   Do not use for ingestion of petroleum distillates, strong acid, base, or other corrosive or caustic agents; not for use in comatose or unconscious patients; caution in CNS depressant overdose.

IPRATROPIUM BROMIDE INHALANT (ATROVENT)

Indications   Bronchospasm associated with COPD.

Dosage   Adults and children older than 12 years: 2–4 puffs qid.

Notes   Not for initial treatment of acute episodes of bronchospasm.

IRON DEXTRAN (IMFERON)

Indications   Iron deficiency when oral supplementation not possible.

Dosage   Based on estimate of iron deficiency (see package insert).

Notes   Must give a test dose since anaphylaxis is common; may be given deep IM using "Z-track" technique although IV route most preferred.

ISOETHARINE (BRONKOSOL, BRONKOMETER)

Indications   Bronchial asthma and reversible bronchospasm.
Dosage   Adults and Peds: Nebulization: 0.25–1.0 mL diluted 1:3 with saline q4–6h;
                   Metered dose inhaler: 1–2 inhalations q4h.

ISONIAZID (INH)

Indications   Treatment of *Mycobacterium* species infections.
Dosage   Adults: Active TB: 5 mg/kg/24h PO or IM qd (usually 300 mg/d).
                   Prophylaxis: 300 mg PO qd for 6–12 months.
                   Peds: Active TB: 10–20 mg/kg/24h PO or IM qd to a maximum of 300 mg/d.
                   Prophylaxis: 10 mg/kg/24h PO qd.
Notes   Can cause severe hepatitis; given with other antituberculous drugs for active tuberculosis; IM route rarely used; to prevent peripheral neuropathy can give pyridoxine 50–100 mg/d.

ISOPROTERENOL (ISUPREL, MEDIHALER-ISO)

Indications   Shock, cardiac arrest, AV nodal block, antiasthmatic.
Dosage   Adults: Emergency cardiac care: 2–20 μg/min IV infusion, titrated to effect.
                   Shock: 1–4 μg/min IV infusion, titrated to effect.
                   AV nodal block: 20–60 μg IV push; may repeat q3–5 min; 1–5 μg/min IV infusion maintenance.
                   Inhalation: 1–2 inhalations 4–6 times daily.
                   Peds: Emergency cardiac care: 0.1–1.5 μg/kg/min IV infusion, titrated to effect.
                   Inhalation: 1–2 inhalations 4–6 times daily.
Notes   Contraindications include tachycardia; pulse > 130 BPM may induce ventricular arrhythmias.

ISOSORBIDE DINITRATE (ISORDIL)

Indications   Angina pectoris.
Dosage   Acute angina: 2.5–10.0 mg PO (chewable tablet) or SL prn q5–10 min; > 3 doses should not be given in 15–30 minute period.
                   Angina prophylaxis: 5–60 mg PO tid.
Notes   Nitrates should not be given on chronic q6h or qid basis due to development of tolerance; can cause headaches; usually need to give a higher oral dose to achieve same results as with sublingual forms.

ISOSORBIDE MONOHYDRATE (ISMO)

Indications   Prevention of angina pectoris.
Dosage   20 mg PO bid, with the 2 doses given 7 hours apart

ISRADIPINE (DYNACIRC)

Indications   Hypertension.
Dosage   2.5–5.0 mg PO bid.

ITRACONAZOLE (SPORANOX)

Indications   Treatment of systemic fungal infections caused by *Aspergillus, Blastomycosis,* and *Histoplasma.*
Dosage   200 mg PO qd-bid.
Notes   Should not be used concurrently with H_2 antagonist, omeprazole, antacids, terfenadine, or astemizole.

KAOLIN-PECTIN

Indications   Treatment of diarrhea.
Dosage   Adults: 60–120 mL PO after each loose stool or q3–4h prn.
Peds: 3–6 years old: 15–30 mL/dose PO prn.
6–12 years old: 30–60 mL/dose PO prn.

KETOCONAZOLE (NIZORAL)

Indications   Treatment of systemic fungal infections: candidiasis, chronic mucocutaneous candidiasis, blastomycosis, coccidioidomycosis, histoplasmosis, and paracoccidioidomycosis; topical cream for localized fungal infections due to dermatophytes and yeast.
Dosage   Adults: Oral: 200 mg PO qd; increase to 400 mg PO qd for very serious infections.
Topical: Apply to affected area once daily.
Peds: 3.3–6.6 mg/kg/24h PO qd.
Notes   Associated with severe hepatotoxicity; monitor LFTs closely throughout course of therapy; drug interaction with any agent increasing gastric pH preventing absorption of ketoconazole; avoid concurrent use with astemizole and terfenadine; may enhance oral anticoagulants; may react with alcohol to produce disulfiram-like reaction.

KETOPROFEN (ORUDIS)

See Table IX–7 on page 457.

KETOROLAC (TORADOL)

See Table IX–7 on page 457.

TABLE IX-7. NONSTEROIDAL ANTI-INFLAMMATORY AGENTS.

Drug (Brand Name)	Maximum Daily Dose (Mg)	Dosing Frequency	Notes
Propionic Acids			
Fenoprofen (Nalfon)	3200	tid, qid	Approval for arthritis and analgesia.
Flurbiprofen (Ansaid)	300	bid, tid, qid	Approval for arthritis.
Ibuprofen (Motrin, Rufen)	3200	bid, tid, qid	Approval for arthritis, analgesia, and dysmenorrhea. Many generic products are available.
Ketoprofen (Orudis)	300	tid, qid	Approval for arthritis and analgesia.
Naproxen (Naprosyn, Anaprox)	1500	bid	Approval for arthritis and analgesia.
Oxaprozin (Daypro)	1200–1800	qd	Very GI irritating.
Indoles			
Indomethacin (Indocin)	200	qd, bid, tid	Approval for arthritis. SR product available.
Ketorolac Tromethamine (Toradol)	40	qid	Approval for pain relief. Parenteral dosage form. IM 60 mg, then 30 q6h up to 120 mg/d.
Sulindac (Clinoril)	400	bid	Approval for arthritis. Least renal toxic.
Tolmetin (Tolectin)	2000	tid, qid	Approval for arthritis.
Etodolac (Lodine)	1600	tid, qid	
Oxicams			
Piroxicam (Feldene)	20	bid	Approval for arthritis. Very GI irritating.
Phenylacetic Acids			
Diclofenac (Voltaren)	200	bid, tid	Approval for arthritis.
Fenamates			
Meclofenamate (Meclomen)	400	tid, qid	Approval for arthritis, analgesia, and dysmenorrhea.
Mefenamic acid (Ponstel)	1000	qid	Approval for analgesia and dysmenorrhea.
Miscellaneous			
Diflusinal (Dolobid)	1500	bid, tid	Approval for arthritis and analgesia
Nambumetone (Relafan)	2000	qd, bid	Approval for arthritis

[1]Childrens ibuprofen dosed at 5–10 mg/kg po q6h

LABETALOL (TRANDATE, NORMODYNE)

Also see Table IX–2 on page 409.

Indications   Hypertension, hypertensive emergencies.
Dosage   Hypertension: 100 mg PO bid initially; then 200–400 mg
                  PO bid.
                  Hypertensive emergency: 20–80 mg IV bolus, then
                  2 mg/min IV infusion titrated to effect.

LACTOBACILLUS (LACTINEX GRANULES)

Indications   Control of diarrhea, especially after antibiotic therapy.
Dosage   Adult and Peds older than 3 years: 1 packet, 2 capsules,
                  or 4 tablets with meals or liquids tid.

LACTULOSE (CHRONULAC, CEPHULAC)

Indications   Hepatic encephalopathy; laxative; constipation.
Dosage   Adult: Acute hepatic encephalopathy: 30–45 mL PO q1h
                  until soft stools are observed, then tid-qid.
                  Chronic laxative therapy: 30–45 mL PO tid-qid; adjust
                  dosage every 1–2 days to produce 2–3 soft stools qd.
                  Peds: Infants: 2.5–10 mL/24 hr divided tid-qid.
                  Children: 40–90 mL/24 hr divided tid-qid.
Notes   Can cause severe diarrhea.

LEUCOVORIN CALCIUM (WELLCOVORIN)

Indications   Overdoses of folic acid antagonist.
Dosage   Adult and Peds: Methotrexate rescue: 10–100 mg/m^2/
                  dose IV or PO q3–6h.
                  Adjunct to antimicrobials: 5–10 mg PO qd.
Notes   Many different dosing schedules exist for Leucovorin res-
                  cue following methotrexate therapy.

LEUPROLIDE (LUPRON)

Indications   Treatment of prostate cancer, endometriosis, and central
                  precocious puberty (CPP).
Dosage   Adults: Prostate: 1 mg s.c. daily or 7.5 mg IM monthly of
                  depot.
                  Endometriosis (depot only): 3.75 mg IM as a single
                  monthly dose.
                  Peds: CPP: 50 μg/kg/d as a daily s.c. injection. May titrate
                  upward by 10 mg/kg/d until total down regulation is
                  achieved.
                  Depot: < 25 kg: 7.5 mg IM every 4 weeks
                  > 25 to 37.5 kg: 11.25 mg IM every 4 weeks
                  > 37.5 kg: 15 mg IM every 4 weeks.

LEVONORGESTREL IMPLANTS (NORPLANT)

Indications   Prevention of pregnancy.
Dosage   Implant 6 capsules in the mid-forearm.
Notes   Prevents pregnancy for up to 5 years; capsules may be
                  removed if pregnancy is desired.

LEVORPHANOL (LEVO-DROMORAN) [C]

Indications   Moderate to severe pain.
Dosage   2 mg PO or s.c. prn.

LEVOTHYROXINE (SYNTHROID)

Indications   Hypothyroidism.
Dosage   Adult: 25–50 μg/d PO or IV initially; increase by 25–
                  50 μg/d every month; usual dose 100–200 μg/d.
                  Peds: 0–1 year old: 8–10 μg/kg/24 hr PO or IV qd.
                  1–5 years old: 4–6 μg/kg/24 hr PO or IV qd.
                  Older than 5 years: 3–4 μg/kg/24 hr PO or IV qd.
Notes   Titrate dosage based on clinical response and thyroid
                  function tests; dosage can be increased more rapidly in
                  young to middle-aged patients.

LIDOCAINE (XYLOCAINE)

Indications   Local anesthesia; treatment of cardiac arrhythmias.
Dosage   Adult: Arrhythmias: 1 mg/kg (50–100 mg) IV bolus, then
                  2–4 mg/min IV infusion, should repeat bolus after 5 min-
                  utes.
                  Local anesthesia: Infiltrate a few mLs of a 0.5–1.0% solu-
                  tion maximum 3 mg/kg/dose.
                  Peds: Arrhythmias: 1 mg/kg dose IV bolus, then 20–
                  50 μg/kg/min IV infusion.
                  Local anesthetic: Infiltrate a few mLs of a 0.5–1.0% solu-
                  tion, with a maximum of 3 mg/kg/dose.
Notes   Epinephrine may be added for local anesthesia to prolong
                  effect and help decrease bleeding; for IV forms, dosage
                  reduction is required with liver disease, CHF; dizziness,
                  paresthesias, and convulsions are associated with tox-
                  icity.

LINDANE (KWELL)

Indications   Head lice, crab lice, scabies.
Dosage   Adults and Peds: Cream or lotion: Apply thin layer after
                  bathing and leave in place for 24 hours; pour on laundry.
                  Shampoo: Apply 30 mL and develop lather with warm wa-
                  ter for 4 minutes; comb out nits.
Notes   Caution with overuse, may be absorbed into blood; wash
                  clothing and bedding as well.

LIOTHYRONINE (CYTOMEL)

Indications Hypothyroidism.
Dosage Adult: Initial dose of 25 μg/24 hr, then titration q1–2 weeks according to clinical response and thyroid function tests to maintenance of 25–75 μg PO qd.
Peds: Initial dose of 5 μg/24 hr, then titration by 5 μg/24 hr increments at 1–2 week intervals; maintenance 25–75 μg/24 hr PO qd.
Notes Reduce dose in elderly; monitor thyroid function test.

LISINOPRIL (PRINIVIL, ZESTRIL)

Indications Hypertension.
Dosage 5–40 mg/24 hr PO qd-bid.
Notes Dizziness, headache, and cough are common side effects.

LITHIUM CARBONATE (ESKALITH, OTHERS)

Indications Manic episodes of manic-depressive illness; maintenance therapy in recurrent disease.
Dosage Acute mania: 600 mg PO tid or 900 mg slow release bid.
Maintenance: 300 mg PO tid-qid.
Notes Dosage must be titrated; follow serum levels (Table IX–12, page 501); common side effects are polyuria, tremor; contraindicated in patients with severe renal impairment; sodium retention or diuretic use may potentiate toxicity.

LOMEFLOXACIN (MAXAQUIN)

Indications Treatment of UTI and lower respiratory tract infections caused by gram-negative bacteria; prophylaxis in transurethral procedures.
Dosage 400 mg PO qd.
Notes May cause severe photosensitivity.

LOPERAMIDE (IMODIUM)

Indications Diarrhea.
Dosage Adult: 4 mg PO initially, then 2 mg after each loose stool, up to 16 mg/d.
Peds: 0.4–0.8 mg/kg/24 hr PO divided q6–12h until diarrhea resolves or for 7 days maximum.
Notes Do not use in acute diarrhea caused by *Salmonella*, *Shigella*, or *Clostridium difficile*.

LORATADINE (CLARITIN)

Indications Treatment of allergic rhinitis.
Dosage 10 mg PO once daily.
Notes: Should be taken on an empty stomach.

LORAZEPAM (ATIVAN, ALZAPAM) [C]

Indications	Anxiety and anxiety mixed with depression; preop sedation; control of status epilepticus.
Dosage	Adult: Anxiety: 0.5–1.0 mg PO bid-tid.
	Preop: 0.05 mg/kg up to max of 4 mg IM 2 hours before surgery.
	Insomnia: 2–4 mg PO qhs.
	Status epilepticus: 2.5–10 mg/dose IV repeated at 15–20 min interval × 2 prn.
	Peds: Status epilepticus: 0.05 mg/kg/dose IV repeated at 15–20 min interval × 2 prn.
Notes	Decrease dosage in elderly; may take up to 10 minutes to see effect when given IV.

LOVASTATIN (MEVACOR)

Indications	Adjunct to diet for the reduction of elevated total and LDL cholesterol levels in patients with primary hypercholesterolemia (types IIa and IIb).
Dosage	20 mg PO daily with the evening meal; may increase at 4 week intervals to maximum of 80 mg/d taken with meals.
Notes	Patient should be maintained on standard cholesterol lowering diet throughout treatment; monitor LFTs every 6 weeks during first year of therapy; headache and gastrointestinal intolerance common.

MAGALDRATE (RIOPAN, LOWSIUM)

Indications	Hyperacidity associated with peptic ulcer; gastritis, and hiatal hernia.
Dosage	1–2 tablets PO or 5–10 mL PO between meals and hs.
Notes	Less than 0.3 mg sodium per tablet or teaspoon; do not use in renal insufficiency.

MAGNESIUM CITRATE

Indications	Vigorous bowel prep; constipation.
Dosage	Adult: 120–240 mL PO prn.
	Peds: 0.5 mL/kg/dose, up to maximum 200 mL PO.
Notes	Do not use in renal insufficiency, intestinal obstruction.

MAGNESIUM HYDROXIDE (MILK OF MAGNESIA)

Indications	Constipation.
Dosage	Adult: 15–30 mL PO prn.
	Peds: 0.5 mL/kg/dose PO prn.
Notes	Do not use in renal insufficiency or intestinal obstruction.

MAGNESIUM OXIDE (URO-MAG, MAG-OX 400, MAOX)

Indications   Replacement for low plasma levels.
Dosage   400–800 mg/d divided qd-qid.
Notes   May cause diarrhea.

MAGNESIUM SULFATE

Indications   Replacement for low plasma levels; refractory hypo-
                    kalemia and hypocalcemia; preeclampsia and premature
                    labor.
Dosage   Adult: Supplement: 1–2 g IM or IV; repeat dosing based
                    on response and continued hypomagnesemia.
                    Preeclampsia, premature labor: 1–4 g/hr IV infusion.
                    Peds: 25–50 mg/kg/dose IM or IV q4–6h for 3–4 doses;
                    may repeat if hypomagnesemia persists.
Notes   Reduce dose with low urine output or renal insufficiency.

MANNITOL

Indications   Osmotic diuresis (cerebral edema, oliguria, anuria, myo-
                    globinuria, etc), bowel prep.
Dosage   Adult: Diuresis: 0.2 g/kg/dose IV over 3–5 min; if no di-
                    uresis within 2 hours, discontinue.
                    Peds: Diuresis: 0.75 g/kg/dose IV over 3–5 minutes; if no
                    diuresis within 2 hours, discontinue.
                    Adult and Peds: Cerebral edema: 0.25 g/kg/dose IV push
                    repeated at 5 min intervals prn; increase incrementally to
                    1 g/kg/dose prn intracranial hypertension.
Notes   Caution with CHF or volume overload.

MAPROTILINE (LUDIOMIL)

Indications   Depressive neurosis; manic-depressive illness; major de-
                    pressive disorder; anxiety associated with depression.
Dosage   75–150 mg/d qhs, maximum of 300 mg/d.
Notes   Contraindicated with MAO inhibitors or seizure history; for
                    patients older than 60 years, give only 50–75 mg/d; anti-
                    cholinergic side effects.

MECLIZINE (ANTIVERT)

Indications   Motion sickness, vertigo associated with diseases of the
                    vestibular system.
Dosage   Adult and Peds older than 12 years: 25 mg PO tid-qid prn.
Notes   Drowsiness, dry mouth, blurred vision commonly occur.

MECLOFENAMATE (MECLOMEN, MECONIUM)

See Table IX–7 on page 457.

MEDROXYPROGESTERONE (PROVERA)

Indications   Secondary amenorrhea and abnormal uterine bleeding owing to hormonal imbalance, and endometrial cancer.

Dosage   Secondary amenorrhea: 5–10 mg PO qd for 5–10 days. Abnormal uterine bleeding: 5–10 mg PO qd for 5–10 days beginning on the 16th or 21st day of menstrual cycle. Cancer: 400–1000 mg IM/wk.

Notes   Contraindicated with past thromboembolic disorders or with hepatic disease.

MEFENAMIC ACID (PONSTEL)

See Table IX–7 on page 457.

MEGESTROL ACETATE (MEGACE)

Indications   Treatment of breast and endometrial cancer; appetite stimulation in HIV-related cachexia.

Dosage   Cancer: 40–320 mg/d PO in divided doses. Appetite: 80 mg PO qid.

MELPHALAN (ALKERAN)

Indications   Treatment of breast and ovarian cancer, and multiple myeloma.

Dosage   6 mg/d PO as single dose or 16 mg/m^2 IV every 2 weeks for 4 doses.

Notes   Monitor blood counts closely.

MEPERIDINE (DEMEROL) [C]

Indications   Relief of moderate to severe pain.

Dosage   Adult: 50–100 mg PO or IM q3–4h prn. Peds: 1–1.5 mg/kg/dose PO or IM q3–4h prn.

Notes   75 mg IM equivalent to 10 mg morphine IM; beware of respiratory depression; a useful preprocedure sedative, particularly in children, is a so-called "cardiac cocktail" consisting of (per 30 lb body weight) 30 mg Demerol, 6.25 mg Thorazine, and 6.25 mg Phenergan given IM.

MEPROBAMATE (EQUINIL, MILTOWN)

Indications   Short-term relief of anxiety.

Dosage   200–400 mg PO tid-qid; sustained release 400–800 mg PO bid.

Notes   May cause drowsiness.

MERCAPTOPURINE (PURINETHOL)

Indications   Treatment of leukemia.

Dosage   Adults and Peds: 2.5 mg/kg/d PO.

MESALAMINE (ROWASA)

Indications   Treatment of mild to moderate distal ulcerative colitis, proctosigmoiditis, or proctitis.
Dosage   Retention enema at bedtime daily.

MESNA (MESNEX)

Indications   Reduce the incidence of ifosfamide-induced hemorrhagic cystitis.
Dosage   20% of the ifosfamide dose (w/w) IV at the time of ifosfamide infusion and 4 and 8 hours after, for a total dose equal to 60% of the ifosfamide dose.

MESORIDAZINE (SERENTIL)

Indications   Schizophrenia; acute and chronic alcoholism; chronic brain syndrome.
Dosage   25–50 mg PO or IV tid initially; titrate to maximum of 300–400 mg/d.
Notes   Low incidence of extrapyramidal side effects.

METAPROTERENOL (ALUPENT, METAPREL)

Indications   Bronchodilator for asthma and reversible bronchospasm.
Dosage   Adult: Inhalation: 1–3 inhalations q3–4h to maximum of inhalations 12 per 24 hrs; allow at least 2 min between inhalations.
Oral: 20 mg q6–8h.
Peds: Inhalation: 0.5 mg/kg/dose up to max of 15 mg/dose inhaled q4–6h by nebulizer or 1–2 puffs q4–6h.
Oral: 0.3–0.5 mg/kg/dose q6–8h.
Notes   Fewer beta-1 effects than isoproterenol and longer acting.

METARAMINOL (ARAMINE)

Indications   Prevention and treatment of hypotension due to spinal anesthesia.
Dosage   Adult: Prevention: 2–10 mg IM q10–15min prn.
Treatment: 0.5–5 mg IV bolus followed by IV infusion of 1–4 μg/kg/min titrated to effect.
Peds: Prevention: 0.1 mg/kg/dose IM prn.
Treatment: 0.01 mg/kg IV bolus followed by IV infusion of 5 μg/kg/min titrated to effect.
Notes   Allow 10 minutes for maximal effect; employ other shock management techniques such as fluid resuscitation as needed; may cause cardiac arrhythmias.

METAXALONE (SKELAXIN)

Indications   Relief of painful musculoskeletal conditions.
Dosage   800 mg PO 3–4 times a day.

METHADONE (DOLOPHINE) [C]

Indications   Severe pain; detoxification and maintenance of narcotic addiction.

Dosage   Adult: 2.5–10 mg IM q8h or 5–15 mg PO q8h (titrate as needed).
Peds: 0.7 mg/kg/24 hr PO or IM divided q8h.

Notes   Equianalgesic with parenteral morphine; long half-life; increase dose slowly to avoid respiratory depression.

METHICILLIN (STAPHCILLIN)

See Table IX–1 on page 398.

METHIMAZOLE (TAPAZOLE)

Indications   Hyperthyroidism; preparation for thyroid surgery or radiation.

Dosage   Adult: Initially, 15–60 mg/d PO divided tid; maintenance of 5–15 mg PO qd.
Peds: Initially, 0.4–0.7 mg/kg/24hr PO divided tid; maintenance of ⅓ to ⅔ the initial dose PO qd.

Notes   Follow patient clinically and with thyroid function tests.

METHOCARBAMOL (ROBAXIN)

Indications   Relief of discomfort associated with painful musculoskeletal conditions.

Dosage   Adult: 1.5 g PO qid for 2–3 days, then 1 g PO qid maintenance therapy; IV form rarely indicated.
Peds: 60 mg/kg/24h PO divided qid.

Notes   Can discolor urine; may cause drowsiness or gastrointestinal upset; contraindicated with myasthenia gravis.

METHOTREXATE (FOLEX)

Indications   Treatment of breast, gestational trophoblastic disease, ovarian, lung, and head and neck cancer, and leukemia; psoriasis; rheumatoid arthritis.

Dosage   Cancer: Dosage varies with type of cancer and individual protocols.
Rheumatoid arthritis: 7.5 mg/wk PO as a single dose or 2.5 mg q12h PO for 3 doses each week.

Notes   Utilize Leucovorin rescue with high doses; monitor blood counts and methotrexate levels carefully.

METHOXAMINE (VASOXYL)

Indications   Support, restoration, or maintenance of blood pressure during anesthesia; for termination of some episodes of paroxysmal supraventricular tachycardia.

Dosage   Adults: Anesthesia: 10–15 mg IM; if emergency exists, 3–5 mg by slow IV push.
Paroxysmal SVT: 10 mg by slow IV push.
Peds: 0.25 mg/kg/dose IM or 0.08 mg/kg/dose slow IV push.

Notes   IM dose requires 15 minutes to act; use 5–10 mg phentolamine locally in case of extravasation; interaction with MAO inhibitors and tricyclic antidepressants to potentiate methoxamine effect.

METHYLDOPA (ALDOMET)

Indications Essential hypertension.
Dosage   Adult: 250–500 mg PO bid-tid (maximum 2–3 g/d) or between 250 mg and 1 g IV q4–8h.
Peds: 10 mg/kg/24 hr PO in 2–3 divided doses (maximum of 40 mg/kg/24 hr divided q6–12h) or 5–10 mg/kg/dose IV q6–8h to a total dose of 20–40 mg/kg/24 hr.

Notes   Do not use in presence of liver disease; can discolor urine; initial transient sedation or drowsiness occurs frequently.

METHYLERGONOVINE (METHERGINE)

Indications Prevention and treatment of postpartum hemorrhage caused by uterine atony.
Dosage   0.2 mg IM after delivery of placenta, may repeat at 2–4 hour intervals or 0.2–0.4 mg PO q6–12h for 2–7 days.
Notes   IV doses should be given over a period of not less than 1 minute with frequent BP monitoring.

METHYLPREDNISOLONE (SOLU-MEDROL)

See "Steroids," page 490.

METOCLOPRAMIDE (REGLAN, CLOPRA)

Indications Relief of diabetic gastroparesis; symptomatic gastroesophageal reflux; relief of cancer chemotherapy-induced nausea and vomiting.
Dosage   Adult: Diabetic gastroparesis: 10 mg PO 30 minutes a.c. and hs for 2–8 weeks prn; or same dose given IV for 10 days, then switch to PO.
Reflux: 10–15 mg PO 30 minutes a.c. and hs.
Antiemetic: 1–3 mg/kg/dose IV 30 minutes before antineoplastic agent, then q2h for 2 doses, then q3h for 3 doses.
Peds: Reflux: 0.1 mg/kg/dose PO qid.
Antiemetic: 2 mg/kg/dose IV on same schedule as adults.
Notes   Dystonic reactions common with high doses that can be treated with IV Benadryl; can also be used to facilitate

small bowel intubation and radiological evaluation of the upper gastrointestinal tract.

METOLAZONE (DIULO, ZAROXOLYN)

Indications Mild to moderate essential hypertension; edema of renal disease or cardiac failure.

Dosage Adults: Hypertension: 2.5–5 mg PO daily. Edema: 5–20 mg PO daily.
Peds: 0.2–0.4 mg/kg/d PO divided q12h–qd.

Notes Monitor fluid and electrolyte status of patient during treatment.

METOPROLOL (LOPRESSOR)

See Table IX–2 on page 409.

METRONIDAZOLE (FLAGYL)

Indications Amebiasis, trichomoniasis, *C difficile*, and anaerobic infections.

Dosage Adult: Anaerobic infections: 500 mg IV q6–8h.
Amebic dysentery: 750 mg PO qd for 5–10 days.
Trichomoniasis: 250 mg PO tid for 7 days or 2 g PO in 1 dose.
C difficile: 500 mg PO or IV q8h for 7–10 days.
Peds: Anaerobic infections: 30 mg/kg/24 hr PO or IV divided q6h.
Amebic dysentery: 35–50 mg/kg/24 hr PO in 3 divided doses for 5–10 days.

Notes For *Trichomonas* infections, also treat partner; reduce dose in hepatic failure; no activity against aerobic bacteria; use in combination in serious mixed infections; may cause disulfiram-like reaction.

METYRAPONE (METOPIRONE)

Indications Diagnostic test for hypothalamic-pituitary ACTH function.

Dosage Metapyrone test:
Day 1: Control period–collect 24-hour urine to measure 17-hydroxycorticosteroids (17-OHCS) or 17-ketogenic steroids (17-KSG).
Day 2: ACTH test–50 units ACTH infused over 8 hours and measure 24-hour urinary steroids.
Days 3–4: Rest period.
Day 5: Administer metyrapone with milk or snack.
Adult: 750 mg PO q4h for 6 doses.
Peds: 15 mg/kg q4h for 6 doses (min 250 mg dose).
Day 6: Determine 24-hour urinary steroids.

Notes   Normal 24-hour urine 17-OHCS is 3–12 mg; following
                 ACTH, it increases to 15–45 mg/24hr; normal response to
                 metyrapone is between a two- and fourfold increase in 17-
                 OHCS excretion; drug interactions with phenytoin, cypro-
                 heptadine, and estrogens may lead to subnormal re-
                 sponse.

MEXILETINE (MEXITIL)

Indications Suppression of symptomatic ventricular arrhythmias.
Dosage   Administer with food or antacids; 200–300 mg PO q8h, do
                 not exceed 1200 mg/d.
Notes   Not to be used in cardiogenic shock, second or third de-
                 gree AV block if no pacemaker; may worsen severe ar-
                 rhythmias; monitor liver function during therapy; drug in-
                 teractions with hepatic enzyme inducers and suppressors
                 requiring dosage changes.

MEZLOCILLIN (MEZLIN)

See Table IX–8 on page 469.

MICONAZOLE (MONISTAT)

Indications Severe systemic fungal infections including coccidioido-
                 mycosis, candidiasis, *Cryptococcus,* and others; various
                 tinea forms; cutaneous candidiasis; vulvovaginal candidi-
                 asis; tinea versicolor.
Dosage   Adult: Systemic: Dosage range from 200–3600 mg/24 hr
                 IV based on diagnosis divided into 3 doses.
                 Topical: Apply to affected area twice daily for 2–4 weeks.
                 Intravaginally: Insert 1 full applicator or suppository at
                 bedtime for 7 days.
                 Peds: 20–40 mg/kg/24 hr IV divided q8h.
Notes   Antagonistic to amphotericin-B in vivo; rapid IV infusion
                 may cause tachycardia or arrhythmias; may potentiate
                 warfarin drug activity.

MIDAZOLAM (VERSED) [C]

Indications Preoperative sedation; conscious sedation for short pro-
                 cedures; induction of general anesthesia.
Dosage   Adult: 1–5 mg IV or IM, titrate dose to effect.
                 Peds: Conscious sedation: 0.08 mg/kg IM × 1.
                 General anesthesia: 0.15 mg/kg IV followed by 0.05 mg/
                 kg/dose q 2 min × 1–3 doses as needed to induce anes-
                 thesia.
Notes   Monitor patient for respiratory depression; may produce
                 hypotension in conscious sedation.

TABLE IX–8. ANTIPSEUDOMONAL PENICILLINS.

Drug (Brand Name)	Daily Dosage Range Adult Interval	Usual Dosing	Peds	mEq Na$^+$ per gram	Supplied	Notes
Carbenicillin (Geopen, Pyopen)	8–40 g[1]	4 hr		4.7	Injection Oral[2]	When used alone, resistant gram (−) bacteria may occur. Hypokalemia and bleeding may occur with high doses.
Ticarcillin (Ticar)	2–24 g[1]	4–6 hr	200–300 mg/kg/d divided q4–6	5.4	Injection	See above Hypokalemia, bleeding and Na$^+$ loading less than with carbenicillin.
Ticarcillin-potassium clavulanate (Timentin)	9–12 g	4–6 hr	300 mg/kg/d divided q6h	5.4	Injection	Clavulanate is a β-lactamase inhibitor.
Mezlocillin (Mezlin)	2–24 g[1]	4–6 hr	225 mg/kg/d divided q8h	1.85	Injection	More active than ticarcillin against Enterobacteriacae, same activity against P. aeruginosa.
Piperacillin	2–24 g[1]	4–6 hr	300 mg/kg/d divided q6h	1.85	Injection	Good activity against P. aeruginosa, B. fragilis and Enterobacteriacae
Piperacillin/ Tazobactam (Zosyn)	12 g[3]	6 hr				Not recommended for *Pseudomonas*.

[1] Reduce dose in renal failure.
[2] The oral form of this drug is only to be used for simple urinary tract infections and never to be used for serious infections of any type.
[3] Based on piperacillin component (combination of 3 g piperacillin and 375 mg tazobactam).

469

MILRINONE (PRIMACOR)

Indications   Treatment of congestive heart failure
Dosage   Loading dose of 50 μg/kg, followed by a continuous infu-
                  sion of 0.375–0.75 μg/kg/min.
Notes   Carefully monitor fluid and electrolyte status.

MINERAL OIL

Indications   Constipation.
Dosage   Adult: 15–45 mL PO prn.
                  Peds older than 6 years: 10–20 mL PO bid.

MINOXIDIL (LONITEN)

Indications   Severe hypertension; treatment of male and female pat-
                  tern baldness.
Dosage   Adult: Oral: 2.5–10 mg PO bid-qid.
                  Topical: Apply twice daily to affected area.
                  Peds: 0.2–1 mg/kg/24 hr divided PO q12–24h.
Notes   Pericardial effusion and volume overload may occur; hy-
                  pertrichosis after chronic use.

MISOPROSTOL (CYTOTEC)

Indications   Prevention of NSAID-induced gastric ulcers.
Dosage   200 μg PO qid.
Notes   **Do not** take if pregnant, can cause miscarriage with po-
                  tentially dangerous bleeding; gastrointestinal side effects
                  are common.

MITOMYCIN (MUTAMYCIN)

Indications   Treatment of breast, cervical, and ovarian cancer, and
                  adenocarcinoma.
Dosage   20 mg/m^2 IV as a single dose every 6–8 weeks.
Notes   May cause cumulative myelosuppression.

MITOXANTRONE (NOVANTRONE)

Indications   Treatment of leukemia, lymphoma, and breast cancer.
Dosage   12 mg/m^2/d IV infusion for 2–3 days of each chemother-
                  apy cycle.
Notes   Causes severe myelosuppression.

MIVACURIUM (MIVACRON)

Indications   Adjunct to general anesthesia or mechanical ventilation.
Dosage   Adults: 0.15 mg/kg/dose IV, may need to repeat at 15
                  minute intervals.
                  Peds: 0.2 mg/kg/dose IV, may need to repeat at 10 minute
                  intervals.

MOLINDONE (MOBAN)

Indications   Management of psychotic disorders.
Dosage   5–100 mg PO tid-qid.

MORICIZINE (ETHMOZINE)

Indications   Treatment of ventricular arrhythmias.
Dosage   200–300 mg PO tid.

MORPHINE SULFATE [C]

Indications   Relief of severe pain.
Dosage   Adult: Oral: 10–30 mg q4h prn; sustained release tablets 30–60 mg q8–12h.
IV/IM: 2.5–15 mg q4h prn.
Peds: 0.1–0.2 mg/kg/dose IM/IV q2–4h prn up to maximum 15 mg/dose.
Notes   Large number of narcotic side effects; may require scheduled dosing to relieve severe chronic pain.

MUROMONAB-CD3 (ORTHOCLONE OKT3)

Indications   Treatment of acute rejection following organ transplantation.
Dosage   5 mg IV qd for 10–14 days.
Notes   Is a murine antibody; may cause significant fever and chills after the first dose.

NABUMETONE (RELAFEN)

See Table IX–7 on page 457.

NADOLOL (CORGARD)

See Table IX–2 on page 409.

NAFCILLIN (NAFCIL, UNIPEN)

See Table IX–1 on page 398.

NALBUPHINE (NUBAIN)

Indications   Moderate to severe pain.
Dosage   10–20 mg IM, IV, s.c. q4–6h prn.
Notes   Causes CNS depression and drowsiness; use with caution in patients receiving opiate drugs.

NALIDIXIC ACID (NEGGRAM)

Indications   Urinary tract infections caused by susceptible strains of *Proteus, Klebsiella, Enterobacter,* and *Escherichia coli* but not *Pseudomonas.*

Dosage   Adult: 1 g PO qid for 7–14 days.
                Peds: 55 mg/kg/24 hr in 4 divided doses.
Notes   Resistance emerges within 48 hours in significant per-
                centage of trials; may enhance effect of oral anticoagu-
                lants; may cause CNS adverse effects which reverse on
                discontinuation of the drug.

NALOXONE (NARCAN)

Indications Reversal of narcotic effect.
Dosage   Adult: 0.4–2.0 mg IV, IM or s.c. every 5 min, maximum to-
                tal dose of 10 mg.
                Peds: 0.01 mg/kg/dose IV, IM, or s.c.; may repeat IV every
                3 min for 3 doses prn.
Notes   May precipitate acute withdrawal in addicts; if no re-
                sponse after 10 mg, suspect a non-narcotic cause.

NAPROXEN (NAPROSYN, ANAPROX)

See Table IX–7 on page 457.

NEOMYCIN-POLYMYXIN BLADDER IRRIGANT SOLUTION

Indications Continuous irrigant for prophylaxis against bacteriuria and
                gram-negative bacteremia associated with indwelling
                catheter use.
Dosage   1 mL irrigant added to 1 L 0.9% NaCl; continuous irriga-
                tion of the bladder with 1–2 L of solution per 24 hours.
Notes   Potential for bacterial or fungal superinfection; possibility
                for neomycin-induced ototoxicity or nephrotoxicity.

NEOMYCIN SULFATE

Indications Hepatic coma; preop bowel prep.
Dosage   Adult: 3–12 g/24hr PO in 3–4 divided doses.
                Peds: 50–100 mg/kg/24hr PO in 3–4 divided doses.
Notes   Part of Condon bowel prep.

NIACIN (NICOLAR)

Indications Adjunctive therapy in patients with significant hyperlipid-
                emia who do not respond adequately to diet and weight
                loss.
Dosage   1–2 g PO tid with meals; up to 8 g/d.
Notes   Upper body and facial flushing and warmth following
                dose; may cause gastrointestinal upset and pruritus.

NICARDIPINE (CARDENE)

Indications Chronic stable angina, hypertension.

Dosage   Oral: 20–40 mg PO tid.
Sustained release: 30–60 mg PO bid.
Intravenous: 0.5–15 mg/hr continuous IV infusion. Titrate to desired blood pressure.

Notes   Oral to IV conversion: 20 mg tid = 0.5 mg/hr; 30 mg tid = 1.2 mg/hr; 40 mg tid = 2.2 mg/hr.

NIFEDIPINE (PROCARDIA, PROCARDIA XL, ADALAT, ADALAT CC)

Indications Vasospastic or chronic stable angina; hypertension.
Dosage   Adult: 10–30 mg PO q8h, maximum 180 mg/d, or sustained release tablets 30–90 mg once daily
Peds: 0.6–0.9 mg/kg/24h divided tid-qid.
Notes   Headaches common on initial treatment; reflex tachycardia may occur; Adalat CC and Procardia XL are not interchangeable dosage forms.

NIMODIPINE (NIMOTOP)

Indications Prevention of vasospasms following subarachnoid hemorrhage.
Dosage   60 mg PO q4h for 21 days.
Notes   Contents of capsule may be extracted and administered down an NG tube if the capsule cannot be swallowed whole.

NITROFURANTOIN (MACRODANTIN, FURADANTIN)

Indications Urinary tract infections.
Dosage   Adult:
Suppression: 50–100 mg PO qd.
Treatment: 50–100 mg PO qid.
Peds: 5–7 mg/kg/24 hr in 4 divided doses.
Notes   Gastrointestinal side effects common; should be taken with food, milk, or antacid; macrocrystals (Macrodantin) cause less nausea than other forms of drug, may cause pulmonary fibrosis.

NITROGLYCERIN (NITROSTAT, NITROLINGUAL, NITRO-BID OINTMENT, NITRO-BID IV, NITRODISC, TRANSDERM-NITRO)

Indications Angina pectoris; acute and prophylactic therapy; congestive heart failure, blood pressure control.
Dosage   Adult:
Sublingual: 1 tablet SL q5 min prn × 3 doses.
Translingual: 1–2 metered doses sprayed onto oral mucosa.
Oral: 2.5–9 mg tid.
Intravenous: 5–20 μg/min titrated to effect.
Topical: 1-2 inches ointment to chest wall q6h, then wipe off at night.

Transdermal: 5–20 cm patch qd.
Peds: 1 μg/kg/min IV titrated to effect.

Notes   Tolerance to nitrates develops with chronic use after 1–2 weeks; this can be avoided by providing a nitrate-free period each day; shorter acting nitrates should be used on a tid basis and long-acting patches and ointment should be removed before bedtime in order to prevent the development of tolerance.

NITROPRUSSIDE (NIPRIDE, NITROPRESS)

Indications   Hypertensive emergency, aortic dissection, pulmonary edema.

Dosage   Adult and Peds: 0.5–10 μg/kg/min IV infusion titrated to desired effect.

Notes   Thiocyanate, the metabolite, is excreted by the kidney; thiocyanate toxicity occurs at plasma levels of 5–10 mg/dL; if used to treat aortic dissection, a β-blocker must be used concomitantly.

NIZATIDINE (AXID)

Indications   Treatment of duodenal ulcers.

Dosage   Active ulcer: 150 mg PO bid or 300 mg PO qhs.
Maintenance: 150 mg PO qhs.

NOREPINEPHRINE (LEVOPHED)

Indications   Acute hypotensive states.

Dosage   Adult: 8–12 μg/min IV titrated to desired effect.
Peds: 0.1 μg/kg/min IV titrated to desired effect.

Notes   Correct blood volume depletion as much as possible before initiation of vasopressor therapy; drug interaction with tricyclic antidepressants leading to severe profound hypertension; infuse into large vein to avoid extravasation; phentolamine 5–10 mg/10 mL NSS injected locally is antidote to extravasation.

NORFLOXACIN (NOROXIN)

Indications   Treatment of complicated and uncomplicated urinary tract infections resulting from a wide variety of gram-negative bacteria, and prostatitis.

Dosage   Adult: 400 mg PO bid.
Peds: Not recommended for use in patients younger than 18 years.

Notes   Not for use in pregnancy; drug interactions with antacids, theophylline, and caffeine.

NORTRIPTYLINE (AVENTYL, PAMELOR)

Indications   Endogenous depression.
Dosage   25 mg PO tid to qid; doses above 100 mg/d are not recommended.
Notes   Many anticholinergic side effects including blurred vision, urinary retention, dry mouth.

NYSTATIN (MYCOSTATIN, NILSTAT)

Indications   Treatment of mucocutaneous *Candida* infections (thrush, vaginitis).
Dosage   Adult: Oral: 400,000–600,000 units PO "swish and swallow" qid.
Vaginal: 1 tablet inserted into vagina qhs.
Topical: Apply 2–3 times daily to affected area.
Peds: Infants: 200,000 units PO q6h.
Children: See adult dosage.
Notes   Not absorbed orally, therefore not effective for systemic infections.

OCTREOTIDE ACETATE (SANDOSTATIN)

Indications   Suppresses or inhibits severe diarrhea associated with carcinoid and vasoactive intestinal tumors.
Dosage   Adult: 100–600 μg/d s.c. in 2–4 divided doses.
Peds: 1–10 μg/kg/24 hr s.c. in 2–4 divided doses.
Notes   May cause nausea, vomiting, and abdominal discomfort.

OFLOXACIN (FLOXIN)

Indications   Treatment of infections of the lower respiratory tract, skin and skin structure, and urinary tract, prostatitis, uncomplicated gonorrhea, and chlamydia infections.
Dosage   Adult: 200–400 mg PO bid or IV q12h.
Peds: Should not be used in children younger than 18 years.
Notes   May cause nausea, vomiting, diarrhea, insomnia and headache; drug interactions with antacids, sucralfate, and iron and zinc containing products that decrease the absorption of ofloxacin; may increase theophylline levels.

OLSALAZINE (DIPENTUM)

Indications   Maintenance of remission of ulcerative colitis.
Dosage   500 mg PO bid.
Notes   Take with food; may cause diarrhea.

OMEPRAZOLE (PRILOSEC)

Indications   Treatment of duodenal ulcers, ZE syndrome, and gastro-esophageal reflux (GERD).
Dosage   20–40 mg qd.

ONDANSETRON (ZOFRAN)

Indications   Prevention of nausea and vomiting associated with cancer chemotherapy and postoperative nausea and vomiting.
Dosage   Adult and Peds:
                  Chemotherapy: 0.15 mg/kg/dose IV before chemotherapy, then repeated 4 and 8 hours after the first dose or 4–8 mg PO tid, administer first dose 30 minutes before chemotherapy.
                  Adults: Postop: 4 mg IV immediately before induction or postop.
Notes   May cause diarrhea and headache.

OXACILLIN (BACTOCILL, PROSTAPHLIN)

See Table IX–1 on page 398.

OXAPROZIN (DAYPRO)

See Table IX–7 on page 457.

OXAZEPAM (SERAX) [C]

Indications   Anxiety; acute alcohol withdrawal; anxiety with depressive symptoms.
Dosage   10–15 mg PO tid-qid; severe anxiety and alcohol withdrawal may require up to 30 mg qid.
Notes   Oxazepam is one of the metabolites of diazepam (Valium).

OXYBUTYNIN (DITROPAN)

Indications   Symptomatic relief of urgency, nocturia, and incontinence associated with neurogenic or reflex neurogenic bladder.
Dosage   Adult and Peds: 5 mg PO bid-qid.
Notes   Anticholinergic side effects.

OXYCODONE (PERCOCET, PERCODAN, TYLOX) [C]

Indications   Moderate to severe pain.
Dosage   1–2 tablets/capsules PO q4–6h prn.
                  (Percocet tablet: 5 mg oxycodone, 325 mg acetaminophen. Percodan tablet: 4.5 mg oxycodone, 325 mg aspirin. Tylox capsule: 5 mg oxycodone, 500 mg acetaminophen).

OXYTOCIN (PITOCIN, SYNTOCINON)

Indications   Induction of labor; control of postpartum hemorrhage.
Dosage   0.001–0.002 U/min IV infusion titrate to desired effect to a maximum of 0.02 U/min.
Notes   Can cause uterine rupture and fetal death; monitor vital signs closely.

PACLITAXEL (TAXOL)

Indications   Treatment of ovarian cancer.
Dosage   135 mg/m^2 IV every 3 weeks.
Notes   May cause severe neutropenia.

PANCREATIN
PANCRELIPASE (PANCREASE, COTAZYME)

Indications   For patients deficient in exocrine pancreatic secretions (cystic fibrosis, chronic pancreatitis, other pancreatic insufficiency), and for steatorrhea of malabsorption syndrome.
Dosage   Adult and Peds: 1–3 capsules (tablets) with meals and snacks; dosage may be increased up to 8 capsules (tablets).
Notes   Avoid antacids; may cause nausea, abdominal cramps, or diarrhea; do not crush or chew enteric-coated products.

PANCURONIUM (PAVULON)

Indications   Aid in the management of patients on mechanical ventilator.
Dosage   Adult: 2–4 mg IV q2–4h prn.
Peds: 0.02–0.10 mg/kg/dose q2–4h prn.
Notes   Patient must be intubated and on controlled ventilation; use adequate amount of sedation or analgesia.

PAROXETINE (PAXIL)

Indications   Treatment of depression.
Dosage   20–50 mg PO as a single daily dose.

PENBUTOLOL (LEVATOL)

See Table IX–2 on page 409.

PENICILLIN G AQUEOUS (POTASSIUM OR SODIUM) (PFIZERPEN, PENTIDS)

Indications   Most gram-positive infections (except penicillin-resistant staphylococci) including streptococci, *Neisseria meningitidis,* syphilis, clostridia, corynebacteria, and some coliforms.

Dosage   Adult: 400,000–800,000 units PO qid; IV doses vary
                  greatly depending on indications, range from 1.2–24 mil-
                  lion U/d.
                  Peds: Newborns younger than 1 week: 25,000–50,000
                  U/kg/dose IV q12h.
                  Infants 1 week–1 month: 25,000–50,000 U/kg/dose IV
                  q8h.
                  Children: 100,000–300,000 U/kg/24h IV divided q4h.
Notes   Beware of hypersensitivity reactions; drug of choice for
                  group A streptococcal infections and syphilis.

PENICILLIN G BENZATHINE (BICILLIN)

Indications   Useful as a single dose treatment regimen for streptococ-
                  cal pharyngitis, rheumatic fever and glomerulonephritis
                  prophylaxis, and syphilis.
Dosage   Adult: 1.2–2.4 million units deep IM injection q2–4 weeks.
                  Peds: 50,000 U/kg/dose to a maximum of 2.4 million
                  U/dose deep IM injection q2–4wk.
Notes   Sustained action with detectable levels up to 4 weeks;
                  considered drug of choice for treatment of noncongenital
                  syphilis; Bicillin L-A contains the benzathine salt only;
                  Bicillin C-R contains a combination of the benzathine and
                  procaine salts and is used for most acute strep infections
                  (300,000 units procaine with 300,000 units benzathine/mL
                  or 900,000 units benzathine with 300,000 units procaine/
                  2 mL).

PENICILLIN G PROCAINE (WYCILLIN, OTHERS)

Indications   Moderately severe infections caused by penicillin G-
                  sensitive organisms that respond to low persistent serum
                  levels (syphilis, uncomplicated pneumococcal pneumonia).
Dosage   Adult: 300,000–1.2 million U/d IM divided qd-bid.
                  Peds: 25,000–50,000 U/kg/d IM divided qd-bid.
Notes   A long-acting parenteral penicillin; blood levels up to 15
                  hours; give probenecid at least 30 minutes before admin-
                  istration of penicillin to prolong action.

PENICILLIN V (PEN-VEE K, VEETIDS, OTHERS)

Indications   Most gram-positive infections (except penicillin-resistant
                  staphylococci) including streptococci, *Neisseria meningi-
                  tidis*, syphilis, clostridia, corynebacteria, and some col-
                  iforms.
Dosage   Adult: 250–500 mg PO q6h.
                  Peds: 25–50 mg/kg/24 hr PO in 4 divided doses.
Notes   A well-tolerated oral penicillin; 250 mg = 400,000 units
                  Penicillin G.

PENTAMIDINE ISETHIONATE (PENTAM 300, NEBUPENT)

Indications Treatment and prevention of *Pneumocystis carinii* pneumonia.

Dosage Adult and Peds: 4 mg/kg/24 hr IV daily for 14–21 days.
Adult: Prevention: 300 mg once every 4 weeks, administered via Respirgard II nebulizer.

Notes Monitor patient for severe hypotension following IV administration; associated with pancreatic islet-cell necrosis leading to hypoglycemia and hyperglycemia; monitor hematology labs for leukopenia and thrombocytopenia.

PENTAZOCINE (TALWIN) [C]

Indications Moderate to severe pain.

Dosage 30 mg IM or IV; 50–100 mg PO q3–4h prn.

Notes 30–60 mg IM equianalgesic to 10 mg morphine IM; associated with considerable dysphoria.

PENTOBARBITAL (NEMBUTAL, OTHERS) [C]

Indications Insomnia, convulsions, induced coma following severe head injury.

Dosage Adult: Sedative: 20–40 mg PO or PR q6–12h.
Hypnotic: 100–200 mg PO or PR qhs prn.
Induced coma: load 3–5 mg/kg IV × 1, then maintenance 2–3.5 mg/kg/dose IV q1h prn to keep level between 25–40 µg/mL.
Peds: Hypnotic: 2–6 mg/kg/dose PO qhs prn.
Induced coma: See adult.

Notes Can cause respiratory depression; may produce profound hypotension when used aggressively IV for cerebral edema; tolerance to sedative-hypnotic effect acquired within 1–2 weeks.

PENTOXIFYLLINE (TRENTAL)

Indications Intermittent claudication.

Dosage 400 mg PO tid with meals.

Notes Treat for at least 8 weeks to see full effect.

PERGOLIDE (PERMAX)

Indications Parkinson's disease.

Dosage Initially 0.05 mg PO tid, titrated every 2–3 days to desired effect.

Notes May cause hypotension during initiation of therapy.

PERINDOPRIL (ACEON)

Indications Treatment of essential hypertension

Dosage 4–16 mg PO qd.

PERMETHRIN (NIX)

Indications   Eradication of lice.
Dosage   Adult and Peds: Saturate hair and scalp; allow to remain in hair for 10 minutes before rinsing out.

PERPHENAZINE (TRILAFON)

Indications   Psychotic disorders, intractable hiccups, severe nausea.
Dosage   Antipsychotic: 4–8 mg PO tid, maximum 64 mg/d.
                  Hiccups: 5 mg IM q6h prn or 1 mg IV at not less than 1–2 mg/min intervals up to 5 mg.

PHENAZOPYRIDINE (PYRIDIUM)

Indications   Symptomatic relief of discomfort from lower urinary tract irritation.
Dosage   Adult: 200 mg PO tid.
                  Peds 6–12 years old: 12 mg/kg/24 hr PO in 3 divided doses.
Notes   Gastrointestinal disturbances; causes red-orange urine color, which can stain clothing.

PHENOBARBITAL [C]

Indications   Seizure disorders, insomnia, anxiety.
Dosage   Adult: Sedative-hypnotic: 30–120 mg PO or IM qd prn.
                  Anticonvulsant: Loading dose of 10–12 mg/kg in 3 divided doses, then 1–3 mg/kg/24 hr PO, IM, or IV.
                  Peds: Sedative-hypnotic: 2–3 mg/kg/24 hr PO or IM qhs prn.
                  Anticonvulsant: Loading dose of 15–20 mg/kg divided into 2 equal doses 4 hours apart, then 3–5 mg/kg/24 hr PO divided in 2–3 doses.
Notes   Tolerance develops to sedation; paradoxical hyperactivity seen in pediatric patients; long half-life allows single daily dosing; see Table IX–12, page 501.

PHENYLEPHRINE (NEO-SYNEPHRINE)

Indications   Treatment of vascular failure in shock, hypersensitivity, or drug-induced hypotension; nasal congestion; mydriatic.
Dosage   Adult: Mild to moderate hypotension: 2–5 mg IM or s.c. elevates BP for 2 hours; 0.1–0.5 mg IV elevates BP for 15 min.
                  Severe hypotension or shock: Initiate continuous infusion at 100–180 μg/min; after BP stabilized, maintenance rate of 40–60 μg/min.
                  Nasal congestion: 1–2 sprays into each nostril prn.

Peds: Hypotension: 5–20 μg/kg/dose IV q10–15 minutes or 0.1–0.5 μg/kg/minute IV infusion titrated to desired effect.

Nasal congestion: 1 spray into each nostril q3–4h prn.

Notes   Promptly restore blood volume if loss has occurred; use with extreme caution in patients with hyperthyroidism, bradycardia, partial heart block, myocardial disease, or severe arteriosclerosis; use large veins for infusion to avoid extravasation; phentolamine 10 mg in 10–15 mL saline for local injection as antidote for extravasation; activity potentiated by oxytocin, MAOIs, and tricyclic antidepressants.

PHENYTOIN (DILANTIN)

Indications   Tonic-clonic and partial seizures.

Dosage   Adult and Peds: Load: 15–20 mg/kg, IV at a maximum infusion rate of 25 mg/min or orally in 400 mg doses at 4 hour intervals.

Adult: Maintenance: 200 mg PO or IV bid or 300 mg qhs initially then follow serum concentrations.

Peds: Maintenance: 4–7 mg/kg/24 hr PO or IV divided qd-bid.

Notes   Caution with cardiac depressant side effects, especially with IV administration; follow levels as needed (see Table IX–12, page 501); nystagmus and ataxia are early signs of toxicity; gum hyperplasia occurs with long term use; avoid use of oral suspension if possible due to erratic absorption; avoid use in pregnancy.

PHYSOSTIGMINE (ANTILIRIUM)

Indications   Antidote for tricyclic antidepressant, atropine, and scopolamine overdose.

Dosage   Adult: 2 mg IV/IM q15min.

Peds: 0.01–0.03 mg/kg/dose IV q15–30 min.

Notes   Rapid IV administration associated with convulsions; cholinergic side effects; may cause asystole.

PHYTONADIONE [VITAMIN K] (AQUAMEPHYTON, OTHERS)

Indications   Coagulation disorders caused by faulty formation of factors II, VII, IX, and X, hyperalimentation.

Dosage   Adults and Peds:

Anticoagulant-induced prothrombin deficiency: 2.5–10.0 mg PO or IV slowly.

Hyperalimentation: 10 mg IM or IV every week.

Infants: 0.5–1.0 mg/dose IM, s.c., or PO.

Notes   With parenteral treatment, usually see first change in pro-
                   thrombin in 12–24 hours; anaphylaxis can result from IV
                   dosage; should be administered slowly IV.

PINDOLOL (VISKEN)

See Table IX–2 on page 409.

PIPECURONIUM (ARDUAN)

Indications   Adjunct to general anesthesia.
Dosage   Adults: 50–100 µg/kg IV.
                   Peds: 40–57 µg/kg IV.

PIPERACILLIN (PIPRACIL)

See Table IX–8 on page 469.

PIPERACILLIN/TAZOBACTAM (ZOSYN)

See Table IX–8 on page 469.

PIRBUTEROL (MAXAIR)

Indications   Prevention and reversal of bronchospasm.
Dosage   Adults and Peds older than 12 years: 2 inhalations q4–6h,
                   maximum of 12 inhalations/day.

PIROXICAM (FELDENE)

See Table IX–7 on page 457.

PLASMA PROTEIN FRACTION (PLASMANATE, OTHERS)

Indications   Shock and hypotension.
Dosage   Adult: 250–500 mL IV initially (not >10 mL/min); subse-
                   quent infusions should depend on clinical response.
                   Peds: 10–15 mL/kg/dose IV; subsequent infusions should
                   depend on clinical response.
Notes   Hypotension associated with rapid infusion; 130–160 mEq
                   sodium/L; **not** a substitute for red cells.

PLICAMYCIN (MITHRACIN)

Indications   Treatment of hypercalcemia of malignancy.
Dosage   25 µg/kg/d IV for 3–4 days.

PNEUMOCOCCAL VACCINE, POLYVALENT (PNEUMOVAX)

Indications   Immunization against pneumococcal infections in patients
                   predisposed to or at high risk of acquiring these infections.
Dosage   Adult and Peds: 0.5 mL IM.
Notes   Do not vaccinate during immunosuppressive therapy.

POLYETHYLENE GLYCOL-ELECTROLYTE SOLUTION (GO-LYTLEY, COLYTE)

Indications   Bowel cleansing before examination or surgery.

Dosage   Following 3–4 hour fast, the patient must drink 240 mL of solution every 10 minutes until 4 L consumed.

Notes   First bowel movement should occur in approximately **1** hour; may cause some cramping or nausea.

POTASSIUM SUPPLEMENTS

Indications   Prevention or treatment of hypokalemia.

Dosage   Adult: 8–24 mEq/d PO divided qd-bid.
Peds: Calculate potassium deficit.

Notes   See Table IX–9 on page 483. Can cause gastrointestinal irritation; powder and liquids must be mixed with beverage (unsalted tomato juice very palatable); use cautiously in renal insufficiency, and along with NSAIDs and ACE inhibitors.

PRAVASTATIN (PRAVACHOL)

Indications   Reduction of elevated cholesterol levels.

Dosage   10–40 mg PO qhs.

TABLE IX–9. ORAL POTASSIUM SUPPLEMENTS.

Brand Name	Salt	Form	mEq Potassium/Dosing Unit
Kaochlor 10%	KCl	Liquid	20 mEq/15 mL
Kaochlor S-F 10% (sugar-free)	KCl	Liquid	20 mEq/15 mL
Kaon Elixir	K^+gluconate	Liquid	20 mEq/15 mL
Kaon	K^+gluconate	Tablets	5 mEq/tablet
Kaon-Cl	KCl	Tablet, SR	6.67 mEq/tablet
Kaon-Cl 20%	KCl	Liquid	40 mEq/15 mL
KayCiel	KCl	Liquid	20 mEq/15 mL
K-Lor	KCl	Powder	15 or 20 mEq/packet
Klorvess	KCl	Liquid	20 mEq/15 mL
Klotrix	KCl	Tablet, SR	10 mEq/tablet
K-Lyte	K^+bicarbonate	Effervescent tablet	25 mEq/tablet
K-Tab	KCl	Tablet, SR	10 mEq/tablet
Micro-K	KCl	Capsules	8 mEq/capsule
Slow-K	KCl	Tablet, SR	8 mEq/tablet

PRAZEPAM (CENTRAX) [C]

Indications Anxiety disorders.
Dosage   5–10 mg PO 3 or 4 times a day, or 20–50 mg PO as single bedtime dose to minimize daytime drowsiness.

PRAZOSIN (MINIPRES)

Indications Hypertension.
Dosage   Adult: 1 mg PO tid; can increase to a total daily dose of 5 mg qid.
Peds: 25–150 µg/kg/24 hr divided q6h.
Notes   Can cause orthostatic hypotension, therefore, patient should take first dose at bedtime; tolerance develops to this effect; tachyphylaxis may result.

PREDNISONE

See "Steroids," page 490.

PREDNISOLONE

See "Steroids," page 490.

PROBENECID (BENEMID)

Indications Gout, maintenance of serum levels of penicillins or cephalosporins.
Dosage   Adult: Gout: 0.25 g bid for 1 week; then 0.5 g PO bid.
Antibiotic effect: 1–2 g PO 30 minutes before dose of antibiotic.
Peds: 25 mg/kg, then 40 mg/kg/d PO divided qid.

PROBUCOL (LORELCO)

Indications Adjunctive therapy for reduction of serum cholesterol.
Dosage   500 mg PO bid with morning and evening meals.
Notes   May note prolongation of QT interval on ECG; diarrhea or loose stools common; may also lower HDL.

PROCAINAMIDE (PRONESTYL, PROCAN)

Indications Treatment of supraventricular and ventricular arrhythmias.
Dosage   Adult: Emergency cardiac care: 100–200 mg/dose IV q5min until dysrhythmia resolves, hypotension ensues, or dose totals 1 g; then maintenance of 1–4 mg/min IV infusion.
Chronic dosing: 50 mg/kg/d PO in divided doses q4–6h.
Peds: Emergency cardiac care: 3–6 mg/kg/dose IV over 5 minutes, then 20–80 µg/kg/min IV infusion.
Maintenance: 15–50 mg/kg/24 hr PO divided q3–6h.

Notes   Can cause hypotension and a lupus-like syndrome; dosage adjustment required with renal impairment; see Table IX–12, page 501.

PROCHLORPERAZINE (COMPAZINE)

Indications   Nausea, vomiting, agitation, psychotic disorders.
Dosage   Adult: Antiemetic: 5–10 mg PO tid-qid or 25 mg PR bid or 5-10 mg deep IM q4–6h.
Antipsychotic: 10–20 mg IM acutely or 5–10 mg PO tid-qid for maintenance.
Peds: 0.1–0.15 mg/kg/dose IM q4–6h or 0.4 mg/kg/24 hr PO divided tid-qid.
Notes   Much larger dose may be required for antipsychotic effect; extrapyramidal side effects common; treat acute extrapyramidal reactions with diphenhydramine.

PROMETHAZINE (PHENERGAN)

Indications   Nausea, vomiting, motion sickness.
Dosage   Adult: 12.5–50 mg PO, PR, or IM bid-qid prn.
Peds: 0.1–0.5 mg/kg/dose PO or IM q4–6h prn.
Notes   High incidence of drowsiness.

PROPAFENONE (RYTHMOL)

Indications   Treatment of life-threatening ventricular arrhythmias.
Dosage   150–300 mg PO q8h.
Notes   May cause dizziness, unusual taste, and first degree heart block.

PROPANTHELINE (PRO-BANTHINE)

Indications   Symptomatic treatment of small intestine hypermotility, spastic colon, ureteral spasm, bladder spasm, pylorospasm.
Dosage   Adult: 15 mg PO a.c. and 30 mg PO hs.
Peds: 1.5–3.0 mg/kg/24 hr PO divided tid-qid.
Notes   Anticholinergic side effects such as dry mouth, blurred vision are common.

PROPOXYPHENE (DARVON, DARVOCET) [C]

Indications   Mild to moderate pain.
Dosage   32–65 mg PO q4h prn. Darvon (Propoxyphene HCl) 32 mg, 65 mg Darvon-N (Propoxyphene Napsylate) 100 mg = 65 mg of Propoxyphene HCl. Darvocet-N: Propoxyphene Napsylate/acetaminophen. Darvon Compound: Propoxyphene HCl/aspirin/caffeine.

PROPRANOLOL (INDERAL)

See Table IX–2 on page 409.

PROPYLTHIOURACIL [PTU]

Indications Hyperthyroidism.
Dosage Adult: Begin at 100 mg PO q8h (may need up to 1200 mg/d for control); after patient is euthyroid (6–8 weeks), taper dose by ⅓ every 4–6 weeks to a maintenance dose of 50–150 mg/24h; treatment is usually able to be discontinued in 2–3 years.
Peds: Initial 5–7 mg/kg/24 hr PO divided q8h, then maintenance of ⅓–⅔ of initial dose.
Notes Follow patient clinically; monitor thyroid function tests.

PROTAMINE SULFATE

Indications Reversal of heparin effect.
Dosage Adult and Peds: Based on amount of heparin reversal desired; given slow IV, 1 mg will reverse approximately 100 units of heparin given in the preceding 3–4h to max dose of 50 mg.
Notes Follow coagulation studies; may have anticoagulant effect if given without heparin.

PSEUDOEPHEDRINE (SUDAFED, NOVAFED, AFRINOL)

Indications Decongestant.
Dosage Adult: 30–60 mg PO q6–8h; sustained release capsules 120 mg PO q12h.
Peds: 4 mg/kg/24 hr PO divided qid.
Notes Contraindicated in patients with hypertension or coronary artery disease, and patients taking MAO inhibitors; an ingredient in many cough and cold preparations.

PSYLLIUM (METAMUCIL, SERUTAN, EFFER-SYLLIUM)

Indications Constipation, diverticular disease of the colon.
Dosage 1 teaspoon (7 g) in a glass of water qd-tid.
Notes Do not use if suspect bowel obstruction; one of the safest laxatives; psyllium in effervescent (Effer-syllium) form usually contains potassium and should be used with caution in patients with renal failure.

PYRAZINAMIDE

Indications Treatment of active tuberculosis.
Dosage Adults: 20–35 mg/kg/24 hr PO divided tid-qid, maximum dose is 3 g/d.
Peds: 15–30 mg/kg/d PO divided bid or qd.

Notes   May cause hepatotoxicity; use in combination with other antituberculosis drugs.

PYRIDOXINE (VITAMIN B$_6$)

Indications   Treatment and prevention of vitamin B$_6$ deficiency.
Dosage   Deficiency: 2.5–10.0 mg PO qd.
                 Drug-induced neuritis: 50 mg PO qd.

QUAZEPAM (DORAL) [C]

Indications   Insomnia.
Dosage   7.5–15 mg PO qhs prn.
Notes   Reduce dose in the elderly.

QUINAPRIL (ACCUPRIL)

Indications   Treatment of hypertension.
Dosage   10–80 mg PO qd in single dose.

QUINIDINE (QUINIDEX, QUINAGLUTE)

Indications   Prevention of tachydysrhythmias.
Dosage   Adult: PAC, PVCs: 200–300 mg PO tid-qid.
                 Conversion of atrial fibrillation or flutter: Use after digital-ization, 200 mg q2–3h for 8 doses; then increase daily dose to maximum of 3–4 g or until normal rhythm.
                 Peds: 30 mg/kg/24 hr PO 4-5 divided doses.
Notes   Contraindicated in digitalis toxicity, AV block; follow serum levels if available (see Table IX–12, page 501); extreme hypotension seen with IV administration.
                 Sulfate salt: Contains 83% quinidine.
                 Gluconate salt: Contains 62% quinidine.

RAMIPRIL (ALTACE)

Indications   Treatment of hypertension.
Dosage   2.5–20 mg/d PO divided qd-bid.
Notes   May use in combination with diuretics; may cause a non-productive cough.

RANITIDINE (ZANTAC)

Indications   Duodenal ulcer, active benign ulcers, hypersecretory con-ditions, gastroesophageal reflux.
Dosage   Adult: Ulcer: 150 mg PO bid, 300 mg PO qhs, or 50 mg IV q6–8h; or 400 mg IV/day continuous infusion.
                 Maintenance: 150 mg PO qhs.
                 Hypersecretion: 150 mg PO bid.
                 Peds: 0.1–0.8 mg/kg/dose IV q6–8h or 1.25–2.0 mg/kg/dose PO q12h.

Notes   Reduce dose with renal failure; note oral and parenteral doses different.

RIBAVIRIN (VIRAZOLE)

Indications   Treatment of infants and children with RSV infection.
Dosage   6 g in 300 mL of sterile water inhaled over 12–18 hours.
Notes   Aerosolized by a SPAG generator; may accumulate on soft contact lenses.

RIFABUTIN (MYCOBUTIN)

Indications   Prevention of *Mycobacterium avium* complex infection in AIDS patients with a CD4 count <100.
Dosage   300 mg PO qd.
Notes   Has similar adverse effects and drug interactions as rifampin.

RIFAMPIN (RIFADIN)

Indications   Tuberculosis, treatment, and prophylaxis of *Neisseria meningitidis, Haemophilus influenzae,* or *Staphylococcus aureus* carriers.
Dosage   Adult: *Neisseria meningitidis* and *Haemophilus influenzae* carrier: 600 mg PO qd × 4 days.
                   Tuberculosis: 600 mg PO or IV qd or twice weekly with combination therapy regimen.
                   Peds: 10–20 mg/kg/dose PO or IV qd-bid.
Notes   Multiple side effects; causes orange-red discoloration of bodily secretions including tears; never used as a single agent to treat active tuberculosis infections.

RIMANTADINE (FLUMADINE)

Indications   Prophylaxis and treatment of influenza A virus infections.
Dosage   Adults: 100 mg PO bid.
                   Peds: 5 mg/kg PO qd, not to exceed 150 mg/d.

RISPERIDONE (RISPERDAL)

Indications   Management of psychotic disorders.
Dosage   1–8 mg PO bid

SARGRAMOSTIM [GM-CSF] (PROKINE, LEUKINE)

Indications   Treatment of myeloid recovery following bone marrow transplantation.
Dosage   Adult and Peds: 250 mg/m^2/d IV for 21 days.
Notes   May cause bone pain.

SCOPOLAMINE, TRANSDERMAL (TRANSDERM-SCOP)

Indications Prevention of nausea and vomiting associated with motion sickness.
Dosage Apply 1 patch behind the ear every 3 days.
Notes May cause dry mouth, drowsiness, and blurred vision.

SECOBARBITAL (SECONAL) [C]

Indications Insomnia.
Dosage Adult: 100 mg PO, or IM qhs prn.
Peds: 3–5 mg/kg/dose PO or IM qhs prn.
Notes Beware of respiratory depression; tolerance acquired within 1–2 weeks.

SELEGILINE (ELDEPRYL)

Indications Parkinson's disease.
Dosage 5 mg PO bid.
Notes May cause nausea and dizziness.

SERTRALINE (ZOLOFT)

Indications Treatment of depression.
Dosage 50–200 mg PO qd.
Notes Can activate manic/hypomanic state; has caused weight loss in clinical trials.

SILVER SULFADIAZINE (SILVADENE)

Indications Prevention of sepsis in second-degree and third-degree burns.
Dosage Adult and Peds: Aseptically cover affected area with 1/16 inch coating bid.
Notes Can have systemic absorption with extensive application.

SIMETHICONE (MYLICON)

Indications Symptomatic treatment of flatulence.
Dosage Adult and Peds: 40–125 mg PO p.c. and hs prn.

SIMVASTATIN (ZOCOR)

Indications Reduction of elevated cholesterol levels.
Dosage 5–40 mg PO qhs.

SODIUM BICARBONATE

Indications Alkalinization of urine, treatment of metabolic acidosis.
Dosage Adult and Peds: Titrate to effect based on blood gases or urine pH.
Notes 1 gram neutralizes 12 mEq of acid.

SODIUM POLYSTYRENE SULFONATE (KAYEXALATE)

Indications Treatment of hyperkalemia.
Dosage Adult: 15–60 g PO or 30–60 g PR q6h based on serum K^+.
Peds: 1 g/kg/dose PO or PR q6h based on serum K^+.
Notes Can cause hypernatremia; given with agent such as sorbitol to promote movement through bowel.

SORBITOL

Indications Constipation.
Dosage 30–60 mL of a 20–70% solution prn.

SOTALOL (BETAPACE)

See Table IX–2 on page 409.

SPIRONOLACTONE (ALDACTONE)

Indications Treatment of hyperaldosteronism, essential hypertension, edematous states (CHF, cirrhosis), polycystic ovary.
Dosage Adult: 25–100 mg PO qid.
Peds: 1–3.3 mg/kg/24 hr PO divided bid-qid.
Notes Can cause hyperkalemia and gynecomastia; avoid prolonged use; diuretic of choice for cirrhotic edema and ascites.

STEROIDS

The following relates only to the commonly used systemic glucocorticoids:

Indications Endocrine disorders (adrenal insufficiency), rheumatoid disorders, collagen-vascular diseases, dermatologic diseases, allergic states, edematous states (cerebral, nephrotic syndrome), immunosuppression for transplantation, hypercalcemia, malignancies (breast, lymphomas), preoperatively (in any patient who has been on steroids in the previous year, known hypoadrenalism, preop for adrenalectomy).
Dosage Varies with indications and institutional protocols. Some commonly used dosages are listed below:
Acute adrenal insufficiency (Addisonian crisis): Hydrocortisone 100 mg IV q8h.
Chronic adrenal insufficiency: Hydrocortisone 20 mg PO q AM, 10 mg PO q PM; may need mineralocorticoid supplementation such as DOCA.
Perioperative steroid coverage: Hydrocortisone 100 mg IV night before surgery, 1 hour preop, intraoperatively, and 4, 8, and 12 hours postoperatively; POD No. 1 100 mg IV

q6h; POD No. 2 100 mg IV q8h; POD No. 3 100 mg IV q12h; POD No. 4 50 mg IV q12h; POD No. 5 25 mg IV q12h; then, resume prior oral dosing if chronic use or discontinue if only perioperative coverage required.

Cerebral edema: Dexamethasone 10 mg IV; then 4 mg IV q4–6h.

Notes
See Table IX–10, below. All can cause hyperglycemia, adrenal suppression; never acutely stop steroids, especially if chronic treatment; taper dose.

STREPTOKINASE (STREPTASE, KABIKINASE)

Indications
Coronary artery thrombosis; acute massive pulmonary embolism; deep vein thrombosis; some occluded vascular grafts.

Dosage
Pulmonary embolus: Loading dose of 250,000 IU IV through a peripheral vein over 30 minutes, then 100,000 IU/hr IV for 24–72 hours.

Deep vein thrombosis or arterial embolism: Load as with pulmonary embolus, then 100,000 IU/hr for 72 hours.

Notes
If maintenance infusion not adequate to maintain thrombin clotting time 2–5 times control, refer to package insert, PDR, or Hospital Formulary Service for adjustments.

TABLE IX–10. COMPARISON OF GLUCOCORTICOIDS.

Drug	Equivalent Dose (mg)	Relative Mineral Activity	Duration	Route
Cortisone (Cortone)	25.00	2	8–12 hr	PO, IM
Dexamethasone (Decadron)	0.75	0	36–72 hr	PO, IV
Hydrocortisone (Solu-Cortef)	20.00	2	8–12 hr	PO, IM, IV
Methylprednisolone (Depo-Medrol, Solu-Medrol)	4.00	0	36–72 hr	PO, IM, IV
Prednisone (Deltasone)	5.00	1	12–36 hr	PO
Prednisolone (Delta-Cortef)	5.00	1	12–36 hr	PO, IM, IV

SUCCINYLCHOLINE (ANECTINE, QUELICIN, SUCOSTRIN)

Indications   Adjunct to general anesthesia to facilitate endotracheal intubation and to induce skeletal muscle relaxation during surgery or mechanically supported ventilation.

Dosage   Adult: 0.6 mg/kg IV over 10–30 seconds followed by 0.04–0.07 mg/kg as needed to maintain muscle relaxation.
Peds: 1–2 mg/kg/dose IV followed by 0.03–0.06 mg/kg/dose at intervals of 10–20 minutes.

Notes   May precipitate malignant hyperthermia; respiratory depression or prolonged apnea may occur; many drug interactions potentiating activity of succinylcholine; observe for cardiovascular effects; use only freshly prepared solutions.

SUCRALFATE (CARAFATE)

Indications   Treatment of duodenal ulcers, gastric ulcers.
Dosage   1 g PO qid, 1 hour before meals and hs.
Notes   Treatment should be continued for 4–8 weeks unless healing demonstrated by x-ray or endoscopy; constipation most frequent side effect.

SUFENTANIL (SUFENTA) [C]

Indications   Analgesic adjunct to maintain balanced general anesthesia.

Dosage   Adjunctive: 1–8 μg/kg with nitrous oxide/oxygen; maintenance of 10–50 μg as needed.
General anesthesia: 8–30 μg/kg with oxygen and a skeletal muscle relaxant; maintenance of 25–50 μg as needed.

Notes   Respiratory depressant effects persisting longer than the analgesic effects; 80 times more potent than morphine.

SULFACETAMIDE

Indications   Conjunctival infections.
Dosage   10% ointment apply qid and qhs; 10, 15, 30% solution for keratitis apply q2–3h depending on severity.

SULFASALAZINE (AZULFIDINE)

Indications   Ulcerative colitis.
Dosage   Adult: 1–2 g PO initially, increase to maximum of 8 g/d in 3–4 divided doses; maintenance 500 mg PO qid.
Peds: 40–60 mg/kg/24 hr PO divided q4–6h initially; maintenance 20–30 mg/kg/24 hr PO divided q6h.

Notes   Can cause severe gastrointestinal upset; discolors urine.

SULFINPYRAZONE (ANTURANE)

Indications Acute and chronic gout.
Dosage 100–200 mg PO bid for 1 week, then increase as needed to maintenance of 200–400 mg bid.

SULINDAC (CLINORIL)

See Table IX–7 on page 457.

SULFISOXAZOLE (GANTRISIN, OTHERS)

Indications Acute uncomplicated urinary tract infections.
Dosage Adult: Between 500 mg and 1 g PO qid.
Peds older than 2 months: 120–150 mg/kg/24 hr PO divided q4–6h.
Notes Avoid use in last half of pregnancy (causes fetal hyperbilirubinemia).

SUMATRIPTAN (IMITREX)

Indications Acute treatment of migraine attacks.
Dosage 6 mg s.c. as a single dose, may be repeated in 1 hour, for a maximum dose of 12 mg per 24-hour period.
Notes May cause pain and bruising at injection site.

TACRINE (COGNEX)

Indications Treatment of mild to moderate dementia.
Dosage 10–40 mg PO qid.
Notes May cause elevations in transaminases; LFTs should be monitored regularly.

TAMOXIFEN (NOLVADEX)

Indications Adjuvant treatment of breast cancer.
Dosage 10–20 mg PO bid.
Notes May increase the risk of secondary uterine cancer.

TEMAZEPAM (RESTORIL) [C]

Indications Insomnia.
Dosage 15–30 mg PO qhs prn.
Notes Reduce dose in elderly.

TENIPOSIDE (VUMON)

Indications Treatment of leukemia.
Dosage 165 mg/m^2 IV twice weekly for 8–9 doses.

TERAZOSIN (HYTRIN)

Indications   Treatment of hypertension and benign prostatic hyperplasia.

Dosage   Initially 1 mg PO hs; titrate up to maximum of 20 mg PO qhs.

Notes   Hypotension and syncope following first dose; dizziness, weakness, nasal congestion, peripheral edema common; must be used with thiazide diuretic.

TERBUTALINE (BRETHINE, BRICANYL)

Indications   Reversible bronchospasm (asthma, COPD); inhibition of labor.

Dosage   Adult: Bronchodilator: 2.5–5 mg PO qid or 0.25 mg s.c., may repeat in 15 minutes (maximum 0.5 mg in 4 hours).
Metered dose inhaler: 2 inhalations q4–6h.
Premature labor: 10–80 μg/min IV infusion for 4 hours, then 2.5 mg PO q4–6h until term.
Peds: Oral: 0.05–0.15 mg/kg/dose PO tid; max of 5 mg/24 hr.

Notes   Caution with diabetes, hypertension, hyperthyroidism; high doses may precipitate β-1-adrenergic effects.

TERCONAZOLE (TERAZOL 7)

Indications   Vaginal fungal infections.
Dosage   1 applicator intravaginally qhs for 7 days.

TERFENADINE (SELDANE)

Indications   Seasonal allergic rhinitis.
Dosage   Adults and Peds older than 12 years: 60 mg PO bid.
Peds: 3–5 years: 15 mg PO bid; 6–12 years: 30–60 mg PO bid.

Notes   Life-threatening arrhythmias reported. Do **not** use concurrently with ketoconazole, itraconazole, or the macrolide antibiotics.

TETANUS IMMUNE GLOBULIN

Indications   Passive immunization against tetanus for any person with a suspect contaminated wound and unknown immunization status (see Appendix).

Dosage   Adults and Peds: 250–500 U IM (higher doses if delay in initiation of therapy).

Notes   May begin active immunization series at different injection site if required.

TETANUS TOXOID

Indications   Protection against tetanus.
Dosage   See Appendix for tetanus prophylaxis.

TETRACYCLINE (ACHROMYCIN V, SUMYCIN)

Indications   Broad-spectrum antibiotic treatment against *Staphylo-coccus, Streptococcus, Chlamydia, Rickettsia,* and *Myco-plasma.*
Dosage   Adult: 250–500 mg PO bid-qid.
                    Peds older than 8 years: 25–50 mg/kg/24 hr PO q6–12h.
                    Do not use in children younger than 8 years old.
Notes   Can stain enamel and depress bone formation in children; caution with use in pregnancy; do not use in presence of impaired renal function (see "Doxycycline," page 436).

THEOPHYLLINE (THEOLAIR, THEO-DUR, SOMOPHYLLIN, OTHERS)

Indications   Asthma, bronchospasm.
Dosage   Adult: 24 mg/kg/24 hr PO divided q6h; sustained release products may be divided q8–12h.
                    Peds: 16 mg/kg/24 hr PO divided q6h; SR products may be divided q8–12h.
Notes   See drug levels in Table IX–12 on page 501. Has many drug interactions; side effects include nausea, vomiting, tachycardia, and seizures.

THIAMINE (VITAMIN B$_1$)

Indications   Thiamine deficiency (beriberi); alcoholic neuritis; Wer-nicke's encephalopathy.
Dosage   Adult: Deficiency: 100 mg IM qd for 2 weeks, then 5–10 mg PO qd for 1 month.
                    Wernicke's encephalopathy: 100 mg IV × 1 dose, then 100 mg IM qd for 2 weeks.
                    Peds:10–25 mg IM qd for 2 weeks, then 5–10 mg/24 hr PO qd for 1 month.
Notes   IV thiamine administration associated with anaphylactic reaction; must be given slowly IV.

THIETHYLPERAZINE (TORECAN)

Indications   Nausea and vomiting.
Dosage   10 mg PO, PR or IM qd-tid.
Notes   Extrapyramidal reactions may occur.

THIORIDAZINE (MELLARIL)

Indications   Psychotic disorders; short-term treatment of depression, agitation, organic brain syndrome.

Dosage   Adult: Initially 50–100 mg PO tid; maintenance 200–800 mg/24 hr PO in 2–4 divided doses.
Peds older than 2 years: 1–2.5 mg/kg/24 hr PO divided bid-tid.

Notes   Low incidence of extrapyramidal effects.

THIOTEPA

Indications   Treatment of breast and ovarian cancer.
Dosage   0.3–0.4 mg/kg IV at 1 to 4 week intervals

THIOTHIXENE (NAVANE)

Indications   Psychotic disorders.
Dosage   Adults and Peds older than 12 years: Mild to moderate psychosis: 2 mg PO tid.
Severe psychosis: 5 mg PO bid; increase to maximum dose of 60 mg/24 hr prn.
Intramuscular use: 16–20 mg/24 hr divided bid-qid; maximum 30 mg/d.
Peds younger than 12 years: 0.25 mg/kg/24 hr PO divided q6–12h.

Notes   Drowsiness and extrapyramidal side effects most common.

TICARCILLIN (TICAR)

See Table IX–8 on page 469.

TICARCILLIN/POTASSIUM CLAVULANATE (TIMENTIN)

See Table IX–8 on page 469.

TICLOPIDINE (TICLID)

Indications   Reduce the risk of thrombotic stroke.
Dosage   250 mg PO bid.
Notes   Should be administered with food.

TIMOLOL (BLOCADREN)

See Table IX–2 on page 409.

TIOCONAZOLE (VAGISTAT)

Indications   Vaginal fungal infections.
Dosage   1 applicator intravaginally at bedtime (single dose).

TOBRAMYCIN (NEBCIN)

Indications   Serious gram-negative infections, especially *Pseudomonas.*
Dosage   Based on renal function; refer to Aminoglycoside Dosing on page 503.
Notes   Nephrotoxic and ototoxic; decrease dose with renal insufficiency; monitor creatinine clearance and serum concentrations for dosage adjustments; see Table IX–12, page 501.

TOCAINIDE (TONOCARD)

Indications   Suppression of ventricular arrhythmias including PVCs, and ventricular tachycardia.
Dosage   400–600 mg PO q8h.
Notes   Properties similar to lidocaine; reduce dose in renal failure; CNS and gastrointestinal side effects common.

TOLAZAMIDE (TOLINASE)

See Table IX–11 on page 497.

TOLBUTAMIDE (ORINASE)

See Table IX–11 on page 497.

TABLE IX–11. ORAL HYPOGLYCEMIC AGENTS (SULFONYLUREAS).

Drug (Brand Name)	Duration of Activity (hr)	Equivalent Dose (mg)	Maximum Daily Dose (mg)
First Generation			
Acetohexamide (Dymelor)	12–18	500	1500
Chlorpropamide (Diabinese)	36–72	250	500
Tolazamide (Tolinase)	24	250	1000
Tolbutamide (Orinase)	6–8	1000	3000
Second Generation			
Glyburide (DiaBeta, Micronase)	24	5	20
Glipizide (Glucotrol)	12–24	10	40

Contraindicated in pregnancy.

TOLMETIN (TOLECTIN)

See Table IX–7 on page 457.

TORSEMIDE (DEMADEX)

Indications	Edema, hypertension, congestive heart failure, and hepatic cirrhosis.
Dosage	5–20 mg PO or IV once daily.

TRAZODONE (DESYREL)

Indications	Major depression.
Dosage	50–150 mg PO qd-qid; maximum 600 mg/d.
Notes	May take 1–2 weeks for symptomatic improvement; anticholinergic side effects.

TRIAMTERENE (DYRENIUM)

Indications	Edema associated with CHF, cirrhosis.
Dosage	100–300 mg/24 hr PO divided qd-bid.
Notes	Can cause hyperkalemia; blood dyscrasias, liver damage, and other reactions.

TRIAZOLAM (HALCION) [C]

Indications	Insomnia.
Dosage	0.125–0.5 mg PO qhs prn.
Notes	Additive CNS depression with alcohol and other CNS depressants.

TRIFLUOPERAZINE (STELAZINE)

Indications	Psychotic disorders.
Dosage	Adult: 2–10 mg PO bid.
	Peds 6–12 years old: 1 mg PO qd-bid initially then gradually increase up to 15 mg/d.
Notes	Decrease dosage in elderly and debilitated patients; oral concentrate must be diluted to 60 mL or more before administration.

TRIHEXYPHENIDYL (ARTANE)

Indications	Parkinson's disease.
Dosage	2–5 mg PO qd-qid.
Notes	Contraindicated in narrow angle glaucoma.

TRIMETHAPHAN (ARFONAD)

Indications	Production of controlled hypotension during surgery; treatment of hypertensive crisis; treatment of pulmonary

edema with pulmonary hypertension and systemic hypertension; in cases of dissecting aortic aneurysm.

Dosage Adult: 0.3–6 mg/min IV infusion titrated to effect.

Peds: 50–150 μg/kg/min IV infusion.

Notes Additive effect with other antihypertensive agents; vasopressors may be used to reverse hypotension if required; phenylephrine is vasopressor of choice for reversal of effects.

TRIMETHOBENZAMIDE (TIGAN)

Indications Nausea and vomiting.

Dosage Adult: 250 mg PO or 200 mg PR or IM tid-qid prn.

Peds: 20 mg/kg/24 hr PO or 15 mg/kg/24 hr PR or IM in 3–4 divided doses (not recommended for infants).

Notes In the presence of viral infections, may contribute to Reye's syndrome; may cause parkinsonian-like syndrome.

TRIMETHOPRIM (TRIMPEX, PROLOPRIM)

Indications Urinary tract infections owing to susceptible gram-positive and gram-negative organisms.

Dosage 100 mg PO bid or 200 mg PO qd.

Notes Reduce dose in renal failure.

TRIMETHOPRIM-SULFAMETHOXAZOLE (CO-TRIMOXAZOLE BACTRIM, SEPTRA)

Indications Urinary tract infections, otitis media, sinusitis, bronchitis, *Shigella, Pneumocystis carinii, Nocardia.*

Dosage Adult: 1 double strength (DS) tablet PO bid or 5–10 mg/kg/24 hr (based on trimethoprim component) IV in 3–4 divided doses.

Pneumocystis carinii: 15–20 mg/kg/d IV or PO (trimethoprim component) in 4 divided doses.

Peds: 8–10 mg/kg/24 hr (trimethoprim) PO divided into 2 doses or 3–4 doses IV; do not use in newborn.

Notes Synergistic combination; reduce dosage in renal failure.

TRIMIPRAMINE (SURMONTIL)

Indications Treatment of depression.

Dosage 75–300 mg PO qhs.

UROKINASE (ABBOKINASE)

Indications Pulmonary embolism, deep venous thrombosis, restore patency to IV catheters, coronary artery thrombosis.

Dosage   Adult and Peds: Systemic effect: 4400 IU/kg IV over 10 minutes, followed by 4400 IU/kg/hr for 12 hours.
Restore catheter patency: Inject 5000 IU into catheter and gently aspirate.

Notes   Do not use systemically within 10 days of surgery, delivery, or organ biopsy.

VALPROIC ACID AND DIVALPROEX (DEPAKENE AND DEPAKOTE)

Indications   Absence seizures; in combination for tonic/clonic seizures.

Dosage   Adult and Peds: 30–60 mg/kg/24 hr PO divided tid.

Notes   Monitor liver functions and follow serum levels (see Table IX–12, page 501); concurrent use of phenobarbital and phenytoin may alter serum levels of these agents.

VANCOMYCIN (VANCOCIN, VANCOLED)

Indications   Serious infections resulting from methicillin-resistant staphylococci and in enterococcal endocarditis in combination with aminoglycosides in penicillin allergic patients; oral treatment of *C difficile* pseudomembranous colitis.

Dosage   Adults: 1 g IV q12h; for colitis 250–500 mg PO q6h.
Peds (not neonates): 40 mg/kg/24 hr IV in divided doses q12–6h.

Notes   Ototoxic and nephrotoxic; not absorbed orally, provides local effect in gut only; IV dose must be given slowly over 1 hour to prevent "red-man syndrome"; adjust dose in renal failure; see Table IX–12 page 501.

VASOPRESSIN (ANTIDIURETIC HORMONE) (PITRESSIN)

Indications   Treatment of diabetes insipidus; gaseous gastrointestinal tract distention; severe gastrointestinal bleeding.

Dosage   Adult and Peds: Diabetes insipidus: 2.5–10 U s.c. or IM tid-qid or 1.5–5.0 U IM q1–3d of the tannate.
Gastrointestinal hemorrhage: 20 U in 50–100 mL D5W or NS given IV over 15–30 minutes.

Notes   Should be used with caution with any vascular disease.

VECURONIUM (NORCURON)

Indications   Skeletal muscle relaxation during surgery or mechanical ventilation.

Dosage   Adult and Peds: 0.08–0.1 mg/kg IV bolus; maintenance of 0.010–0.015 mg/kg after 25–40 minutes followed with additional doses every 12–15 minutes.

Notes   Drug interactions leading to increased effect of vecuronium include aminoglycosides, tetracycline, and succinylcholine; less cardiac effects then pancuronium.

TABLE IX–12. DRUG LEVELS.[1]

Drug	Therapeutic Level	Toxic Level
Carbamazepine	8.0–12.0 μg/mL	>15.0 μg/mL
Digoxin	0.8–2.0 ng/mL	>2.4 ng/mL
Ethanol		100–200 mg/100 mL (legally drunk, labile behavior)
		150–300 mg/100 mL (confusion)
		250–400 mg/100 mL (stupor)
		350–500 mg/100 mL (coma)
		>450 mg/100 mL (death)
Ethosuximide	40.0–100.0 μg/mL	>150.0 μg/mL
Lidocaine	1.5–6.5 μg/mL	>6.0–8.0 μg/mL
Lithium	0.6–1.2 mmol/L	>2.0 mmol/L
Phenobarbital	15.0–40.0 μg/mL	>45.0 μg/mL
Phenytoin	10.0–20.0 μg/mL	>25.0 μg/mL
Procainamide	4.0–10.0 μg/mL	>16.0 μg/mL
Quinidine	3.0–7.0 μg/mL	>7 μg/mL
Theophylline	10.0–20.0 μg/mL	>20.0 μg/mL
Valproic acid	50–100 μg/mL	>150 μg/mL

Antibiotic	Trough (μg/mL) (maintain below upper limit)	Peak (μg/mL)
Amikacin	5.0–7.5	25–35
Gentamicin	1.5–2.0	5–8
Tobramycin	1.5–2.0	5–8
Netilmicin	0.5–2.0	6–10
Vancomycin	5.0–10.0	20–40

[1]Each lab may have its own set of values that may vary slightly from those given.

VENLAFAXINE (EFFEXOR)

Indications   Treatment of depression.
Dosage   75–225 mg/d divided into 2–3 equal doses.

VERAPAMIL (CALAN, ISOPTIN)

Indications   Supraventricular tachyarrhythmias (PAT, Wolff-Parkinson-White syndrome, atrial flutter or fibrillation); vasospastic (Prinzmetal's) and unstable (crescendo, preinfarction) angina; chronic stable angina (classical effort-associated); hypertension.
Dosage   Adult: Tachyarrhythmias: 5–10 mg IV over 2 minutes (may repeat in 30 minutes).
Angina: 240–480 mg/24 hr divided in 3–4 doses.
Hypertension: 80–180 mg PO tid or SR tablet 240 mg PO qd.

Peds: Younger than 1 year: 0.1–0.2 mg/kg IV over 2 minutes (may repeat in 30 minutes).
1–15 years old: 0.1–0.3 mg/kg IV over 2 minutes (may repeat in 30 minutes); **Do not exceed 5 mg.**

Notes   Caution with elderly patients; reduce dose in renal failure; constipation is a common side effect.

VINBLASTINE (VELBAN)

Indications   Treatment of Hodgkin's disease, lymphoma, and testicular and ovarian cancer.
Dosage   Varies with individual protocol.
Notes   May cause severe neutropenia.

VINCRISTINE (ONCOVIN)

Indications   Treatment of cervical and ovarian cancer, sarcoma, leukemia, and Hodgkin's disease.
Dosage   1.4–2 mg/m^2 IV once a week.
Notes   May cause severe extravasation.

VITAMIN B$_{12}$

See "Cyanocobalamin," page 427.

VITAMIN K

See "Phytonadione," page 481.

WARFARIN SODIUM (COUMADIN)

Indications   Prophylaxis and treatment of pulmonary embolism and venous thrombosis, atrial fibrillation with embolization, other postop indications.
Dosage   Adult: Need to individualize dosage to keep prothrombin time at 1.12–2.0 times control (INR 2–4.5); initially, 10–15 mg PO, IM, or IV qd for 1–3 days; then maintenance, 2–10 mg PO, IV, or IM qd; follow daily PT (prothrombin time) during initial phase to guide dosage.
Peds: 0.05–0.34 mg/kg/24 hr PO, IM, or IV qd. Follow PT closely to adjust dosage.
Notes   PT needs to be checked periodically while on maintenance dose; beware of bleeding caused by over anticoagulation (PT > 3 times control); caution patient on effects of taking Coumadin with other medications, especially aspirin; to rapidly correct over coumadinization, use vitamin K or fresh frozen plasma or both; highly teratogenic, do not use in pregnancy.

ZALCITABINE (HIVID)

Indications	Management of patients with HIV infection who are intolerant to zidovudine and didanosine.
Dosage	0.75 mg PO tid.
Notes	May be used in combination with zidovudine; may cause peripheral neuropathy.

ZIDOVUDINE (RETROVIR)

Indications	Management of patients with HIV infections.
Dosage	Adults: 100 mg PO 5 times per day or 200 mg PO tid or 1–2 mg/kg/dose IV q4h.
	Peds: 720 mg/m^2/24 hr PO divided 5 times/d.
Notes	Not a cure for HIV infections.

ZOLPIDEM (AMBIEN) [C]

Indications	Short-term treatment of insomnia.
Dosage	5–10 mg PO qhs prn.

TABLE IX–13. AMINOGLYCOSIDE DOSING.

See Table IX-12, page 501, "Drug Levels" for the trough and peak levels of the aminoglycosides gentamicin, tobramycin, and amikacin. Peak levels should be drawn 30 minutes after the dose is completely infused; trough levels should be drawn 30 minutes before the dose. As a general rule, draw the peak and trough around the fourth maintenance dose.

Therapy can be initiated with the recommended guidelines that follow. The following calculations are not valid for netilmicin.

Procedure (Adult)

1. Calculate the estimated creatinine clearance (CrCl) based on serum creatinine (SCr), age, and weight (kg) or a formal creatinine clearance can also be ordered, if time permits.

$$CrCl: male = \frac{(140\ 2\ age)\ 3\ (weight\ in\ kg)}{(ScCr)\ 3\ (72)}$$

   CrCl: female = 0.85 3 (CrCl male)

2. Select the loading dose:
   Gentamicin: 1.5–2.0 mg/kg   Tobramycin: 1.5–2.0 mg/kg
   Amikacin: 5.0–7.5 mg/kg

3. By using the following table you can now select the maintenance dose (as a percentage of the chosen loading dose) most appropriate for the renal function of the patient based on CrCl and dosing interval. Shaded areas are the suggested percentages and intervals for any given creatinine clearance.

TABLE IX–13. PERCENTAGE OF LOADING DOSE REQUIRED FOR DOSAGE INTERVAL
SELECTED (continued).[1]

CrCl (ml/min)	Dosing Interval		
	8 hr	12 hr	24 hr
90	90	—	—
90	86	—	—
70	84	—	—
60	79	91	—
50	74	87	—
40	66	80	—
30	57	72	92
25	51	66	88
20	45	59	83
15	37	50	75
10	29	40	64
7	24	33	55
5	20	28	48
2	14	20	35
0	9	13	25

[1]Based on data, with permission, from Hull JH, Sarubbi FA: Gentamicin serum concentrations: Pharmacokinetic predictions. Ann Intern Med 1976; 85: 183.

Shaded areas indicate suggested dosage intervals.

This is only an empirical dose to begin therapy. Serum levels should be monitored routtinely for optimal therapy. Use the previous table, "Drug Levels."

Appendix

BODY SURFACE AREA: ADULT

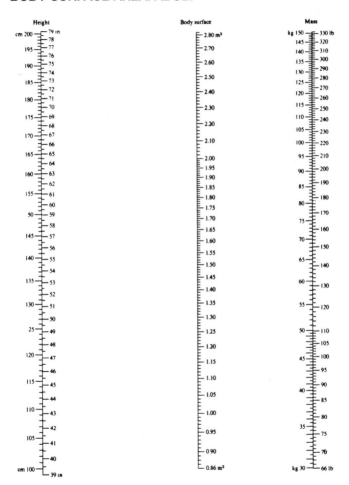

Figure A–1. To determine the body surface area in an adult, use a straight edge to connect the height and mass. The point of intersection on the body surface line gives the area in m². (From Geigy Scientific Tables, 8/e. Lentner C (editor). CIBA-GEIGY 1981;1:226.)

BODY SURFACE AREA: CHILDREN

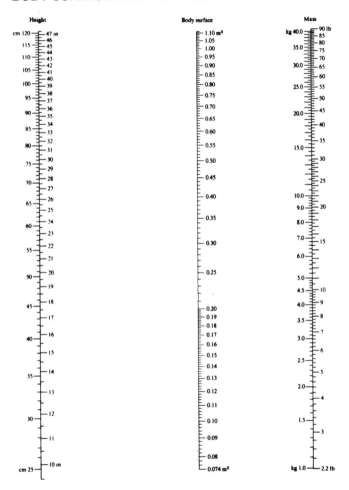

Figure A–2. To determine the body surface area in a child, use a straight edge to connect the height and mass. The point of intersection on the body surface line gives the area in m². (From Geigy Scientific Tables, 8/e. Lentner C (editor). CIBA-GEIGY 1981;1:227.)

BOWEL PREPS

The purpose of a bowel preparation is to remove all solid and most liquid from the bowel and to reduce the bacterial population in anticipation of procedures or complications of procedures that may contaminate the wound or the peritoneal cavity.

A. Noncolonic surgery.
   1. Stomach decompression before induction of anesthesia by remaining NPO after midnight before surgery or by NG suction.
   2. Bowel preparation required if any of the upper or lower gastrointestinal tract is to be opened.
       a. Surgery may involve colon, eg, extensive surgery for gynecologic malignancy or abdominal masses that impinge on the colon or where there is a potential for mechanical or ischemic bowel damage (aneurysmectomy).
       b. Achlorhydria, gastric carcinoma, prolonged H_2-receptor blocker use, and obstructive peptic ulcer disease will allow bacterial growth in the stomach. One should consider using an oral antibiotic prep (ie, neomycin) for gastric surgery in these patients (see below).

B. Colonic surgery mechanical or whole gut lavage prep with or without oral antibiotic prep. Many variations exist.
   1. Mechanical prep.
       a. Day 1–clear liquid diet, laxative of choice (castor oil 60 mL, Milk of Magnesia (MOM) 30 mL, magnesium citrate 250 mL) tap water or soap-suds enema until clear.
       b. Day 2–clear liquid diet, IV fluids, laxative of choice.
       c. Day 3–operation.
OR
       d. Day 1–clear liquid diet, IV fluids, Fleets, Phospho-soda 1–2 oz with water (repeat × 1), Dulcolax suppository in the evening.
       e. Day 2–operation.
   2. Whole gut lavage GoLYTELY (a polyethylene glycol base electrolyte balanced solution).
       a. Day 1–GoLYTELY 4 L PO or per NG tube over 5 hours.
       b. Metoclopramide 10 mg PO to reduce bloating and nausea.
       c. Day 2–operation.
   3. Oral antibiotic prep, mechanical prep, or whole gut lavage should be completed before the administration of the oral antibiotic prep.
       a. Nichols-Condon prep–on day before surgery neomycin 1 g and erythromycin base I 1 PO at 1 PM, 2 PM, 11 PM for case scheduled at 8 AM.
       b. Metronidazole (500 mg) PO–may be substituted for erythromycin base in the Nichols-Condon prep (less nausea than with erythromycin base).
   4. Perioperative IV antibiotics may be used in conjunction with, or in place of, the oral antibiotic prep.

a. These antibiotics should be administered immediately preoperatively (see above) and intraoperatively for prolonged operations. Any further doses postoperatively have not been shown to be effective in the prevention of wound infection; however, most surgeons administer at least one dose of antibiotic postoperatively and it is common to continue the antibiotic for 24 hours postoperatively.

b. Choice of antibiotic–need broad coverage of enteric organisms (gram-negatives, anaerobes), eg, gentamicin and clindamycin, cefazolin and metronidazole, or cefotetan.

(From Preoperative Preparation in *The Mont Reid Surgical Handbook.* Koutlas TC (editor). Mosby, 1994, with permission.)

COMMONLY USED RESUSCITATION DRUGS AND TECHNIQUES[1]

Drug	Adult dosage	Pediatric dosage	Indications	Notes
Adenosine	6 mg bolus over 1–3 sec, followed by 20 ml saline flush Repeat 12 mg bolus, 1–3 sec after 1–2 min	.05 mg/kg, titrate by .05 q 2 min to max .25 mg/kg.	Narrow complex SVT	
Atropine	Asystole 1 mg IV q 3–5 min; bradycardia, 0.5–1.0 mg IV q 3–5 min to max .04 mg/kg	0.01–0.3 mg/kg IV	Sinus bradycardia, AV block, asystole	If no response to 2 mg total, use isoproterenol Total dose 3 mg causes full vagal blockade
Bretylium tosylate	VF 5 mg/kg IV bolus then 10 mg/kg q 5 min to max 30–35 mg/kg VT 5–10 mg/kg diluted in 50 mL D5W, IV over 8–10 min infusion	5 mg/kg, additional boluses at 10 mg/kg	Recurrent ventricular tachycardia or ventricular fibrillation (after epi & lido failure)	After loading dose, give infusion in adult of 1–2 mg/min.
Calcium chloride	2–4 mg/kg of 10% solution IV q 10 min	0.3 mL/kg IV (10% solution)	Hypocalemia, hyperkalemia, calcium channel blocker toxicity	Flush line before giving sodium bicarbonate
Dopamine	2.5–5 µg/kg/min, infusion titration	As for adults	Nonthypovolemic shock (cardiogenic, septic) Hypotension with SIG-brady	Add Norepi if more than 20 µg/kg needed to maintain blood pressure Flush line before NaHCO₃
Epinephrine	1.0 mg IV q 3–5 min (10 mL of 1 : 10,000) follow with 20 mL flush	0.1 mL/kg of 1 : 10,000 IV q 5 min	Asystole, ventricular fibrillation	Flush line before giving sodium bicarbonate; can give ET tube if no IV ET tubes need at least 2–2.5× the peripheral dose
Isoproterenol	2–10 µg/min IV titration	Start 0.1 µg/kg/min, titrate to effect	Significant bradycardia, refractory torsades de pointes	Add 1 mg to 500 mL D5W to get 2 µg/mL Use with caution
Lidocaine	1.0–1.5 mg/kg IV bolus, then 0.5–1.5 mg/kg q 5–10 min to total 3 mg/kg	1 mg/kg dose IV, then 30 µg/kg/min drip	PVC, ventricular fibrillation, tachycardia, wide SVT	Give drip after bolus to maintain effect (adult 2–4 mg/kg) Use more aggressive dosing in cardiac arrest Stop/decrease immediately with signs of toxicity
Sodium bicarbonate	1 mEq/kg IV initially, then .5 mEq/kg q 10 min after	1–2 mEq/kg/IV, then 1 mEq/kg q 10 min	Hyperkalemia; no longer recommended for routine use; preexisting metabolic acidosis, tricyclic/phenobarb overdose	Flush line before giving calcium or epinephrine Do not completely correct the acidosis
Verapamil	2.5–5 mg IV over 2 min, repeat 5–10 mg q 15–30 min to max 20 mg	0.1–0.3 mg/kg IV, repeat dose in 30 min; if needed, 0.1–0.2 mg/kg	Atrial fibrillation, or flutter, MAT narrow SVT	Give slowly over 1 min (3 min in elderly); use carotid massage before Verapamil
Defibrillation	1st attempt 200 joules, 2nd attempt 200–300 J, 3rd attempt 360 J immediately	2 joules/kg, advance to 6 joules/kg maximum	Ventricular fibrillation; pulseless ventricular tachycardia	Synchronizer off or unit may not fire If initial 3 shocks fail to defib, continue CPR, IVF, drugs, then repeat

[1]See Figures I–4 through I–12. ET = endotracheal; PVC = premature ventricular contractions; SVT = supraventricular tachycardia; NS = normal saline.

509

CHARTWORK

Preoperative Note

The specific items in the preoperative note are dependent on institutional guidelines, the nature of the procedure, and the age and health of the patient. For example, an ECG and blood set-up may not be necessary for a 2-year-old child for a herniorrhaphy but essential for a 70-year-old scheduled for vascular surgery.

Preop diagnosis: Such as "Acute appendicitis."

Procedure: What the planned procedure is, such as "Exploratory laparotomy."

Labs: Results of complete blood count (CBC), electrolytes, prothrombin time (PT), partial thromboplastin time (PTT), urinalysis, etc.

Chest x-ray (CXR): Note results.

ECG: Note results.

Blood: Type and cross (T&C) 2 units packed red cells, blood not needed, etc.

History and physical: Should be "on chart."

Orders: Note special preop orders written, such as preoperative colon preps, vaginal douches, prophylactic antibiotics.

Permit: If completed, write "Signed and on chart."

Operative Note

The operative note is written immediately after surgery to summarize the operation for those who were not present and is meant to complement the formal operative summary that is dictated by the surgeon.

Preop diagnosis: Why the patient was taken to surgery such as "Acute appendicitis."

Postop diagnosis: Based on the operative findings such as "Mesenteric lymphadenitis."

Procedure: What procedure was performed: "Exploratory laparotomy."

Surgeons: List the attending, residents, and students who scrubbed on the case along with titles (eg, MD, CCIV, MSII). It is often helpful to identify the dictating surgeon.

Findings: Briefly note operative findings, such as "normal appendix with marked lymphadenopathy."

Anesthesia: Local, spinal, general, endotracheal, etc.

Fluids: Amount and type during case, eg, normal saline, blood, albumin. This is usually obtained for the anesthesia records.

Estimated Blood Loss (EBL): Usually obtained from the anesthesia or nursing records.

Drains: State location and type of drain, such as "Jackson-Pratt drain in left upper quadrant," "T-tube in midline," etc.

Specimens: State any specimens sent to pathology lab and the results of any intraoperative frozen sections.

Complications: Hopefully, "None."

Condition: Note where the patient is taken immediately after surgery and the condition, for example, "transferred to the recovery room in stable condition."

Night of Surgery Note (Postoperative Note)

This is a specific type of progress note written several hours after or the night of surgery.

Procedure: Indicate the operation performed.

Level of consciousness: Note if the patient is alert, drowsy, etc.

Vital signs: Blood pressure, pulse, respiration.

Intake and output (I&O): Calculate IV fluids, urine output, other drainage and attempt to assess fluid balance.

Labs: Review results, if any were obtained since surgery.

Physical exam: Examine and note the findings of the chest, heart, abdomen, extremities, and any other part as needed; examine the dressing for bleeding.

Assessment: Evaluate the postop course thus far (stable, etc).

Plan: Any changes in orders.

PROPHYLACTIC ANTIBIOTICS IN SURGERY

Nature of Operation	Likely Pathogens	Recommended Drugs	Adult Dosage before Surgery[1]
Clean			
Cardiac			
Prosthetic valve, coronary artery bypass, other open-heart surgery, pacemaker implant	*Staphylococcus epidermidis, S aureus, Corynebacterium,* enteric gram-negative bacilli	cefazolin or cefuroxime OR vancomycin[3]	1–2 g IV[2] 1 g IV
Vascular			
Arterial surgery involving the abdominal aorta, a prosthesis, or a groin incision	*S aureus, S epidermidis,* enteric gram-negative bacilli	cefazolin OR vancomycin[3]	1–2 g IV 1 g IV
Lower extremity amputation for ischemia	*S aureus, S epidermidis,* enteric gram-negative bacilli, clostridia	cefazolin OR vancomycin[3]	1 g IV 1 g IV
Neurosurgery			
Craniotomy	*S aureus, S epidermidis*	cefazolin OR vancomycin[3]	1 g IV 1 g IV
Orthopedic			
Total joint replacement, internal fixation of fractures	*S aureus, S epidermidis*	cefazolin OR vancomycin[3]	1–2 g IV 1 g IV
Ophthalmic	*S aureus, S epidermidis,* streptococci, enteric gram-negative bacilli, *Pseudomonas*	gentamicin OR tobramycin OR neomycin-gramicidin-polymyxin B cefazolin	multiple drops topically over 2–24 hours 100 mg subconjunctivally at end of procedure
Clean-contaminated			
Head and neck			
Entering oral cavity or pharynx	*S aureus,* streptococci, oral anaerobes	cefazolin OR clindamycin	1–2 g IV 600–900 mg IV
Abdominal			
Gastroduodenal	Enteric gram-negative bacilli, gram-positive cocci	High risk, gastric bypass, or percutaneous endoscopic gastrostomy only: cefazolin	1 g IV
Biliary tract	Enteric gram-negative bacilli, enterococci, clostridia	High risk only: cefazolin	1 g IV

Colorectal	Enteric gram-negative bacilli, anaerobes	Oral: neomycin + erythromycin base[4]	
		Parenteral: cefoxitin OR cefotetan	1 g IV
Appendectomy	Enteric gram-negative bacilli, anaerobes	cefoxitin OR cefotetan	1 g IV
Gynecologic			
Vaginal or abdominal hysterectomy	Enteric gram-negatives, anaerobes, Gp B strep, enterococci	cefazolin	1 g IV
Cesarean section	Same as for hysterectomy	High risk only: cefazolin	1 g IV after cord clamping
Abortion	Same as for hysterectomy	First trimester high risk:[5] aqueous penicillin G	1 million units IV
		OR doxycycline	300 mg PO[6]
		Second trimester: cefazolin	1 g IV
Dirty surgery			
Ruptured viscus[7]	Enteric gram-negative bacilli, anaerobes, enterococci	cefoxitin	2 g IV q6h
		OR cefotetan	1-2 g IV q12h
		either with or without gentamicin	1.5 mg/kg IV q8h
		OR clindamycin with	600 mg IV q6h
		gentamicin	1.5 mg/kg IV q8h
		cefazolin	1-2 g IV q8h
Traumatic wound[7,8]	S aureus, Gp A strep, clostridia		

[1]Parenteral prophylactic antimicrobials can be given as a single intravenous dose just before the operation. Cefazolin can also be given intramuscularly. For prolonged operations, additional intraoperative doses should be given q4-8h for the duration of the procedure.

[2]Some consultants recommend an additional dose when patients are removed from bypass during open-heart surgery.

[3]For hospitals in which methicillin-resistant S aureus and S epidermidis frequently cause wound infection, or for patients allergic to penicillins or cephalosporins. Rapid IV administration may cause hypotension, which could be especially dangerous during induction of anesthesia. Even if the drug is given over 60 minutes, hypotension may occur; treatment with diphenhydramine (Benadryl, and others) and further slowing of the infusion rate may be helpful (DG Maki et al: J Thorac Cardiovasc Surg 1992;104:1423). For procedures in which enteric gram-negative bacilli are likely pathogens, such as vascular surgery involving a groin incision, cefazolin should be included in the prophylaxis regimen.

[4]After appropriate diet and catharsis, 1g of each at 1 PM, 2 PM, and 11 PM the day before an 8 AM operation.

[5]Patients with previous pelvic inflammatory disease, previous gonorrhea, or multiple sex partners.

[6]Divided into 100 mg one hour before the abortion and 200 mg one-half hour after.

[7]For "dirty" surgery, therapy should usually be continued for 5-10 days.

[8]For bite wounds, in which likely pathogens may also include oral anaerobes, Eikenella corrodens (human), and Pasteurella multocida (dog and cat), some Medical Letter consultants recommend use of amoxicillin-clavulanic acid (Augmentin) or ampicillin-subactam (Unasyn).

(Reproduced, with permission, from: The Medical Letter 1993;35:94.)

Glasgow Coma Scale

The Glasgow Coma Scale (EMV Scale) gives a fairly reliable, objective way to monitor changes in levels of consciousness. It is based on eye opening, motor responses, and verbal responses (EMV). A person's EMV score is based on the total of the three different responses. The score ranges from three (lowest) to 15 (highest).

Parameter	Response		Score
Eyes	Open: spontaneously		4
	To verbal command		3
	To pain		2
	No response		1
Best motor response	To verbal command	Obeys	6
	To painful stimulus	Localizes pain	5
		Flexion-withdrawal	4
		Decorticate (flex)	3
		Decerebrate (extend)	2
		No response	1
Best verbal response	Oriented, converses		5
	Disoriented, converses		4
	Inappropriate responses		3
	Incomprehensible sounds		2
	No response		1

SBE Prophylaxis

(This section based on guidelines published by the American Heart Association in JAMA December 12, 1990, Vol 264, pages 2919–2922.) Various surgical and dental procedures can result in transient bacteremia and can result in subacute bacterial endocarditis (SBE). SBE prophylaxis is recommended for patients with congenital heart malformations, prosthetic heart valves, rheumatic and other valvular dysfunction, hypertrophic cardiomyopathy, mitral valve prolapse **with** mitral regurgitation, and a history of SBE in the absence of heart disease.

Procedures for which prophylaxis is recommended include: dental procedures that can cause gingival or mucosal bleeding (including cleaning), tonsillectomy, surgery on the respiratory or gastrointestinal tract, gallbladder surgery, cystoscopy, urethral dilatation, prostate surgery, incision and drainage of infected tissues, vaginal hysterectomy or delivery. Tables below outline current recommendations.

Recommended standard oral SBE prophylaxis for dental, oral, or upper respiratory tract procedures (see text).

Drug	Regimen
Adult patients	
Amoxicillin	3 g, PO 1 hr before procedure, then 1.5 g 6hr after first dose.
	If Amoxicillin/Penicillin allergic:
Erythromycin	Erythromycin ethylsuccinate 800 mg or erythromycin stearate, 1 g PO 2 hr before procedure then 1/2 dose 6 hr after initial dose.
	or
Clindamycin	300 mg PO 1 hr before procedure and 150 mg 6 hr after initial dose.
Pediatric patients (total dose not to exceed adult)	
Amoxicillin	50 mg/kg PO 1 hr before procedure, 1/2 dose 6 hr after first dose.
	If Amoxicillin/Penicillin allergic:
Erythromycin	20 mg/kg PO 1 hr before procedure, 1/2 dose 6 hr after first dose.
	or
Clindamycin	10 mg/kg before procedure, 1/2 dose 6 hr after first dose.

Recommended SBE prophylaxis for dental, oral or upper respiratory tract procedures for patients unable to take oral medications before the procedure (see text).

Drug	Regimen
Adult patients	
Ampicillin	2 g IM/IV 30 min before procedure, then 1 g IM/IV or 1.5 g PO 6 hr after initial dose.
	If Ampicillin/Amoxicillin/Penicillin allergic:
Clindamycin	300 mg IV 30 min before procedure, then 150 mg IV or PO 6 hr after initial dose.
	If high risk[1] and not candidate for above regimen:
Ampicillin	Ampicillin 2 g IM/IV with gentamicin 1.5 mg/kg (80 gentamicin & mg max) 30 min before procedure; then amoxicillin 1.5 g amoxicillin PO 6 hr after first dose or repeat parenteral dose 8 hr later.
	If Ampicillin/Amoxicillin/Penicillin allergic and high risk:[1]
Vancomycin	1 g IV over 1 hr, 1 hr before procedure; no follow up dose.

Pediatric patients

Follow above guidelines using the following dosages, with follow-up doses ½ initial dose. Do not exceed adult dose levels.

> ampicillin 50 mg/kg
> amoxicillin 25 mg/kg
> gentamicin 10 mg/kg
> clindamycin 10 mg/kg
> vancomycin 20 mg/kg

---

[1]Some practitioners feel that patients with prosthetic valves, history of endocarditis, or surgically reconstructed congenital defects are at increased risk for infection and should be treated with parenteral treatment.

Recommended SBE prophylaxis for genitourinary or gastrointestinal procedures (see text).

Drug	Regimen
Adult patients	
Ampicillin:	Ampicillin 2 g IM/IV with gentamicin 1.5 mg/kg (80 gentamicin mg max) 30 min before procedure; then amoxicillin 1.5 g amoxicillin PO 6 hr after first dose or repeat parenteral dose 8 hr later.
	If Ampicillin/Amoxicillin/Penicillin allergic:
Vancomycin & Gentamicin:	Vancomycin 1 g IV over 1 hr with gentamicin IV/IM (1.5 mg/kg, 80 mg max) 1 hr before and repeated 8 hr later.
	Alternate regimen for low risk patient:
Amoxicillin:	3 g PO 1 hr before procedure, then 1.5 g 6 hr after dose.

Pediatric patients

Follow above guidelines using the following dosages, with follow-up doses ½ initial dose. Do not exceed adult dose levels.

> ampicillin 50 mg/kg
> amoxicillin 25 mg/kg
> gentamicin 10 mg/kg
> clindamycin 10 mg/kg
> vancomycin 20 mg/kg

SPECIMEN TUBES FOR VENIPUNCTURE[1]

Tube Color	Additives	General Use
Red	None	Clot tube to collect serum for chemistry, crossmatching, serology
Red and black (hot pink)	Silicone gel for rapid clot	As above, but not for osmolality or blood bank work
Blue	Sodium citrate (binds calcium)	Coagulation studies (best kept on ice, not for fibrin split products)
Blue/yellow label		Fibrin split products
Royal blue		Heavy metals, arsenic
Purple	Disodium EDTA (binds calcium)	Hematology, not for lipid profiles
Green	Sodium heparin	Ammonia, cortisol, ionized calcium (best kept on ice)
Green/glass beads		LE prep
Grey	Sodium fluoride	Lactic acid
Yellow	Transport media	Blood cultures

[1]Individual labs may vary slightly from these listings.

TETANUS PROPHYLAXIS

Tetanus prophylaxis, based on guidelines from the Centers for Disease Control and Prevention and reported in MMWR 1990:39, [No. 3].

History Adsorbed Tetanus Toxoid Immunization	Clean, Minor Wounds		All Other Wounds	
	Td[2]	TIG[3]	Td[2]	TIG[3]
Unknown or <3 doses	Yes	No	Yes	Yes
> or = 3 doses[4]	No[5]	No	No[6]	No

[1]Such as, but not limited to, wounds contaminated with dirt, feces, soil, saliva, etc; puncture wounds; avulsions; and wounds resulting from missiles, crushing, burns, and frostbite.

[2]Td = tetanus-diphtheria toxoid, (Adult type) dose: 0.5 mL IM. For children younger than 7 years DPT (DT, if pertussis vaccine contraindicated) is preferred to tetanus toxoid alone. For persons 7 years of age or older, Td is preferred to tetanus toxoid alone. DT = diptheria-tetanus toxoid (Pediatric) used for those who cannot receive pertussis.

[3]TIG = tetanus immune globulin, 250 units IM.

[4]If only three doses of fluid toxoid have been received, then a fourth dose of toxoid, preferably an adsorbed toxoid, should be given.

[5]Yes, if more than 10 years since last dose.

[6]Yes, if more than 5 years since last dose.

TEMPERATURE CONVERSION TABLE[1]

F	C	C	F
0	-17.7	0	32.0
95.0	35.0	35.0	95.0
96.0	35.5	35.5	95.9
97.0	36.1	36.0	96.8
98.0	36.6	36.5	97.7
98.6	37.0	37.0	98.6
99.0	37.2	37.5	99.5
100.0	37.7	38.0	100.4
101.0	38.3	38.5	101.3
102.0	38.8	39.0	102.2
103.0	39.4	39.5	103.1
104.0	40.0	40.0	104.0
105.0	40.5	40.5	104.9
106.0	41.1	41.0	105.8

$C = (F - 32) \times \frac{5}{9}$ $F = (C \times \frac{9}{5}) + 32$

[1] F = degrees Fahrenheit; C = degrees Celsius.

Index